DISORGANIZED ATTACHMENT AND CAREGIVING

DISORGANIZED ATTACHMENT AND CAREGIVING

Edited by

JUDITH SOLOMON
CAROL GEORGE

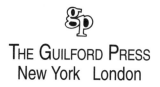

THE GUILFORD PRESS
New York London

© 2011 The Guilford Press
A Division of Guilford Publications, Inc.
72 Spring Street, New York, NY 10012
www.guilford.com

Printed in the United States of America

This book is printed on acid-free paper.

Last digit is print number: 9 8 7 6 5 4 3 2 1

Library of Congress Cataloging-in-Publication Data

Disorganized attachment and caregiving / edited by Judith Solomon, Carol George.
    p. ; cm.
Includes bibliographical references and index.
ISBN 978-1-60918-128-4 (hardcover : alk. paper)
1. Attachment disorder.   2. Parent and child—Psychological aspects.
I. Solomon, Judith.   II. George, Carol.
[DNLM: 1. Reactive Attachment Disorder.   2. Maternal Behavior.   3. Mother–
Child Relations.   4. Object Attachment.   5. Personality Development.
WS 350.6]
RC455.4.A84D57 2011
616.85′88—dc22
                                                                2010052859

About the Editors

Judith Solomon, PhD, is Director of Training for the Child FIRST Program at Bridgeport Hospital in Bridgeport, Connecticut. She is internationally recognized for her pioneering research in attachment and caregiving, including (with Mary Main) the discovery and delineation of the disorganized attachment classification group and the first longitudinal study of infants in separated and divorced families. With Carol George, she developed key representational measures of caregiving and child attachment, including the Caregiving Interview and the Attachment Doll Play Projective Assessment. In addition to her research and theoretical contributions, Dr. Solomon is also a practicing clinical psychologist, providing consultation, supervision, and training in attachment-based assessment and intervention for infants and young children.

Carol George, PhD, is Lee Mirmow Professor of Psychology at Mills College in Oakland, California. The author of numerous research articles and book chapters on adult and child attachment and caregiving, Dr. George has been at the forefront of developing attachment assessments for children and adults, including the Attachment Doll Play Projective Assessment, the Caregiving Interview, the Adult Attachment Interview, and the Adult Attachment Projective Picture System. She teaches courses in development and attachment, codirects a master's degree program in infant mental health, and trains and consults on the application of attachment assessment in research and clinical settings.

Contributors

Sydnye Allen, PhD, is an early childhood professional who has experience in laboratory schools, child development centers, Head Start, and private child care. Along with colleagues, she has published several articles on implementation of positive guidance in early childhood education. More recently, she has investigated the impact of HIV-related loss on surviving family members.

Douglas Barnett, PhD, is Professor, researcher, and clinical psychologist in the Department of Psychology at Wayne State University. He is especially interested in applying developmental psychopathology to the prevention and treatment of mental health problems.

Julie Braciszewski, PhD, completed her doctorate in clinical psychology at Wayne State University. She is continuing her interests in attachment research, intervention, and community psychology as a postdoctoral fellow in the Psychiatry and Human Behavior Training Program at Brown University.

Anna Buchheim, PhD, is Professor of Clinical Psychology at the University of Innsbruck, Austria. A psychoanalyst and full member of the International Psychoanalytic Association, she is also a guest professor at the International Psychoanalytic University in Berlin. Her research interests include attachment, psychotherapy, psychoanalysis, neurobiology, and neuroendocrinology.

Jean-François Bureau, PhD, is Associate Professor in the School of Psychology at the University of Ottawa, Canada. His research focuses on the determinants of attachment in the preschool and early school years and the role of family dynamics in the development of psychopathologies in young adulthood.

Christine M. Butler, PhD, is a clinical psychologist serving in Connellys Springs, North Carolina.

Glen Cooper, MA, is a cofounder of the Circle of Security early intervention protocol and the Circle of Security parenting program. A licensed marriage and family therapist and a mental health counselor, Mr. Cooper also is a designated child mental health specialist. He and his colleagues have authored several professional articles and chapters regarding early intervention with parents and children, and they received the Washington State Governor's Child Abuse Prevention Award in 2000 for their work on the Circle of Security Project.

Daryn H. David, PhD, is a postdoctoral fellow at the Program for Recovery and Community Health in the Department of Psychiatry at the Yale University School of Medicine. Her research focuses on the parenting needs and strengths of mothers diagnosed with severe mental illness.

Michelle DeKlyen, PhD, is Associate Research Scholar at the Office of Population Research at Princeton University, where she is also a child clinical psychologist and visiting faculty in the Department of Psychology.

Carol George. *See* "About the Editors."

Rachelle Kisst Hackett, PhD, is Associate Professor in the Educational and School Psychology Department at the Gladys L. Benerd School of Education at the University of the Pacific. She teaches courses in the doctoral program that focus on research design, applied statistics, and measurement. Her research interests include the teaching and learning of quantitative research methods and statistical analysis.

Wendy Haight, PhD, is Professor of Social Work at the University of Illinois at Urbana–Champaign. Her research focuses on socialization practices in vulnerable families, most recently rural, methamphetamine-involved families.

Nancy L. Hazen, PhD, is Associate Professor of Human Development and Family Sciences at the University of Texas at Austin. Her research focuses on the role of parenting and family relationships in the development of children's social competence, with a particular focus on attachment, peer relationships, and the role of fathers. She teaches classes in child development, peer relationships, and family relationships.

Katherine H. Hennighausen, PhD, is Clinical Instructor of Psychology at Harvard Medical School. She helped create observational measures of relationships for three major longitudinal studies and she researches how family and peer relationships influence romantic relationships. Dr. Hennighausen also is a licensed clinician who works with children, parents, and educators.

Lesley Hetterscheidt, MA, is finishing her doctorate in clinical psychology at Wayne State University. She has broad interests in child and adult assessment and psychotherapy research and practice. She hopes to serve in the Grand Rapids, Michigan, area.

Kristina N. Higgins, PhD, is a lead teacher at Loyola University Preschool in Chicago. Her research focuses on infant attachment, parental limit setting on young children, and children's compliance and defiance with limits. She also is interested in the relationship between attachment, limit setting, and the prevention of behavioral and emotional problems in early and middle childhood.

Kent Hoffman, RelD, is Adjunct Professor in the Department of Psychology at Gonzaga University in Spokane, Washington, and a cofounder of the Circle of Security Project. He also is a clinical consultant for attachment-related issues to several organizations and universities. He was awarded the 2010 Excellence in Advocacy Award by the Washington State Counseling Association.

Bjarne M. Holmes, PhD, is Senior Lecturer in Psychology and Director of the Family and Personal Relationships Laboratory at Heriot–Watt University in Edinburgh, Scotland. His research focuses on understanding how dysfunctional beliefs and attitudes about relationships bias attachment-related behavior across different types of relationships—from mother–infant, to parent–teenager, to spouse–spouse.

Jaclyn Issner, MA, is finishing her doctorate in clinical psychology at Wayne State University. She has interests in research and practice combining pediatric and family psychology.

Deborah Jacobvitz, PhD, is Professor of Human Development and Family Sciences at the University of Texas at Austin. She teaches classes in child development, attachment across the lifespan, theories of child and family development, and infancy. Her research focuses on the transmission of attachment relationships across generations, parent–child relationships, relationships within the family, and developmental outcomes from infancy to middle childhood.

Mi Kyoung Jin, PhD, is Assistant Professor of Child Welfare at Namseoul University, Korea. Her research interests include the intergenerational transmission of attachment and its effects on the development of children's social and emotional competence. She also is interested in cross-cultural studies of attachment relationships and interventions to enhance parent–child attachment relationships.

Sandra N. Jolley, PhD, ARNP, is a Pediatric and Psychiatric Mental Health Nurse Practitioner at the University of Washington Medical Center Pediatric Care Center, and Clinical Assistant Professor, Family and Child Nursing, at the University of Washington.

Melissa Kaplan-Estrin, PhD, is retired from four decades of teaching and research on infant assessment and development at Wayne State University. She is enjoying other adventures in Southeast Michigan.

Giovanni Liotti, MD, is a psychiatrist and psychotherapist. He teaches in the APC School of Cognitive Psychotherapy and in the Postgraduate School of Clinical Psychology of the Salesian University, Rome, Italy. Many of his publications address his interest in the clinical applications of attachment theory, in particular the links between dissociation, trauma-related mental disorders, and disorganization of attachment.

Karlen Lyons-Ruth, PhD, is Associate Professor of Psychiatry at Harvard Medical School. Her research has focused on the assessment of attachment relationships in high-risk environments over the infancy, childhood, and adolescent periods and has been supported by the National Institute of Mental Health, the National Institute of Child Health and Human Development, and private foundations. She is the author of numerous research articles and book chapters on infant social development, maternal trauma and depression, and infant–parent disorganized attachment relationships.

Lisa Mennet, MEd, is a doctoral candidate in Infant Mental Health at the University of Washington, and in private practice in Seattle.

Ellen Moss, PhD, is Full Professor of Developmental Psychology at the University of Quebec at Montreal, where she teaches courses on child development, family relations, and evaluation and treatment of behavior problems. She is also Director of the Centre for Study of Attachment and the Family, a research center that is presently conducting longitudinal studies on the developmental effects of parent–child attachment relationships as well as clinical-outcome studies evaluating attachment-based intervention programs with maltreated children and their families. She is active in training professionals who work with troubled youth and their families and in conducting workshops in divorce prevention and parent–child relationships.

Elizabeth M. Nelson, EdD, is a researcher and lecturer in the Center on Infant Mental Health and Development at the University of Washington.

Teresa Ostler, PhD, is Associate Professor of Social Work at the University of Illinois at Urbana–Champaign, and a clinical psychologist. Her research focuses on the effects of mental illness on parenting and on children's mental health and development.

Bert Powell, MA, is Adjunct Assistant Professor in the Graduate School of Counseling Psychology at Gonzaga University in Spokane, Washington, and one of the cofounders of the Circle of Security early intervention program for at-risk parents. He also is an International Advisor to the Editorial Board of the *Journal of Attachment and Human Development*, and licensed in Washington State as a marriage and family therapist and a mental health counselor. In 2000, the Circle of Security Project received the Washington State Governor's Child Abuse Prevention Award and in 2005, Head Start Region 10 gave the Project its Regional Award of Honor for work in early intervention.

Judith Solomon. *See* "About the Editors."

Gottfried Spangler, PhD, is Professor of Psychology at the University of Erlangen–Nuremberg, Germany. His research focuses on development of attachment and emotional regulation, psychobiological processes, genetic and environmental influences, attachment and developmental risk, and psychobiology of parental behavior.

Susan Spieker, PhD, is Director of the Center on Infant Mental Health and Development and Professor of Family and Child Nursing at the University of Washington.

Diane St-Laurent, PhD, is Associate Professor of Developmental Psychology at the University of Quebec at Trois-Rivières, where she holds a Canada Research Chair on children and their environment. Her work focuses on the role of parent–child relationships in the cognitive and socioaffective development of at-risk children, including maltreated children and children from socioeconomically disadvantaged families.

George M. Tarabulsy, PhD, is a developmental research psychologist at Laval University in Quebec City, Canada. His research has focused on identifying relations between developmental ecology, the developmental process, and outcome during infancy and early childhood. His recent work has used intervention strategies in high-risk groups to address issues of developmental process related to attachment and emotion regulation.

Linda Webster, PhD, is Associate Professor and Department Chair of the School Psychology Program at the Gladys L. Benerd School of Education at the University of the Pacific. Her research interests include attachment and child maltreatment. She maintains a private practice and training program that focuses on foster children and families.

Caroline A. Zanetti, MB, BS, FRANZCP, is Director of Psychiatry at the Raphael Centre of St. John of God Hospital, Subiaco, in Western Australia, and Adjunct Associate Professor at Notre Dame University, Perth, in Western Australia. She has considerable experience in working with the Circle of Security protocol and is an accredited Circle of Security supervisor. Her clinical work focuses on treatment of perinatal mental health disorders and parent–child relationship problems. Her research interests include theoretical understanding of the psychodynamic etiology of perinatal mood disorders and comprehensive treatment program development.

Preface

Since Main and Solomon's discovery of disorganized attachment 20 years ago, this category of at-risk parent–child relationships has achieved a central position in studies of development and psychopathology and in intervention for children and adults. The current volume presents significant advances in the study of disorganization, with particular emphasis on clinical applications. Over 10 years ago, when our first edited volume, *Attachment Disorganization,* was published, only a small group of specialists were aware that attachment relationships could be disorganized as well as insecure. Today the construct of disorganized attachment is a familiar one. Empirical research has been taken up by an expanding group of developmental psychologists and practitioner-scientists in the clinical realm, leading to new discoveries and applications that allow us to better understand the complexity of this construct and refine and revise earlier theories.

Disorganized Attachment and Caregiving is a follow-up to the first volume, yet goes well beyond being an update to or revision of its predecessor. It expands on some features of the first volume and adds new perspectives and state-of-the-art theory building and research. The title reflects what we hope will become accepted wisdom in the field—that disorganized infant and child attachment develops in the context of caregiving that is itself disorganized and dysregulated. This statement may have the ring of being, at once, self-evident and surprising. We have contributed three chapters to this volume that explore its meaning and implications. The remaining chapters represent studies and clinical applications across the lifespan by contributing authors who are prominent in the field for their interdisciplinary interests and creativity. In addition to presenting original research, authors were invited to provide, where possible, expanded case descriptions that make attachment concepts accessible and underline the clinical relevance of their work.

The 14 chapters in this volume are organized into three parts. The first part, "Core Questions: Etiology, Continuity, and Developmental Transformation," includes chapters that address fundamental and enduring questions related to disorganization. In Chapter 1, Judith Solomon and Carol George provide a framework for understanding disorganized attachment and caregiving as the products of dysregulation of adaptive systems at the levels of behavior, biological substrates, and representation. In Chapter 2, this framework is employed to interpret new data and revise long-standing hypotheses regarding the intergenerational transmission of disorganized attachment and caregiving. In Chapter 3, Ellen Moss and her colleagues provide a much-needed developmental perspective on disorganized attachment through the childhood years. This chapter integrates research on the etiology and transformations of disorganized behavior, featuring discussions of the correlates and sequelae for children and their mothers in the controlling–punitive, controlling–caregiving, and insecure–other (or unclassifiable) dyads in this age group. In Chapter 4, Susan Spieker and her colleagues address stability and change in Strange Situation and Adult Attachment Interview (AAI) classifications and the suitability of the AAI for predicting disorganization in a sample of high-risk adolescent mothers and their infants. Illustrated by case examples, this chapter tackles important questions about how attachment assessment, especially experiences discussed during the AAI, are related to mothers' life experiences. In Chapter 5, Gottfried Spangler focuses on the genetic and environmental precursors of attachment disorganization in infancy. This chapter reviews studies in this area, both his own and that of others, and raises important questions about the study of gene–environment interaction.

The second part, "New Directions," as the title suggests, is a collection of chapters that represent new ideas and approaches to the study of disorganization. In Chapter 6, Carol George and Judith Solomon describe their research on maternal helplessness and present a new questionnaire for research and clinical settings to evaluate helplessness in mothers of children ages 3–11. In Chapter 7, Nancy L. Hazen and her colleagues take on the question of the impact of gender on the development of disorganized attachment. Rich with case examples, this chapter examines whether boys and girls in middle childhood develop different approaches to manage helpless, dissociated, and hostile mothers. In Chapter 8, Katherine H. Hennighausen and her colleagues present pioneering research on disorganized attachment in adolescence. This chapter presents an intriguing new methodological approach to assessing attachment in this age group, using case examples to illuminate the nuances of this coding system. In Chapter 9, Douglas Barnett and his colleagues bring a fresh approach to thinking about attachment disorganization in children with special needs. This chapter introduces the concepts of maternal overinvolvement and overprotection, qualities of maternal behavior that are especially relevant to dyads in which the child is at significant developmental risk.

The final part presents chapters on "Clinical Applications" of disorganization across the lifespan from infancy to adulthood. In Chapter 10, Teresa Ostler and Wendy Haight discuss caregiving and attachment patterns in mothers who have lost custody of their children. They weave Bion's concept of maternal containment into an attachment-focused clinical approach, resulting in an elegant integration of attachment theory and Bion's influential clinical construct. In Chapter 11, Linda Webster and Rachelle Kisst Hackett present a study of maltreated children in foster care. Rather than relying on the Strange Situation, these authors use the Attachment Doll Play Assessment (Solomon & George, 2008; Solomon, George, & De Jong, 1995) to examine the mental representations of these young children. The results and case study highlight the importance of children's representation of attachment figures as protectors and havens of safety, a theme that echoes the intergenerational findings we present in Chapter 1. Chapter 12 presents a case study using the acclaimed Circle of Security method of intervention with families of young children (Hoffman, Marvin, Cooper, & Powell, 2006; Marvin, Cooper, Hoffman, & Powell, 2002). Caroline A. Zanetti and her colleagues demonstrate how this model of intervention can facilitate change from disorganized attachment and caregiving to security. The focus of the last two chapters in this part shifts to adults. In Chapter 13, Anna Buchheim and Carol George describe using the Adult Attachment Projective Picture System (AAP) to understand attachment dysregulation in patients with borderline personality disorder and anxiety disorder. These authors discuss how the AAP can be used to "look inside" the overarching attachment classification to provide important attachment information for diagnosis and treatment. In Chapter 14, Giovanni Liotti presents new thinking and case material on the place of disorganization in trauma and dissociative disorders. He also discusses how mentalization-based treatment, an approach commonly used in treatment for individuals with dissociating symptoms, enhances the therapist's understanding of the mechanisms associated with attachment disorganization.

It has been a privilege to work with these authors. As with our first book, most chapters were sent out for blind peer reviews. Our contributing authors, therefore, were challenged not only to organize their ideas, but also to engage in a dialogue with reviewers and ourselves, in the role of editors. The creativity and expertise of our reviewers added greatly to the dialogue and our own understanding of disorganization. We are grateful to the following colleagues for providing reviews: Zeynip Birengen, Preston Britner, Keith Crnic, Judith Crowell, Diana Diamond, Martha Erikson, Gabi Gloger-Tippelt, John Gunderson, Carolee Howes, Klaus Minde, Katherine Rosenblum, Arietta Slade, Douglas Teti, Ross Thompson, Sheree Toth, Everett Waters, and Malcolm West.

REFERENCES

Hoffman, K., Marvin, R., Cooper, G., & Powell, B. (2006). Changing toddlers' and preschoolers' attachment classifications: The Circle of Security Intervention. *Journal of Clinical and Consulting Psychology, 74*, 1017–1026.

Marvin, R., Cooper, G., Hoffman, K., & Powell, B. (2002). The Circle of Security project: Attachment-based intervention with caregiving–pre-school child dyads. *Attachment and Human Development, 4*, 107–124.

Solomon, J., & George, C. (2008). The measurement of attachment security and related constructs in infancy and early childhood. In J. Cassidy & P. R. Shaver (Eds.), *Handbook of attachment: Theory, research, and clinical applications* (2nd ed., pp. 383–416). New York: Guilford Press.

Solomon, J. George, C., & De Jong, A. (1995). Children classified as controlling at age six: Evidence of disorganized representational strategies and aggression at home and at school. *Development and Psychopathology, 7*, 447–463.

Contents

I. CORE QUESTIONS: ETIOLOGY, CONTINUITY,
AND DEVELOPMENTAL TRANSFORMATION

Chapter 1   The Disorganized Attachment–Caregiving System: 1
Dysregulation of Adaptive Processes at Multiple Levels
Judith Solomon and Carol George

Chapter 2   Disorganization of Maternal Caregiving across Two Generations: 25
The Origins of Caregiving Helplessness
Judith Solomon and Carol George

Chapter 3   Understanding Disorganized Attachment at Preschool   52
and School Age: Examining Divergent Pathways of Disorganized
and Controlling Children
*Ellen Moss, Jean-François Bureau, Diane St-Laurent,
and George M. Tarabulsy*

Chapter 4   Continuity and Change in Unresolved Classifications of Adult   80
Attachment Interviews with Low-Income Mothers
*Susan Spieker, Elizabeth M. Nelson, Michelle DeKlyen,
Sandra N. Jolley, and Lisa Mennet*

Chapter 5   Genetic and Environmental Determinants   110
of Attachment Disorganization
Gottfried Spangler

II. NEW DIRECTIONS

Chapter 6 Caregiving Helplessness: The Development of a Screening Measure 133
for Disorganized Maternal Caregiving
Carol George and Judith Solomon

Chapter 7 Pathways from Disorganized Attachment to Later 167
Social–Emotional Problems: The Role of Gender
and Parent–Child Interaction Patterns
*Nancy L. Hazen, Deborah Jacobvitz, Kristina N. Higgins,
Sydnye Allen, and Mi Kyoung Jin*

Chapter 8 Disorganized Attachment Behavior Observed in Adolescence: 207
Validation in Relation to Adult Attachment Interview Classifications
at Age 25
*Katherine H. Hennighausen, Jean-François Bureau,
Daryn H. David, Bjarne M. Holmes, and Karlen Lyons-Ruth*

Chapter 9 Maternal Solicitousness and Attachment Disorganization 245
among Toddlers with a Congenital Anomaly
*Douglas Barnett, Melissa Kaplan-Estrin, Julie Braciszewski,
Lesley Hetterscheidt, Jaclyn Issner, and Christine M. Butler*

III. CLINICAL APPLICATIONS

Chapter 10 Viewing Young Foster Children's Responses to Visits 269
through the Lens of Maternal Containment:
Implications for Attachment Disorganization
Teresa Ostler and Wendy Haight

Chapter 11 An Exploratory Investigation of the Relationships 292
among Representational Security, Disorganization,
and Behavior Ratings in Maltreated Children
Linda Webster and Rachelle Kisst Hackett

Chapter 12 The Circle of Security Intervention: Using the Therapeutic 318
Relationship to Ameliorate Attachment Security
in Disorganized Dyads
*Caroline A. Zanetti, Bert Powell, Glen Cooper,
and Kent Hoffman*

Chapter 13 Attachment Disorganization in Borderline Personality Disorder 343
and Anxiety Disorder
Anna Buchheim and Carol George

Chapter 14 Attachment Disorganization and the Clinical Dialogue: 383
Theme and Variations
Giovanni Liotti

Index 415

PART I
CORE QUESTIONS
Etiology, Continuity, and Developmental Transformation

Chapter 1

The Disorganized Attachment–Caregiving System
Dysregulation of Adaptive Processes at Multiple Levels

JUDITH SOLOMON and CAROL GEORGE

> For all objects and experiences, there is a quantity that has an
> optimum value. Above that quantity the variable becomes toxic.
> To fall below that value is to be deprived.
> —GREGORY BATESON, *Mind and Nature*

The last two decades have witnessed an extraordinary integration of developmental and clinical theory with knowledge about the psychological and physiological effects of stress and trauma. This integration amounts to a paradigm shift in our understanding of the development of several types of psychopathology (Buchheim & George, Chapter 13, this volume; Lieberman & Van Horn, 2009; Perry, 2008; Siegal, 2001; Tronick, 1989; Van der Kolk & Fisler, 1994). Bowlby's ethological theory of attachment and Ainsworth's concept of attachment security have a central place in this grand synthesis. Secure attachments are now understood to buffer the infant and child from toxic levels of stress and serve a critical role in the organization of the neurophysiologicial substrates responsible for self-regulation (Ainsworth, Blehar, Waters, & Wall, 1978; Bowlby, 1980; Hertsgaard, Gunnar, Erickson, & Nachmias, 1995; Nachmias, Gunnar, Mangelsdorf, Parritz, & Buss, 1996; Shore, 2003). Earlier we proposed that the construct of disorganized attachment provides a bridge between traditional and contemporary

3

areas of interest in attachment theory and research (Solomon & George, 1999b). Our goal in this chapter is to provide a conceptual framework for understanding the disorganized attachment–caregiving system and its pivotal role in developmental maladaptation and psychopathology. To do so, we draw both on John Bowlby's seminal ideas and current models of biobehavioral organization that point to the child–caregiver relationship as a critical component of the homeostatic response to stress. We show why the behavior of both children and mothers in these relationships is described as disorganized, discuss the variety of contexts in which disorganized behavior is observed, and propose that the disorganized infant– or child–parent relationship represents dysregulation of coadaptive processes at the level of behavior, physiology, and representation. We conclude with a brief consideration of the implications of this framework for clinical practices and future research.

ATTACHMENT DISORGANIZATION IN NORMATIVE AND HIGH-RISK CHILD-REARING CONTEXTS

The term "disorganized" as applied to infant attachment originated with Main and Solomon's descriptions of the behavior of infants who were "unclassifiable" with respect to Ainsworth's well-accepted classification system of patterns of infant behavior with the parent in the Strange Situation (Main & Solomon, 1986, 1990). Unclassifiable and/or disorganized infant attachments are most common in maltreatment and other high-risk samples, but also comprise about 15% of cases in normative samples (Lyons-Ruth & Jacobvitz, 2008). In contrast to the organized secure and organized insecure patterns identified by Ainsworth, disorganized attachment behaviors often seem bizarre or inexplicable under the circumstances. They include approach, avoidance, or angry behaviors that are succeeded or interrupted by opposing displays or which are subsequently constricted. Indications of disorientation, confusion, or fear of the parent sometimes accompany these events and are also defined as indices of disorganization. These moments of behavioral disorganization impede the achievement of the functional goal of the attachment system.

In Bowlby's view, the attachment system evolved primarily to promote protection by regulating the child's proximity to the mother. Activation of the child's attachment system results in behavior that ordinarily helps the child establish or maintain proximity to the attachment figure and elicits caregiving and comfort behavior that will soothe distress and reduce fear in response to danger or threats, including the threat of separation (Bowlby, 1982). Main and Solomon (1986, 1990) concluded that despite wide variation in the surface appearance of anomalous behaviors, all of the unclassifiable cases were characterized by a breakdown in the smooth coordination of attachment behavior and were indicative of the absence of a coherent attachment strategy with respect to the parent. Note that the words *organized* and *disorganized* refer both to the immediate organization or control of attachment behavior and to the development of stable patterns of attachment ("strategies") in response to stable variations in maternal sensitivity. That is, the organized insecure patterns may be conceptualized, in sociobiological terms, as *conditional strategies*, the capacity for which is presumed to have evolved through natural selection (Main, 1990).

DISORGANIZED CAREGIVING BEHAVIOR

For some time, we have referred to the maternal behavior that is associated with disorganized infant and child attachment as evidence of a disorganized *caregiving* system (George & Solomon, 1996, 2008; Solomon & George, 1996, 2000). Our usage reflects the context in which we have studied the mother–child relationship, which has been mainly through the study of mothers' representations of the relationship with their kindergarten-age child. At this age, children who were disorganized in toddlerhood may be classified as disorganized or controlling. The controlling subgroup is superficially more organized (Solomon, George, & De Jong, 1995); controlling behavior usually takes the form of a punitive or caregiving (role-reversed) stance with respect to the parent (Main & Cassidy, 1988). The subjective experience of the mothers of disorganized or controlling children is one of helplessness with respect to the child, their own emotions, and the relationship. In some cases, mothers' interactions with the child would objectively be described as hostile or confrontational, in others, constricted and submissive. We concluded that these mothers were experiencing a breakdown in their sense of themselves as the "stronger and wiser" member of the dyad and, at the functional level we described them as "abdicating" the protective function of the caregiving system (see also George & Solomon, Chapter 6, this volume).

Mothers' descriptions of themselves in interaction with their children have been confirmed repeatedly in observational studies. Mothers of controlling children are judged to be more disruptive, conflict-laden, disengaged, and hostile than mothers of children with organized attachments, as well as passive and role-reversed (Britner, Marvin, & Pianta, 2005; Easterbrooks, Biesecker, & Lyons-Ruth, 2000; Humber & Moss, 2005; Macfie, Fitzpatrick, Rivas, & Cox, 2008; Moss, Bureau, Cyr, Mongeau, & St-Laurent, 2004; Moss, Rousseau, Parent, St-Laurent, & Saintonge, 1998; O'Conner, Marvin, Rutter, Olrick, & Britner, 2003). Mothers in punitive dyads also have been found to struggle with cooperation and joint engagement in a variety of structured laboratory contexts (Moss et al., 2004; Moss & St-Laurent, 2001).

Although the interview and observational findings establish that mothers of disorganized and controlling infants are ineffective, it might also be said that their own behavior is disorganized in ways that parallel their children's behavior in laboratory reunions. A profusion of terms has been invoked to capture observations of the mothers of disorganized infants and children. These include "frightening" or "frightened," "atypical," "anomalous," "disruptive" (Goldberg, Benoit, Blokland, & Madigan, 2003; Lyons-Ruth, Yellin, Melnick, & Atwood, 2005; Madigan, Bakermans-Kranenburg, et al., 2006; Madigan, Hawkins, Goldberg, & Benoit, 2006; Main & Hesse, 1990; Moss et al., 2004; Vondra, Hommerding, & Shaw, 1999), and "disconnected" (Out, Bakermans-Kranenburg, & Van IJzendoorn, 2009; but see George & Solomon, 1996, 2008, for a prior and different use of the term "disconnected"). Researchers have not necessarily identified this behavior specifically as disorganized, perhaps because of the focus on identifying what it is about maternal behavior that is *disorganizing* to the infant. For example, when studying videotapes of disorganized infants, Main and Solomon (1990) noted as important a variety of "odd" behaviors on the part of parents, including breathy and exaggerated greetings; sudden attempts to frighten the baby, usually in the guise of play, and evidence of confusion about or deference toward the infant. Main and Hesse (1998) encapsulated these events in a coding system organized around the concept of "frightening or frightened" maternal behavior, which also included unambiguous indices of dissociation (e.g., behavioral freezing and stilling).

These moments reflect a breakdown in the smooth coordination of caregiving behavior that is certainly analogous, and in some cases may be homologous, to the infant or child behaviors that comprise the indices of attachment disorganization. The same may be said for many of the maternal behaviors that constitute evidence for "disrupted communication" in Bronfman and Lyons-Ruth's AMBIANCE system (Lyons-Ruth & Bronfman, 1999). This system encompasses Main and Hesse's (1998) codes, but in addition covers a broader array of apparently dysfunctional maternal behaviors. This reflects the investigators' observation that Main and Hesse's system fails to capture the behavior of mothers of disorganized infants who otherwise appear secure. In the home and in the Strange Situation, these mothers appear to be passive and withdrawn, rather than actively frightening, frightened, or dissociated. Notably, the AMBIANCE system is sensitive to a variety of contradictory cues from the mother (such as inviting approach, then retreating) and withdrawal behaviors (such as holding the infant away from the body with stiff arms) that have direct analogues in disorganized infant behavior (e.g., holding on to the parent while sharply averting gaze).

Recently, Out et al. (2009) demonstrated that it is specifically *disorganized* rather than just "extremely insensitive" maternal behavior that differentiates between mothers of disorganized infants and the mothers of organized infants, at least in structured laboratory situations. Consistent with what is captured in the disorganized infant classifications, these behaviors were characterized by "lack of meta-signals indicating play or affection (e.g., smiling), the absence of any explanation or justification for these behaviors, and their sudden occurrence" (p. 427).

OTHER CONTEXTS IN WHICH DISORGANIZED ATTACHMENT BEHAVIOR MAY BE OBSERVED

In the introduction to our first volume, *Attachment Disorganization* (Solomon & George, 1999a), we argued that disorganized attachment behavior is the empirical "missing link" unifying Bowlby's theory about the effects of major separations and loss on attachment and Ainsworth's identification of normative variations in infant attachment patterns. That is, disorganized attachment, rather than being a recent phenomenon, had been observed, though not necessarily labeled as such, by early investigators of young children's reactions to major separations. A concern with effects of separation was, of course, one of Bowlby's central preoccupations (Bowlby, 1977) and a cornerstone of his argument for the importance of attachment in the emotional development of the infant and young child. His theory of attachment was framed, however, in terms of an ethological approach to the study of motivational systems that had evolved under the pressure of natural selection. Ainsworth's studies of normative mother–child interaction in Uganda, in middle-class homes in the United States, and in the Strange Situation procedure were designed to test Bowlby's theory that infant attachment behavior would increase in response to small increments in stress and would subside when the infant had achieved proximity to the attachment figure (Ainsworth et al., 1978; Ainsworth & Marvin, 1995). Ainsworth concluded that this pattern was indeed normative and reflected the infant's confidence in the psychological availability of the attachment figure (i.e., his or her security). The attachment patterns of a minority of infants were characterized by high levels of behavior that were already familiar to Ainsworth from observations of young children following major separation, that is, avoidance and ambivalent clinging and resistance, which allowed her to readily identify these patterns as insecure.

Main and Solomon's (1986, 1990) identification of indices of disorganization in the Strange Situation provided a new lens with which to view the earlier, "classic" observations of children who had experienced major separation under adverse conditions, especially the absence of a sensitive, alternative mothering figure (Heinicke & Westheimer, 1965; Robertson & Robertson, 1971). The reunion behavior of several of these children was described by observers in terms suggestive of a profound state of disorientation and inhibition of activity, especially with respect to the attachment figure, and lasting hours or days. Family members typically interpreted this behavior as a failure to "recognize" the mother. This clearly was not the case, as these children readily recognized other family members and familiar objects; neither did they treat the mother with the casual, friendly behavior that is typically shown to unfamiliar individuals. This disorientation with respect to the immediate environment is the prime differentiating feature of this behavior both from the avoidance shown by many infants in the Strange Situation and that shown by children who had experienced major separation under more favorable circumstances. It is a "pathonomic" indicator of disorganized attachment in the Main and Solomon system, observable as stilling, freezing, or "disorganized" wandering in response to reunion with the parent. In contrast, simple avoidance, as defined in the Strange Situation, is marked by the child's increased focus on the environment, for example, picking up and manipulating toys, and rarely lasts more than a minute or two. Separated children were frequently observed to combine, in mutually contradictory ways, behavior suggestive of a disorientation with respect to the mother and proximity seeking and contact maintaining. For example, Gillian, age 19 months, refused to take her mother's hand or look at her, then broke into intense sobbing. Afterward, "she lay across her mother's shoulder, still and motionless, with eyes brimming with tears and face averted from her mother" (Heinicke & Westheimer, 1965, p. 217).

Two other salient features of the behavior of children following major separations are more analogous to disorganized behavior than to the "organized" variants of avoidance and resistance. Some children combined anger, resistance, and avoidance in ways that are consistent with the Main and Solomon guidelines for disorganization but differ from that of children with "organized" attachments. For example, John, age 17 months, alternated between attempts to flee from his mother (into the arms of other figures) and close contact with mother, during which he appeared to be asleep. It is noteworthy that apparent "falling asleep" has now also been described by Ostler and Haight (Chapter 10, this volume) during visitations with mother of young children who have been removed by social services from the mother's home. Other separated children displayed delayed anger or out-of-context aggression toward mother. For example, Heinicke and Westheimer (1965, p. 104) described 18-month-old Dawn as apparently calm and accepting of contact and distraction from mother following a brief tussle over a sticky spoon only to "smack" her mother on the face some minutes later. Solomon and George (1999b) frequently observed similar patterns of "out-of-context" anger and provocation among toddlers who were regularly separated overnight from the mother due to visitation with the father.

Disorganized attachment classifications have been found to predominate among infants and young children in foster care or who have been adopted (Chisolm, 1998; Marcovitch et al., 1997; O'Connor et al., 2003; Stovall & Dozier, 2000). To the degree that the children in these samples may have previously experienced maltreatment and/or separation from primary caregivers, fostering and adoption ought not to be considered a unique determinant of disorganized attachment. In a recent meta-analysis of adopted children, however, previously institutionalized children and children adopted later rather than earlier (over 12 months of age) were most likely to be classified as disorganized, suggesting that maternal deprivation (possibly along with other kinds of environmental deprivation) makes a unique contribution to disorganization (van den Dries, Juffer, van IJzendoorn, & Bakermans-Kranenburg, 2009). It is not clear whether disorganization in these contexts directly reflects the consequences of maternal deprivation during a "sensitive period" for the development of the attachment system or problematic responses of foster and adoptive mothers to the challenging behaviors shown by young children whose earlier attachments have been disrupted. Both factors may be relevant. Children adopted after the first 12 months of life are described as requiring more time to organize their attachment behavior around the new mother. Yet this process is facilitated when the mother has an autonomous (secure) state of mind with respect to attachment and is more likely to result in disorganization when the mother has an insecure state of mind (Dozier, Stoval, Albus, & Bates, 2001). We note, as well, that there continues to be debate as to whether institutionalized children can really be labeled as disorganized in attachment because their disordered behaviors are so extreme (Zeanah, Smyke, Koga, & Carlson, 2005; cf. Marvin & Whelan, 2003). Regardless of how currently or formerly institutionalized children ought to be classified in the Strange Situation, what is key for our present discussion is that they undoubtedly show behavior that is disorganized in the sense that Main and Solomon (1986, 1990) outlined in their studies of home-reared infants.

DYSREGULATION OF BIOBEHAVIORAL ADAPTATIONAL PROCESSES

We have now described at least two and possibly three conditions in which disorganized attachment is likely: (1) in home-reared children who may be presumed to be attached to a caregiver whose caregiving behavior is also disorganized—maltreatment may be a feature of these relationships, but not necessarily; (2) following major separation from an adequate caregiver; and

(3) as a consequence of maternal deprivation during the first year of life or beyond. The differences among these caregiving contexts are as salient as their commonalities.

As originally proposed and elaborated by Main (Main & Hesse, 1990; Main & Morgan, 1996), disorganized attachment among home-reared infants is commonly understood to be a product of the infant's experience of "fright without solution." That is, in the laboratory and at home, disorganized attachment behavior results from immediate and/or repeated experiences of fear with the mother, which simultaneously compel the infant toward the parent, due to the action of the attachment system, and drive the infant away. Main has speculated that these incompatible motives result in a "collapse in attention" and the failure of behavioral and representational mechanisms that would ordinarily organize attachment behavior. There is no indication, however, that the mothers in the early, classic studies of separation were alarming before separation, despite the fact that the behavior of the children on reunion might suggest elements of fear (e.g., running away from the mother, dissociation). Furthermore, although it is true that some institutionally reared infants and children appear to become globally frightened or inhibited, the reverse pattern is at least as common, that is, the children become bold and "indiscriminately" sociable (Zeanah et al., 2005).

Following Bowlby (1980), we propose as a unifying explanation that disorganized attachment behavior in all three contexts reflects a failure in the regulating or organizing properties of the attachment–caregiving relationship. Bowlby (1973) emphasized the role that the attachment system plays as part of the infant's overall homeostatic response to stress, that is, he considered the attachment system to be a component in the overall homeostatic system that regulates the organism's response to stress. This construct implies, clearly, that the ongoing regulation of the infant's internal state depends upon maternal coregulation just as the infant's attachment behavior must be supported by the complementary caregiving behavior of the mother. This in turn requires that the mother's caregiving system itself ought to be organized to respond in an effective, coherent way to infant cues and other environmental demands.

Animal studies of the development and organization of attachment behavior and its neurological substrates essentially validate Bowlby's more global concept of the attachment and caregiver systems as coregulating and linked to homeostatic response to stress and threat. At the same time, contemporary studies highlight the fact that the attachment–caregiving system itself reflects an interplay and coordination of several component subsystems (e.g., infant rat responses to contact and separation are each linked to distinct characteristics and behaviors on the part of the mother) (Polan & Hofer, 2008). The notion that the attachment–caregiver system consists of component modules adds an additional potential source of disorganization.

Typically acting in concert, the adequacy or failure of coregulating processes results in developmental variations, at multiple levels, in the infant's immediate responses as well as resilience in the face of future stresses. These levels include epigenetic and molecular functioning; organization of brain structures underlying affect, memory, and information processing, such as the amygdala, hippocampus, and prefrontal cortex; and activation and function of the autonomic and limbic–hypothalamic–pituitary–adrenal systems (L-HPA), which modulate the body's response to both immediate and chronic stress (Buchheim, George, Kächele, Erk, & Walter, 2006; Fox, 1994; Gunnar & Barr, 1998; Porges, 2003). To these levels we would add, for humans, at any rate, representational processes that determine perception and coordinate behavior in response to projections (predictions) about the behavior of both the self and caregiving figures (Bretherton & Munholland, 2008).

For a system to function homeostatically, it must have available at least one, preferably several, adaptive processes that maintain or return the system to an optimal or steady state. In terms of attachment, the normal functioning or regulation of the system depends not only on the well-known attachment behaviors (e.g., calling, crying, searching, following the attachment figure) and their physiological substrates, but also on processes of adaptation to less-than-optimal conditions (e.g., in maternal sensitivity), such as avoidance or displays of anger. When adaptive or defensive processes are unable to maintain a system within minimally adequate limits, the system will tend to function in a dysregulated or unstable state. Dysregulated responses, by definition, are characterized by a lack of coordination with respect to the "set-goal" of the system and will tend to veer between polarized extremes of functioning, that is, the system remains "all on" or "all off" or alternates unpredictably between these extremes. Note that dysregulation is equivalent neither to stress nor, strictly speaking, to the intensity or quality of expressions of distress. Thus, for example, even very intense crying in the mother's absence ought not to be considered evidence of dysregulation. We might infer that crying is dysregulated, however, when the child is oriented away from the source of soothing, crying begins or ends abruptly or "out of context," or is mixed with contradictory communication, such as intense, spasmodic laughter. Note that all of these examples are previously defined indices of disorganized attachment (Main & Solomon, 1990).

In order to avoid circularity, it is important to search for evidence of dysregulated systems in addition to or outside the context of attachment behavior itself. For example, we would expect disorganized attachment or caregiving to be associated both with explosive anger and with its opposite, extreme constriction of anger. This is indeed how mothers of disorganized and controlling children describe both themselves and their children (George & Solomon, 1996, 2008; Solomon & George, 1996, 2008). These dysregulated affective patterns may, at least in part, explain the often replicated finding that children whose attachment to their mother is disorganized (or was assessed as such in infancy) show high levels of externalizing as well as internalizing behavior outside the home (Lyons-Ruth & Jacobvitz, 2008). The dysregulated quality of the disorganized child's anger or constriction has not been demonstrated definitively as yet, however, since the commonly used parent or teacher self-report measures of child social behavior do not differentiate as to context.

Another potentially relevant example of dysregulated anger was reported by George and Main (1979) who found "out-of-context," peer-directed aggression mixed with comforting behavior to be characteristic of abused toddlers. Note also that the extreme, polarized social behaviors shown by institutionalized children (i.e., inhibited or socially indiscriminant behavior) fit well to the construct of dysregulation. A recent study of high-risk, home-reared children is interesting in this light. Lyons-Ruth and colleagues (Lyons-Ruth, Bureau, Ruley, & Atlas-Corbett, 2009) found that even when variation related to disorganized and avoidant attachment was removed, socially indiscriminate behavior was associated with aggression and hyperactivity (i.e., dysregulated affect and activity).

Highly relevant, though still fragmentary, evidence of dysregulation related to disorganized attachment is found in studies of neuroendocrine responses to stress. In the case of disorganized infants living in normative, stable homes and observed in the Strange Situation, the D classification appears to be associated with elevation of cortisol levels, which, unlike the cortisol responses of children with organized attachments, remain high for some time after the end of the Strange Situation (Hertsgaard et al., 1995; Spangler & Schieche, 1998). In a set of elegant studies among recently adopted children, Gunnar and Dozier demonstrated the existence of dysregulation of diurnal cortisol rhythms, which appear to be associated with the well-known "out of control" emotional displays frequently shown by children in these circumstances. Once cortisol levels became regulated through the establishment of daily routines by caregivers, the behavior of these children improved (Dozier et al., 2006; Fisher, Stoolmiller, Gunnar, & Burraston, 2007; Gunnar, Morison, Chisholm, & Schuder, 2001). It is worth noting that the systems underlying dysregulation of cortisol rhythms may be to some degree independent of the organization of the attachment system itself. Thus, dysregulated cortisol rhythms appear to be sensitive to disruptions in care before 6 months of age, whereas maternal deprivation or disrupted attachments do not appear to interfere with the establishment of secure attachment behavior prior to 12 months (Dozier, Albus, Fisher, & Sepulveda, 2002). Finally, in a recent test of polyvagal theory (Porges, 2003), Oosterman, De Schipper, Fisher, Dozier, and Schuengel (2010) demonstrated a stronger effect of disorganized attachment classifications on dysregulated autonomic processes in foster children than earlier experiences of neglect.

DYSREGULATION AT THE LEVEL OF REPRESENTATION

Bowlby proposed the construct of "segregated systems" (Bowlby, 1980; Solomon & George, 1999, 2008; Chapter 2, this volume; Solomon et al., 1995) to characterize and explain dysregulated representational processes. Segregated systems were said to arise when "exclusionary" or defensive representational processes of deactivation and cognitive disconnection were unable to contain intensely painful thoughts and feelings associated with attachment figures. When this occurred, "the specific patterns of behavior that go to make up attachment behavior together with the desires, thoughts, working models and personal memories integral to them" (Bowlby, 1980, p. 348) become a part of this unintegrated system, leading to a separate representational self that under most conditions is unavailable to consciousness. In this way, segregated systems may be said to equate to processes of repression or dissociation. In Bowlby's view, the process of segregation did not entirely preclude memories, thoughts, and feelings associated with the attachment figure from influencing behavior. Rather, these might be elicited by attachment cues or other reminders, sometimes quite idiosyncratic ones. Because they could not be processed in awareness (i.e., by higher integrative functions), previously segregated material was likely to emerge in ways that were out of context and out of control.

We have adapted Bowlby's model to explain variations in the symbolic representation of attachment of kindergarten-age children through doll play (Solomon et al., 1995) and the caregiving representations of their mothers in the course of semistructured interviews (George & Solomon, 1999, 2008). Bowlby defined two types of defensive exclusion of information, which, when not extreme, can be considered to be adaptive: deactivation and cognitive disconnection. Briefly, we find that deactivating defenses (i.e., ways of thinking and symbolically representing parent–child interaction that *preclude* the need for engagement or assistance) to be characteristic of insecure–avoidant children and their mothers. For example, a child might depict in doll play that when the parents return from a trip, the children are asleep in their beds; a mother of an avoidant child in the course of the Caregiving Interview might describe, as a source of pleasure, watching from afar her child in play. We find defenses related to cognitive disconnection to be characteristic of insecure–ambivalent children and their mothers. Disconnecting processes help the individual *circumvent* the expression of attachment by separating feelings from the awareness of what is eliciting them. Often this occurs by distracting one's attention to irrelevant details. For example, an ambivalently attached 5-year-old might in doll play enact a thorough cleaning of the house when the doll parents are away; in the context of an interview, the mother of an ambivalent child might describe doing the same thing as a distraction from worry about her child's first day at school. Consistent with the notion that dysregulated representations (segregated systems) are associated with polarized representations of attachment and caregiving behavior, the symbolic representations of controlling and disorganized children and their mothers are manifested as either affective flooding or constriction. That is, both controlling children and their mothers represent parent–child interaction as wildly frightening, out of control, and dangerous *or* manifest or describe efforts to constrict behavior. Examples of constriction include the child refusing to enact a family scene, or the mother barricading herself in her room rather than display anger toward the child. Other investigators, using our measure or different ones, have reported qualitatively similar indices of disorganization among high-risk, maltreated, and foster children and their parents (Fury, Carlson, & Sroufe, 1997; Jacobsen & Miller, 1999; Katsurada, 2007; Shields, Ryan, & Cicchetti, 2001; Venet, Bureau, Gosselin, & Capuano, 2007; Webster & Hackett, Chapter 11, this volume).

CAUSALITY

As Gregory Bateson so lucidly pronounced, conditions that fall outside the optimum range of a system become either toxic or depriving: they flood the adaptive defenses of the system or they starve the system of essential constituents. Somewhat less eloquently, Bowlby proposed that the attachment system becomes dysregulated when it is chronically or intensely activated (mobilized) but not assuaged. This occurred, he believed, under adverse conditions of separation or loss, as well as when the infant or child was punished for the display of attachment behavior.

Bowlby's formulation applies most easily to disorganization among children who have been separated from parents under adverse conditions, are observed in foster care or following adoption, and, possibly, also to institutionalized children who have never had an opportunity to establish a stable attachment. In all of these cases, an attachment figure is now or always was chronically unavailable to assuage distress or to otherwise coregulate the infant or child. Maternal separation and deprivation are, however, usually not the most common causes of disorganized attachment. A recent meta-analysis of the conditions under which disorganized attachments are most likely points strongly to families in which there has been maltreatment or where there is high cumulative stress (Cyr, Euser, Bakermans-Kranenburg, & van IJzendoorn, 2010). Curiously, as a reflection of the times, there is no direct mention of maltreatment in the original editions of Bowlby's *Attach-*

ment trilogy (Bowlby, 1969, 1973, 1980). Main adapted Bowlby's formulation (based on shock administration research with baby animals; Bowlby, 1979), however, by pointing out that when the caregiver is frightening, the infant is placed in a position of "irresolvable conflict" and the attachment system is activated but cannot be terminated (Hesse & Main, 2006; Main & Hesse, 1990; Main & Morgan, 1996). That is, the attachment figure is present but unable to function as a source of security or coregulation, especially when the infant or child is most frightened or distressed. Clearly, frank physical abuse would function in this way and would be a dysregulating event or condition. Our interviews with mothers of infants and kindergartners in our normative samples convince us that although it may fall short of abuse, mother–child interaction in the homes of these controlling and disorganized children is characterized by unpredictable and intense rage or other negative affect, which is either directly or more covertly expressed. Many mothers also report significant failures to buffer the child or respond protectively to psychological and physical dangers, requiring the child to remain more or less continually vigilant and fearful (George & Solomon, 1996, 2008; Solomon & George, 1996, 2000). Corrrelatively, we have found that mothers of disorganized or controlling children report qualitatively similar experiences during their own childhoods (Solomon & George, 2006; Chapter 2, this volume). That is, they describe caregiving figures as out of control, frightening, and/or failing to buffer or protect them and they describe themselves as frightened and helpless. We hypothesize that these child-rearing circumstances have enduring effects on mothers' ability to self-regulate and coregulate the child.

Do the disorganized caregiving behaviors described earlier actually disorganize infant or child attachment? On this matter there continues to be debate. Main and Hesse (1990) have proposed that the subtle frightened, frightening, or dissociated behaviors shown by some mothers of disorganized infants and children are sufficient to disorganize attachment behavior; presumably, the disrupted communication coded by Lyons-Ruth (Lyons-Ruth & Bronfman, 1999) might also be disorganizing in the moment. Observational studies more-or-less consistently demonstrate support for both Main and Hesse's and Lyons-Ruth's approaches to describing maternal behavior in the laboratory and the home. Significant "transmission gaps" remain with respect to both disrupted and frightened–frightening–dissociative maternal behavior and infant disorganization, however (Madigan, Bakermans-Kranenburg, et al., 2006; Out et al., 2009). An alternative hypothesis to that proposed by Main and Hesse (1990) is that all of these indices of disorganized caregiving behavior, detectable, often, only through microanalysis of interaction, are the behavioral products of dysregulation in parent and child and the relationship, as a consequence of a history of unambiguously (macro) frightening interactions, but are not themselves the source of this dysregulation. Experimental studies comparable to manipulating interaction through the use of the still-face paradigm (Tronick, 1989) would be useful to resolve this question.

Can the infant or child challenge the mother's caregiving system sufficiently to dysregulate the attachment–caregiving system? The preponderance of studies has shown the attachment–caregiving system to be remarkably resilient. Typically, studies reveal that variables such as infant temperament and affect regulatory capacities have an impact on attachment security only when combined with other stressors (Vaughn, Kelly, Bost, & van IJzendoorn, 2008). An intriguing development in recent years are data that appear to show a relation between genetic variations related to neurotransporter efficiency and disorganized attachment, first reported by Gervai and colleagues in a Hungarian sample (Gervai et al., 2007). Results of replication studies have been inconsistent, however, with some studies showing main effects of allelic variants, others finding no effects, and still others showing that these variations result in disorganized attachment only in combination with high levels of maternal sensitivity (for a review, see Spangler, Chapter 5, this volume). If genetically based differences among infants indeed contribute to disorganization, they may do so by affecting the infants' own regulatory abilities or their "set-points" for optimal levels and patterns of maternal behavior and responsiveness.

CLINICAL AND RESEARCH IMPLICATIONS

Twenty years of research involving the disorganized and controlling attachment categories in home-reared children have demonstrated that these infants and children express the most distress and display the most insecure behavior in the home (Lyons-Ruth, Dutra, Schuder, & Bianchi, 2006; Solomon & George, 2008). They are more likely than children who are assigned to the organized classifications to show maladaptive behavior in the classroom and to require clinical services (Lyons-Ruth & Jacobvitz, 2008). Their mothers report the highest levels of parenting stress and helplessness (see George & Solomon, Chapter 6, this volume) and are most likely to receive major mental health diagnoses such as depression and borderline personality disorder (Dozier, Stovall-McClough, & Albus, 2008; Lyons-Ruth & Jacobvitz, 2008). Clearly, these dyads are operating toward the farther reaches of the "expectable" environments within which coregulating mechanisms have evolved. From this perspective, dysregulation of adaptive mechanisms at the levels of behavior, affect, neurophysiological substrates, and representation are hardly surprising.

The construct of disorganization is now well integrated into the lexicon of clinicians, especially those involved in providing infant mental health intervention (Dozier et al., 2002; Hoffman, Marvin, Cooper, & Powell, 2006; Lieberman & Van Horn, 2009; Slade, 2005; Toth, Rogosch, Manly, & Cicchetti, 2006). Evidence-based treatment recommendations incorporate relationship-based approaches to intervention to improve the parent's ability to respond empathically, refrain from frightening the child, repair ruptures quickly, and behave in a protective manner. To our knowledge, only child–parent psychotherapy (Lieberman & Van Horn, 2009) adds to this mix specific techniques to ameliorate the self-regulation difficulties faced by the caregiver. The accumulating research summarized here indicates, however, that the majority of "disorganized" caregivers may benefit from such strategies, whether or not they have directly experienced trauma as it is typically defined (see Solomon & George, Chapter 2, this volume).

Increasingly, research in the field of attachment reflects an awareness of the links between attachment disorganization, affect regulation, and the physiological substrates of regulation. The precise neurophysiological mechanisms through which the dysregulated caregiver influences the child's internal state are largely unknown, however. Furthermore, because the caregiver is so often seen in terms of his or her stimulus value for the child, rather than as an integral part of a coregulating relationship, even less is known about the ways in which the child's behavior regulates or dysregulates the caregiver's adaptive control systems at multiple levels. Investigations into this phenomenon from the perspective of the attachment–caregiving system would parallel the elegant animal research models (Polan & Hofer, 2008). One would like to know, for example, whether the L-HPA and autonomic systems of the mothers of disorganized infants are also dysregulated, in general, and during various kinds of interaction with the child (see Buchheim & George, Chapter 13, this volume).

Attachment researchers have only recently turned their attention to the role of disorganized infant–caregiver relationships in the relational diathesis of psychopathology. Recent work by Lyons-Ruth and colleagues on the development of borderline disorders, examining the interrelations of caregiver behavior and representation with infant genetic vulnerabilities is an inspiring example (Hobson et al., 2009; Lyons-Ruth et al., 2006; Nemoda et al., 2007). Given the failures of the disorganized attachment–caregiving relationship to buffer the infant and child from stress of many kinds, including those generated through the relationship itself, we would expect them to be associated with and potentiating of a wide range of psychological and physical disorders, including those believed to have a genetic or immunological basis. For example, an issue of particular interest to us is the role of disorganized attachment–caregiving relationships in the development of "childhood bipolar disorder," apparently soon be labeled "temper dysregulation disorder with dysphoria" (American Psychiatric Association, 2010). Our clinical experience indicates a link between this diagnosis, disorganized attachment and caregiving, and recent trauma. Disorganized relationships might also be considered a risk factor for stress-related effects on health, including, for example, newly "rediscovered" virus-initiated affective disorders (Bortolato & Godar, 2010).

Though we propose that disorganized attachment–caregiving relationships will provide a powerful model for examining the interplay between dysregulated systems at multiple levels, we also emphasize that a multiplicity of relationships and histories are subsumed under this rubric. We have argued here that all of the contexts in which disorganized attachments are common—home rearing with a disorganized and affectively dysregulated caregiver, following major separation from attachment figures in adverse conditions, and as a consequence of maternal deprivation in institutionalized children—are associated with dysregulated adaptive systems within the child. These conditions represent a continuum of assaults to the attachment and caregiving systems. We can expect to find important qualitative differences among these relationships as a function of etiology, including the presence or absence of regulatory impairments originating with the child. These, in turn, are likely to be associated with differences, as well as commonalities, in the developmental onset, type, and degree of impairment of biobehavioral and representational adaptations.

REFERENCES

Ainsworth, M. D. S., Blehar, M. C., Waters, E., & Wall, S. (1978). *Patterns of attachment: A psychological study of the Strange Situation.* Hillsdale, NJ: Erlbaum.

Ainsworth, M. D. S., & Marvin, R. S. (1995). On the shaping of attachment theory and research: An interview with Mary D. S. Ainsworth. In E. Waters, B. E. Vaughn, G. Posada, & K. Kondo-Ikemura (Eds.), Caregiving, cultural,and cognitive perspectives on secure-base behavior and working models. *Monographs of the Society for Research in Child Development, 60*(2–3, Serial No. 244), 3–12.

American Psychiatric Association (2010). DSM-5 development website. *www.dsm5. org.*

Bortolato, M., & Godar, S. C. (2010, May 18). Animal models of virus-induced neurobehavioral sequelae: Recent advances, methodological issues, and future prospects. *Interdisciplinary Perspectives on Infectious Diseases.* Article ID 380456. doi:10.1155/2010/380456.

Bowlby, J. (1973). *Attachment and loss: Vol. 2. Separation: Anger and anxiety.* New York: Basic Books.

Bowlby, J. (1977). The making and breaking of affectional bonds: II. Some principles of psychotherapy. *British Journal of Psychiatry, 130,* 421–431.

Bowlby, J. (1980). *Attachment and loss: Vol. 3. Loss: Sadness and depression.* New York: Basic Books.

Bowlby, J. (1982). *Attachment and loss: Vol. 1. Attachment.* New York: Basic Books. (Original work published 1969)

Bretherton, I., & Munholland, K. A. (2008). Internal working models in attachment relationships: Elaborating a central construct in attachment theory. In J. Cassidy & P. R. Shaver (Eds.), *Handbook of attachment: Theory, research, and clinical applications* (2nd ed., pp. 102–127). New York: Guilford Press.

Britner, P. A., Marvin, R. S., & Pianta, R. C. (2005). Development and preliminary validation of the Caregiving Behavior System: Association with child attachment classification in the preschool Strange Situation. *Attachment and Human Development, 7,* 83–102.

Buchheim, A., George, C., Kächele, H., Erk, S., & Walter, H. (2006). Measuring adult attachment representation in an fMRI environment: Concepts and assessment. *Psychopathology, 39,* 136–143.

Chisolm, K. (1998). A three year follow-up of attachment and indiscriminate friendliness in children adopted from Romanian orphanages. *Child Development, 69,* 1092–1106.

Cyr, C., Euser, E. M., Bakermans-Kranenburg, M. J., & van IJzendoorn, M. H. (2010). Attachment security and disorganization in maltreating and high-risk families: A series of meta-analyses. *Development and Psychopathology, 22,* 87–108.

Dozier, M., Albus, K., Fisher, P. A., & Sepulveda, S. (2002). Interventions for foster parents: Implications for developmental theory. *Development and Psychopathology, 14,* 843–860.

Dozier, M., Manni, M., Gordon, M. K., Peloso, E., Gunnar, M. R., Stovall-McClough, K. C., et al. (2006). Foster children's diurnal production of cortisol: An exploratory study. *Child Maltreatment, 11,* 189–197.

Dozier, M., Stoval, K. C., Albus, K. E., & Bates, B. (2001). Attachment for infants in foster care: The role of caregiver state of mind. *Child Development, 72,* 1467–1477.

Dozier, M., Stovall-McClough, K. C., & Albus, K. E. (2008). Attachment and psychopathology in adulthood. In J. Cassidy & P. R. Shaver (Eds.), *Handbook of attachment: Theory, research, and clinical applications* (2nd ed., pp. 718–744). New York: Guilford Press.

Easterbrooks, M. A., Biesecker, G., & Lyons-Ruth, K. (2000). Infancy predictors of emotional availability in middle childhood: The roles of attachment security and maternal depressive symptomatology. *Attachment and Human Development, 2,* 170–187.

Fisher, P. A., Stoolmiller, M., Gunnar, M. R., & Burraston, B. O. (2007). Effects of a therapeutic intervention for foster preschoolers on diurnal cortisol activity. *Psychoneuroendocrinology, 32,* 892–905.

Fox, N. (1994). Dynamic cerebral processes underlying emotion regulation. In N. Fox (Ed.), The development of emotion regulation: Biological and behavioral considerations. *Monographs of the Society for Research in Child Development, 59*(Serial No. 240), 152–166.

Fury, G. S., Carlson, E. A., & Sroufe, L. A. (1997). Children's representations of attachment in family drawings. *Child Development, 68,* 1154–1164.

George, C., & Main, M. (1979). Social interactions of young abused children: Approach, avoidance, and aggression. *Child Development, 50,* 306–318.

George, C., & Solomon, J. (1996). Representational models of relationships: Links between caregiving and attachment. *Infant Mental Health Journal, 17,* 18–36.

George, C., & Solomon, J. (2008). The caregiving system: A behavioral systems approach to parenting. In J. Cassidy & P. R. Shaver (Eds.), *Handbook of attachment: Theory, research, and clinical applications* (2nd ed., pp. 833–856). New York: Guilford Press.

Gervai, J., Novak, A., Lakatos, J., Toth, I., Danis, I., Ronai, Z., et al. (2007). Infant genotype may moderate sensitivity to maternal affective communications: Attachment disorganization, quality of care, and the DRD4 polymorphism. *Social Neuroscience, 2,* 307–319.

Goldberg, S., Benoit, D., Blokland, K., & Madigan, S. (2003). Atypical maternal behavior, maternal representations, and infant disorganized attachment. *Development and Psychopathology, 15,* 239–257.

Gunnar, M. R., & Barr, R. G. (1998). Stress, early brain development, and behavior. *Infants and Young Children, 11,* 1–14.

Gunnar, M. R., Morison, S. J., Chisholm, K., & Schuder, M. (2001). Salivary cortisol levels in children adopted from Romanian orphanages. *Development and Psychopathology, 13,* 611–628.

Heinicke, C. M., & Westheimer, I. (1965). *Brief separations.* New York: International Universities Press.

Hertsgaard, L., Gunnar, M., Erickson, M. F., & Nachmias, M. (1995). Adrenocortical responses to the Strange Situation in infants with disorganized/disoriented attachment relationships. *Child Development, 66,* 1100–1106.

Hesse, E., & Main, M. (2006). Frightened, threatening, and dissociative parental behavior in low-risk samples: Description, discussion, and interpretations. *Development and Psychopathology, 18,* 309–343.

Hobson, R. P., Patrick, M. P. H., Hobson, J. A., Crandell, L., Bronfman, E., & Lyons-Ruth, K. (2009). How mothers with borderline personality disorder relate to their year-old infants. *British Journal of Psychiatry, 195,* 325–330.

Hoffman, K. T., Marvin, R. S., Cooper, G., & Powell, B. (2006). Changing toddlers' and preschoolers' attachment classifications: The Circle of Security intervention. *Journal of Consulting and Clinical Psychology, 74,* 1017–1026.

Humber, N., & Moss, E. (2005). The relationship of preschool and early school age attachment to mother–child interaction. *American Journal of Orthopsychiatry, 75,* 128–141.

Jacobsen, T., & Miller, L. J. (1999). Attachment quality in young children of mentally ill mothers: Contribution of maternal caregiving abilities and foster care context. In J. Solomon & C. George (Eds.), *Attachment disorganization* (pp. 347–378). New York: Guilford Press.

Katsurada, E. (2007). Attachment representation of institutionalized children in Japan. *School Psychology International, 28,* 331–345.

Lieberman, A. F., & Van Horn, P. V. (2009). Child–parent psychotherapy: A developmental approach to mental health treatment in infancy and early childhood. In C. H. Zeanah, Jr. (Ed.), *Handbook of infant mental health* (3rd ed., pp. 439–449): New York: Guilford Press.

Lyons-Ruth, K., & Bronfman, E. (1999). Maternal frightened, frightening, or atypical behavior and disorganized infant attachment. *Monographs of the Society for Research in Child Development, 64,* 67–96.

Lyons-Ruth, K., Bureau, J.-F. O., Riley, C. D., & Atlas-Corbett, A. F. (2009). Socially indiscriminate attachment behavior in the Strange Situation: Convergent and discriminant validity in relation to caregiving risk, later behavior problems, and attachment insecurity. *Development and Psychopathology, 21,* 355–372.

Lyons-Ruth, K., Dutra, L., Schuder, M. R., & Bianchi, I. (2006). From infant attachment disorganization to adult dissociation: Relational adaptations or traumatic experiences? *Psychiatric Clinics of North America, 29,* 63–86.

Lyons-Ruth, K., & Jacobvitz, D. (2008). Attachment disorganization: Genetic factors, parenting contexts, and developmental transformation from infancy to adulthood. In J. Cassidy & P. R. Shaver (Eds.), *Handbook of attachment: Theory, research, and clinical applications* (2nd ed., pp. 666–697). New York: Guilford Press.

Lyons-Ruth, K., Yellin, C., Melnick, S., & Atwood, G. (2005). Expanding the concept of unresolved mental states: Hostile/helpless states of mind on the Adult Attachment Interview are associated with disrupted mother–infant communication and infant disorganization. *Development and Psychopathology, 17,* 1–23.

Macfie, J., Fitzpatrick, K. L., Rivas, E. M., & Cox, M. J. (2008). Independent influences upon mother–toddler role reversal: Infant–mother attachment disorganization and role reversal in mother's childhood. *Attachment and Human Development, 10,* 29–39.

Madigan, S., Bakermans-Kranenburg, M. J., Van IJzendoorn, M. H., Moran, G., Pederson, D. R., & Benoit, D. (2006). Unresolved states of mind, anomalous parental behavior, and disorganized attachment: A review and meta-analysis of a transmission gap. *Attachment and Human Development, 8,* 89–111.

Madigan, S., Hawkins, E., Goldberg, S., & Benoit, D. (2006). Reduction of disrupted caregiver behavior using modified interaction guidance. *Infant Mental Health Journal, 27,* 509–527.

Main, M. (1990). Cross-cultural studies of attachment organization: Recent studies, changing methodologies, and the concept of conditional strategies. *Human Development, 33,* 48–61.

Main, M., & Cassidy, J. (1988). Categories of response to reunion with the parent at age 6: Predictable from infant attachment classifications and stable over a 1-month period. *Developmental Psychology, 24,* 415–426.

Main, M., & Hesse, E. (1990). Parents' unresolved traumatic experiences are related to infant disorganized attachment status: Is frightened and/or frightening parental behavior the linking mechanism? In M. T. Greenberg, D. Cicchetti, and E. M. Cummings (Eds.), *Attachment in the preschool years: Theory, research, and intervention* (pp. 161–182). Chicago: University of Chicago Press.

Main, M., & Hesse, E. (1998). *Frightening, frightened, dissociated, deferential, sexualized, and disorganized parental behavior: A coding system for parent–infant interactions* (6th ed). Unpublished manual, University of California at Berkeley.

Main, M., & Morgan, H. (1996). Disorganization and disorientation in infant

Strange Situation behavior: Phenotypic resemblance to dissociative states. In *Handbook of dissociation: Theoretical, empirical, and clinical perspectives* (pp. 107–138). New York: Plenum Press.

Main, M., & Solomon, J. (1986). Discovery of an insecure–disorganized/disoriented attachment pattern. In *Affective development in infancy* (pp. 95-124). Westport, CT: Ablex.

Main, M., & Solomon, J. (1990). Procedures for identifying infants as disorganized/disoriented during the Ainsworth Strange Situation. In T. B. Brazelton & M. Yogman (Eds.), *Attachment in the preschool years: Theory, research, and intervention* (pp. 121–160). Chicago: University of Chicago Press.

Markovitch, S., Goldberg, S., Gold, A., Washington, J., Wasson, C., Krekewich, K., et al. (1997). Determinants of behavioural problems in Romanian children adopted in Ontario. *International Journal of Behavioral Development, 20*, 17–31.

Marvin, R. S., & Whelan, W. F. (2003). Disordered attachments: Toward evidence-based clinical practice. *Attachment and Human Development, 5*, 283–288.

Moss, E., Bureau, J.-F. O., Cyr, C., Mongeau, C., & St-Laurent, D. (2004). Correlates of attachment at age 3: Construct validity of the Preschool Attachment Classification System. *Developmental Psychology, 40*, 323–334.

Moss, E., Rousseau, D., Parent, S., St-Laurent, D., & Saintonge, J. (1998). Correlates of attachment at school age: Maternal reported stress, mother–child interaction, and behavior problems. *Child Development, 69*, 1390–1405.

Moss, E., & St-Laurent, D. (2001). Attachment at school age and academic performance. *Developmental Psychobiology, 37*, 863–874.

Nachmias, M., Gunnar, M., Mangelsdorf, S., Parritz, R. H., & Buss, K. (1996). Behavioral inhibition and stress reactivity: The moderating role of attachment security. *Child Development, 67*, 508–522.

Nemoda, Z., Lyons-Ruth, K., Szekely, A., Bertha, E., Faludi, G., & Sasvari-Szekely, M. (2007). Association between dopaminergic polymorphisms and borderline personality traits among at-risk young adults and psychiatric inpatients. *Behavioral and Brain Functions, 6*.

O'Conner, T. G., Marvin, R. S., Rutter, M., Olrick, J. T., & Britner, P. A. (2003). Child–parent attachment following early institutional deprivation. *Development and Psychopathology, 15*, 19–38.

Oosterman, M., De Schipper, J. C., Fisher, P., Dozier, M., & Schuengel, C. (2010). Autonomic reactivity in relation to attachment and early adversity among foster children. *Development and Psychopathology, 22*, 109–118.

Out, D. E., Bakermans-Kranenburg, M. J., & van IJzendoorn, M. H. (2009). The role of disconnected and extremely insensitive parenting in the development of disorganized attachment: Validation of a new measure. *Attachment and Human Development, 11*, 419–443.

Perry, B. D. (2008). Child maltreatment: A neurodevelopmental perspective on the role of trauma and neglect in psychopathology. In T. Beauchaine & S. P. Hinshaw (Eds.), *Child and adolescent psychopathology* (pp. 93–129). Hoboken, NJ: Wiley.

Polan, H. J., & Hofer, M. A. (2008). Psychobiological origins of infant attachment and its role in development. In J. Cassidy & P. R. Shaver (Eds.), *Handbook of attachment: Theory, research, and clinical applications* (2nd ed., pp. 158–172). New York: Guilford Press.

Porges, S.W. (2003). Social engagement and attachment: A phylogenetic perspective. *Annals of the New York Academy of Science, 1008,* 31–47.

Robertson, J., & Robertson, J. (1971). Young children in brief separation: A fresh look. *Psychoanalytic Study of the Child, 8,* 288–309.

Shields, A., Ryan, R. M., & Cicchetti, D. (2001). Narrative representations of caregivers and emotion dysregulation as predictors of maltreated children's rejection by peers. *Developmental Psychology, 37,* 321–337.

Shore, A. (2003). *Affect dysregulation and disorders of the self.* New York: Norton.

Siegel, D. J. (2001). Toward an interpersonal neurobiology of the developing mind: Attachment relationships, "mindsight," and neural integration. *Infant Mental Health Journal, 22,* 67–94.

Slade, A. (2005). Parental reflective functioning: An introduction. *Attachment and Human Development, 7,* 269–281.

Solomon, J., & George, C. (1996). Defining the caregiving system: Toward a theory of caregiving. *Infant Mental Health Journal, 17,* 3–17.

Solomon, J., & George, C. (Eds.). (1999a). *Attachment disorganization.* New York: Guilford Press.

Solomon, J., & George, C. (1999b). The place of disorganization in attachment theory: Linking classic observations with contemporary findings. In J. Solomon & C. George (Eds.), *Attachment disorganization* (pp. 3–32). New York: Guilford Press.

Solomon, J., & George, C. (2000). Toward an integrated theory of maternal caregiving. In J. D. Osofsky & H. E. Fitzgerald (Eds.), *World Association of Infant Mental Health handbook of infant mental health* (Vol. 3, pp. 323–368). New York: Wiley.

Solomon, J., & George, C. (2006). Intergenerational transmission of dysregulated maternal caregiving: Mothers describe their upbringing and childrearing. In O. Mayseless (Ed.), *Parenting representations: Theory, research, and clinical implications* (pp. 265–295): New York: Cambridge University Press.

Solomon, J., & George, C. (2008). The measurement of attachment security and related constructs in infancy and early childhood. In J. Cassidy & P. R. Shaver (Eds.), *Handbook of attachment: Theory, research, and clinical applications* (2nd ed., pp. 383–416). New York: Guilford Press.

Solomon, J., George, C., & De Jong, A. (1995). Children classified as controlling at age six: Evidence of disorganized representational strategies and aggression at home and at school. *Development and Psychopathology, 7,* 447–463.

Spangler, G., & Schieche, M. (1998). Emotional and adrenocortical responses of infants to the Strange Situation: The differential function of emotional expression. *International Journal of Behavioral Development, 22,* 681–706.

Stovall, K. C., & Dozier, M. (2000). The development of attachment in new relationships: Single subject analyses for 10 foster infants. *Development and Psychopathology, 12,* 133–156.

Toth, S. L., Rogosch, F. A., Manly, J. T., & Cicchetti, D. (2006). The efficacy of tod-dler–parent psychotherapy to reorganize attachment in the young offspring of mothers with major depressive disorder: A randomized preventive trial. *Journal of Consulting and Clinical Psychology, 74,* 1006–1016.

Tronick, E. Z. (1989). Emotions and emotional communication in infants. *American Psychologist, 44,* 112–119.

van den Dries, L., Juffer, F., van IJzendoorn, M. H., & Bakermans-Kranenburg, M. J. (2009). Fostering security?: A meta-analysis of attachment in adopted chil-dren. *Children and Youth Services Review, 31,* 410–421.

Van der Kolk, B. A., & Fisler, R. E. (1994). Childhood abuse and neglect and loss of self-regulation. *Bulletin of the Menninger Clinic, 58,* 145–168.

Vaughn, B. E., Bost, K. K., & van IJzendoorn, M. H. (2008). Attachment and tem-perament: Additive and interactive influences on behavior, affect, and cognition during infancy and childhood. In J. Cassidy & P. R. Shaver (Eds.), *Handbook of attachment: Theory, research, and clinical applications* (2nd ed., pp. 192–216). New York: Guilford Press.

Venet, M., Bureau, J. F., Gosselin, C., & Capuano, F. (2007). Attachment repre-sentation in a sample of neglected preschool age children. *School Psychology International, 28,* 264–293.

Vondra, J. I., Hommerding, K. D., & Shaw, D. S. (1999). Stability and change in infant attachment style in a low-income sample. *Monographs of the Society for Research in Child Development, 64,* 119–144.

Zeanah, C. H., Smyke, A. T., Koga, S. F., & Carlson, E. (2005). Attachment in institutionalized and community children in Romania. *Child Development, 76,* 1015–1028.

Chapter 2

Disorganization of Maternal Caregiving across Two Generations

The Origins of Caregiving Helplessness

JUDITH SOLOMON and CAROL GEORGE

Disorganized infant attachment is identified by behavior that is contradictory, disordered, misdirected, fearful, or disoriented upon reunion with the parent, following a brief laboratory separation (Main & Solomon, 1986, 1990). This behavior indicates that the child, at least temporarily, is unable to use the caregiver as a secure base and haven of safety. By kindergarten age, formerly disorganized infants are quite likely to use behavioral strategies for controlling the parent upon reunion, either in positive or negative ways, but some disorganized infants and children fail to develop this form of control (i.e., they show continued disorientation and disordering of behavior) (Cicchetti & Barnett, 1991; Main & Cassidy, 1988; see also Moss, Bureau, St-Laurent, & Tarabulsy, Chapter 3, this volume). Attachment-based symbolic play that measures these children's "internal working model of attachment" attests to continuing disorganization of representational processes at this later age, whether or not the child has developed a controlling behavioral strategy with the parent (Solomon, George, & De Jong, 1995).

Mothers of disorganized infants and children can also readily be described as disorganized in caregiving behavior, both at the microanalytic and the functional levels. For example, behavior might seem suddenly threatening or frozen; child-directed speech might have a stuttering, stop–start quality; and caregiving behaviors may be misdirected or quickly con-

25

tradicted (Hesse & Main, 2006; Lyons-Ruth & Block, 1996; Lyons-Ruth, Bronfman, & Parsons, 1999; Lyons-Ruth & Spielman, 2004; Madigan et al., 2006; Madigan, Moran, Schuengel, Pederson, & Otten, 2007; Main & Hesse, 1990; Main & Morgan, 1996). At a functional level, mothers not only fail to provide reassurance, but they also passively place the child at risk or directly frighten the child (George & Solomon, 1989, 2008; Hesse & Main, 2006; Lyons-Ruth et al., 1999; Madigan et al., 2006; Solomon & George, 1996, 2000). In describing the experience of the relationship with their children, these caregivers portray themselves as helpless to manage or protect the child and flooded by powerful, negative feelings (George & Solomon, 1989, 2008; Solomon & George, 2000). We have described these mothers as, at least intermittently, "abdicating" their role as the stronger and wiser member of the caregiving–attachment partnership (George & Solomon, 1989, 2008; Solomon & George, 1996; see also George and Solomon, Chapter 6, this volume), a concept that is now firmly established in contemporary attachment theory (e.g., Britner, Marvin, & Pianta, 2005; Hennighausen, Bureau, David, Holmes, & Lyons-Ruth, Chapter 8, this volume). One of the central questions still to be fully determined is what the mother brings from her past to her caregiving that contributes to the child's attachment disorganization (e.g., Bakermans-Kranenburg, Schuengel, & van IJzendoorn, 1999; Bernier & Dozier, 2003; George & Solomon, 2008; Solomon & George, 2006). In this chapter, we present research that explores the intergenerational roots of caregiver helplessness in a normative, middle-class sample of mothers and their kindergarten-age children.

INTERGENERATIONAL TRANSMISSION OF CAREGIVING PATTERNS

It is axiomatic in clinical developmental theory and practice that a mother carries her own attachment experiences into the relationship she establishes with her child. This proposition is fundamental to Selma Fraiberg's approach to infant–parent psychotherapy, which is based on the identification of the "ghosts in the nursery" that disrupt and distort the mother's caregiving (Fraiberg, Adelson, & Shapiro, 1975). It is also an essential element in many of the successful evidence-based models of infant and child mental health intervention (e.g., Lieberman & Van Horn, 2008; Marvin, Cooper, Hoffman, & Powell, 2002; Tarabulsy et al., 2008; Van Zeijl et al., 2006). To one degree or another, all of these intervention approaches focus on helping the mother to be aware of her "ghosts" and her "angels" (Lieberman, 2007) and their effects on her mothering.

Attachment research forms the empirical basis of these interventions. George, Kaplan, and Main's (1984/1985/1996) Adult Attachment Interview

(AAI) has been particularly influential. Classification of the mother's "state of mind with respect to attachment," which is based on the content and mental organization of her descriptions of childhood attachments, losses, and traumas, strongly predicts classification of her infant's or child's attachment to her (Hesse, 2008; Main, Kaplan, & Cassidy, 1985; van IJzendoorn, 1995; see also Spieker, Nelson, DeKlyen, Jolly, & Mennet, Chapter 4, this volume). In this body of research, the actual events of the past are understood to be less important than the mother's current representation of the past in predicting her child's attachment security, especially the fluidity of her thinking and the place that past and current attachment experience and affect hold in her mind.

How does the mother's representation of the past become incorporated into her mothering? Drawing on our research over the past 20 years, we proposed that the mediating link between the mother's attachment "state of mind" and her current relationship with her child is found in her symbolic representation of her relationship with her child, that is, her caregiving representation (George & Solomon, 1996, 2008; Solomon & George, 1996, 1999). Interviews with mothers about their relationship with the child reveal regular and systematic differences in how women remember, describe, and evaluate their interactions with their child, which correspond strongly both to their children's attachment classification and their own adult attachment classification. We have argued that caregiving representations do not reflect a simple "readout" of earlier attachment-related experiences, but incorporate the child's contribution as well. Thus, the mother's current appraisal or thinking about the parent–child relationship reflects her immediate "retranscription" (West & Sheldon-Keller, 1994) or reconstruction of experiences with the child, in part interpreted in light of her representation of herself in interaction with her own attachment figures (George & Solomon, 2008, p. 840).

Elsewhere we describe at length the definitive features of maternal caregiving representation that we found to be significantly associated with all four of the main child attachment classifications (George & Solomon, 2008; Solomon & George, 2000, 2006; see also George & Solomon, Chapter 6, this volume). The representational feature that is associated with disorganized and controlling child attachment is *caregiving helplessness*. These mothers describe themselves as struggling but failing to manage or control both the child and their own emotions. Some mothers describe themselves as enraged and punitive; others portray themselves as constricting their display of anger, for example, by shutting themselves in their rooms; others portray themselves as dependent on their child's care. Correlatively, some of the children are described as "wild," out of control, aggressive, or defiant; others as precociously competent and caregiving or psychologically merged with the mother; and still others as showing elements of both extremes. We have emphasized that both the punitive and the constricted representational positions are indications of *maternal helplessness* because both violate the adaptive function of the caregiving system, a biologically based behavioral system that is reciprocal to the attachment system and has evolved to protect the immature young (Bowlby, 1982).

DISORGANIZED CAREGIVING
AND LACK OF RESOLUTION OF LOSS AND TRAUMA

In the first middle-class sample we studied, we found that the mother's caregiving classification as "helpless" in the Caregiving Interview was associated both with her child's classification as insecure–controlling or disorganized and with lack of resolution of mourning (unresolved status) in the AAI. This seemed to suggest that whatever caused the mother to fail to complete or integrate mourning at the representational level also made her susceptible to experiencing herself as helpless and her child as out of her control. Previous research gives us some idea of what these experiences might be. Both early loss of attachment and other loved figures, especially loss through death, and maltreatment have figured prominently in etiological investigations. It is not clear, however, if these are independent or interrelated causes. That is, do loss and maltreatment contribute independently to caregiving helplessness, or do these two "assaults" to the attachment system tend to interact in their effect on the development of caregiving?

The hypothesis that loss can disorganize caregiving was first suggested by Main, who, in the course of developing the Adult Attachment Classification System (Main & Goldwyn, 1985), detected an association between the peculiar quality of discourse shown by the parent when discussing the death of an attachment figure and the child's earlier classification as insecure–disorganized. Main described these linguistic features as "lapses" in or loss of monitoring of discourse or reasoning. Examples include extreme attention to the details of the loss, odd expressions or voicing patterns, and evidence that the individual felt an enduring sense of guilt for the event. Main speculated that these, typically linguistic, features were major violations of the discourse rules that organize coherent "conversation" (Grice's maxims; see Hesse, 2008). These lapses were therefore interpreted as a sign of failure to resolve the loss, leading to the proposition that, especially in low-risk samples, disorganized infant attachment was an example of a second-generation effect of the mother's unresolved (dissociated) experience of fears related to loss (Hesse & Main, 2006; Hesse & van IJzendoorn, 1998; Main & Hesse, 1990; Main & Morgan, 1996).

Is the mother's experience of loss in itself frightening and disorganizing at the representational level or are there additional factors that potentiate lack of resolution? Main's data initially suggested that early loss of an attachment figure might be causal, but this was not supported in Ainsworth and Eichberg's (1991) subsequent replication study. Although Ainsworth and Eichberg confirmed the link between lack of resolution of mourning and disorganized infant attachment, they found no association between early loss and lack of resolution of mourning. Rather, they noted that parents might display lapses of monitoring when discussing a broad variety of losses, but these losses might have occurred at any time in the life cycle and did not necessarily involve attachment figures. Losses included parents, significant others outside the nuclear family, and even, in one case, a near stranger. Ainsworth and Eichberg observed that many of the mothers in their sample who were judged to be unresolved (U) for loss had histories of abusive or otherwise very insecure relationships with their parents. These observations were consistent with Bowlby's proposal that adverse events such as problematic early attachment might lead to incomplete or "pathological" mourning (Bowlby, 1980; see also Buchheim & George, Chapter 13, this volume). As a consequence of these and other findings, Main and Hesse (1990) reorganized their model so as to emphasize the centrality of the mother's failure to resolve past or recent losses rather than the loss experience itself as a predisposing factor in the development of attachment disorganization. Faced, too, with the empirical reality that some of the disorganized infants in her sample had parents who talked about physical abuse in their AAIs, Main also developed a lack of resolution of abuse scale, paralleling the loss scale, to capture parental lapses of monitoring when discussing physical abuse. Other researchers have extended the application of these scales to a broad variety of attachment-related events such as sexual abuse and miscarriage. Lack of resolution with respect to loss or abuse, broadly defined, repeatedly has been found to be associated with disorganized attachment in a wide variety of studies (Madigan et al., 2006). It does not account for all cases of disorganization, however. Van IJzendoorn (1995) estimated that just over 50% of disorganized infants have mothers judged U for loss or trauma. This means that about half of disorganized attachments are not unresolved; that is, attachment disorganization for 50% of infants is associated with mothers whose representations of adult attachment are resolved or organized with respect to these factors.

Lyons-Ruth's studies of high-risk and maltreating mothers point to a second developmental pathway. She found that maternal early loss predicted disorganized attachment at 12 months but not at 18 months; indeed, there was considerable instability in disorganized classification over this brief time period (Lyons-Ruth, Connell, Zoll, & Stahl, 1987; Lyons-Ruth, Yellin, Melnick, & Atwood, 2003). At the later point of assessment, maternal experiences of abuse and neglect were most predictive of attachment disorganization. Furthermore, she and her colleagues noted that lack of resolution of scores in general were not sufficient to explain the majority of disorganized attachments in her sample by 18 months. Mothers rarely were classified as U with respect to physical abuse; the majority of U mothers were unresolved for loss. To address this problem, Lyons-Ruth developed an additional set of scales for use with the AAI to capture indices of failure to integrate early maltreatment experiences that have resulted in "hostile" versus "helpless" states of mind with respect to attachment figures. Significantly, severity of abuse was not predictive of either of lack of resolution or hostile–helpless scores (Lyons-Ruth et al., 1987; Lyons-Ruth et al., 2003, 2005). These data echo Main and Hesse's (1990) original approach of highlighting the representation of events rather than their objective quality, but do not in themselves indicate precisely what determines those subjective evaluations.

Finally, there are data that suggest that maternal experiences of loss in adulthood, either alone or in combination with early experience of trauma, can produce disorganized infant attachment (and, it is presumed, disorganization of caregiving). Bakersman-Kranenburg et al. (1999) found that lack of resolution of miscarriage predicted infant disorganization. Hughes and colleagues (Hughes, Turton, Hopper, McGauley, & Fonagy, 2004; Hughes, Turton, McGauley, & Fonagy, 2006), classified attachment in 1-year-olds whose mothers had previously had late miscarriages or stillbirths and administered AAIs to the mothers. Maternal childhood trauma or abuse, overall, was the strongest predictor of being classified as U in relation to that stillbirth and of disorganized attachment in the children born subsequently.

HYPOTHESES OF THE STUDY

As described above, the empirical literature on the antecedents of unresolved or other unintegrated states of mind and, by implication, the antecedents of caregiving helplessness and the disorganized/controlling classification are complex and still unclear, particularly for normative, low-risk samples. A pivotal theoretical and methodological question is how to define the kind of family relationship background that alone, or in interaction with loss, might increase the risk for later caregiving helplessness. Previous investigators have relied on objective or consensual definitions of variables such as "early loss" and "maltreatment." To address this question, we turned to what we learned about the experience of caregiving helplessness from our previous research. We reasoned that if caregiving representations mediate between the mother's attachment representations and her mothering behavior, a mother ought to describe her own attachment experiences in much the same language that she uses to describe her relationship with her child.

As applied to the disorganized and controlling group, this leads to the prediction that mothers of disorganized and controlling children will describe themselves as helpless and frightened with respect to one or more attachment figures and describe those figures as out of control, unpredictable, and frightening or frightened. In addition, because the mother's subjective evaluation of her experience is likely to be most important, the objective severity of her fear and the immediate causes of that fear might be less important than her sense of being without protective figures in the face of threat and without strategies for protecting herself. We should note also that, logically, something in the nature of a loss might complicate the mother's capacity to resolve mourning, a question that also has not been investigated. For example, early losses, losses that are sudden, horrifying, or both, and multiple losses in a brief time span might be especially challenging to the normal process of mourning (Bowlby, 1980).

Our previous research and the reasoning above led to four main hypotheses. First, we expected to replicate our findings from our first study of attachment classification in 5-year-olds (George & Solomon, 1989, 1996). We expected the insecure–controlling and disorganized (D) classifications to be associated both with maternal caregiving helplessness at the representational level and with the mother's U classification on the AAI (i.e., U_{loss} and $U_{physical\ abuse}$). Second, we expected that mothers of children with disorganized–controlling classifications would be more likely than other mothers to describe one or more of their childhood caregiving figures as out of control and unpredictably frightening, themselves as helpless and frightened, and other adult figures as failing to protect or buffer them from the threats or assaults to their attachment systems by these out-of-control individuals. Third, we predicted that "complicated losses," as described above, would be important in predicting maternal caregiving helplessness and child disorganized/controlling attachment. Finally, we predicted that loss and the experience of unpredictably frightening caregivers would have an additive effect in predicting maternal caregiving helplessness and disorganized/controlling attachment.

METHODS

Data for this study were based on 57 of 69 mother–child dyads recruited for the Transition to Middle-Childhood Sample. Twelve dyads from the original sample were dropped from the sample because of missing AAI data. Sample characteristics, recruitment, and data collection procedures have been reported fully elsewhere (Solomon et al., 1995) and are summarized briefly here.

The Sample

The mother–child dyads were recruited from public- and private-school kindergarten classrooms in the San Francisco East Bay area through letters or phone calls, depending upon school policies, or based on referrals from other participants. This sample reflected approximately 90% of all those who expressed interest in participation. The children, 27 boys (47%) and 30 girls (53%), were between the ages of 4 and 7 (mean = 70 months) and the mothers were mature (mean = 38 years), predominantly married (82%), middle-income, college-educated, and white (79%).

Procedures

Child attachment and maternal caregiving data were collected during a single, videotaped laboratory session and a follow-up interview session in the home. In the laboratory, mother and child engaged in a reading task and were then separated for approximately 1 hour. During the separation, mothers were administered the Caregiving Interview (George & Solomon, 1996/2002/2008, adapted from the Parent Development Interview, with permission from Slade and Aber, personal communication, 1989) and children completed semistructured tasks, including our Attachment Doll Play Assessment (Solomon et al., 1995) and free play with a female administrator who was previously unknown to them. Following procedures outlined by Main and Cassidy (1988), the first 5 minutes of the mother–child reunion were used for attachment classification purposes. One to 2 weeks later, research assistants visited mothers in their homes to administer the AAI, which was audiorecorded for later transcription.

Measures

Child Attachment Classifications

The child's attachment to mother was classified into one of four patterns—secure (B), avoidant (A), ambivalent (C), and controlling or disorganized/unclassifiable (D)—following instructions provided by Main and Cassidy (1988). Classifications were completed by the first author who was blind to all other information about the dyad. Agreement with Mary Main on a subsample that included difficult-to-classify or problem cases (n = 14) was 71% (kappa = .62). The distribution of patterns was as follows: B = 15 (26%); A = 18 (32%); C = 13 (23%); and D = 15 (26%). Four of the D children were judged to be unclassifiable/disorganized rather than controlling in attachment, but all of these received an alternate controlling classification (either controlling–punitive or controlling–caregiving). Controlling and disorganized children were combined into a single group for the purposes of analysis. For analysis focused on differences between the controlling sub-groups, the alternate controlling classification of the child was used.

Caregiving Helplessness

We were interested in the present study in evaluating caregiving representational helplessness, one of four rating scales developed for classification of maternal caregiving representations using the Caregiving Interview. The other scales represent organized indices, a description of which is beyond the scope of this chapter. In brief, these scales—flexible integration, rejection/deactivation, uncertainty/cognitive disconnection—identify defensive processing elements that we have shown to be related to caregiving representations associated with the organized attachment groups, (secure, avoidant, and ambivalent–resistant attachments, respectively [see George & Solomon, 1996, 2008]).

Ratings of maternal caregiving helplessness were completed from verbatim transcripts of the Caregiving Interview by the senior authors who were blind to identifying information. A full description of the interview and rating system is provided in the rating manual (George & Solomon, 1996/2002/2008). This semistructured interview asks mothers to describe and reflect upon their relationship with the child through questions about interactions and events that evoke a range of positive and negative thoughts and feelings, including typical and unusual separation experiences. The emphasis in administering the Caregiving Interview is on encouraging the mother to describe specific interactions with the child ("vignettes") using only open-ended questions and prompts. Raters begin by searching through the transcript for vignettes in order to develop an interactive picture of the mother–child relationship from the mother's perspective. Raters next examine each vignette for positive indices of helplessness, including describing the self or the child as behaviorally or emotionally out of control (e.g., "I'm way over my head in this one"), confrontations or avoidance of confrontation with the child (e.g., "What happens then is the wrath of Con, and violence is not below her"), and descriptions of merging or role-reversal on the part of mother or child ("We are very, very close. Like I can sit there with her and just tell her, Mommy did this today"). These indices were derived from our previous study of the links between child attachment and maternal caregiving representation in a sample of 32 middle-class mothers and children (George & Solomon, 1989, 1996). Finally, a helplessness score was assigned for the entire interview using a 7-point rating scale (1 = not helpless and 7 = very helpless), based on the proportion and quality of helplessness indices in the vignettes. Evidence that the mother's thinking, as she finishes describing a vignette, ends on a note of helplessness receives greater weight in the final score than signs of helplessness that are followed by other organizing representational indices. These finishing thoughts suggest that she is not able to contain or reintegrate appraisals of the caregiving relationship as helpless and out of control in that particular situation. The more vignettes that indicate lingering helplessness, the higher the rating. Seven caregiving interviews in the present sample could not be rated either due to missing interviews or technical difficulties, leaving a sample of 50 cases for analyses involving this variable. Correlations between the authors' ratings and those of trained student raters on reliability sets drawn from this and other samples range from .80 to .92

Adult Attachment

Adult attachment was assessed using the 1985 version of the AAI (George et al., 1984/1985/1996). The AAI consists of questions about childhood experiences with parents, including experiences of support, rejection, separation, loss, and maltreatment, that ask the individual to describe and think about past and present effects of these experiences. The interview is rated for a variety of attachment-related experiences as well as aspects of the individual's discourse. These ratings are used to generate classifications of the mother's current state of mind with respect to attachment: secure (F), insecure/dismissing (Ds), insecure/preoccupied (E), or insecure/unresolved with respect to loss or physical abuse (U). Classification of an interview as unresolved (U) is based only on the quality of the individual's comments with respect to a particular loss or trauma (see Main & Goldwyn, 1994, and Hesse, 2008, for a complete description of this system). All of the AAI classifications were completed blind by the second author (CG) who helped develop the classification system and has established reliability of 80% on other samples with trained certified judges who completed Main's AAI Training Workshop.

Life Events Coding

Using mothers' AAI transcripts, four categories of life events were coded to represent childhood experiences (before age 18 or leaving home, whichever came first) of failed protection. We defined the presence of one or more of three life event categories—family violence, affect dysregulation, and substance abuse—as the elements of a "rage pattern," though it would also be appropriate to describe these as elements of a "fear pattern." *Family violence* was defined as all forms of harsh physical or verbal treatment, or behavior leading to physical or verbal harm, intimidation, or humiliation. *Affect dysregulation* was defined as behavior of any household member that was characterized as unpredictable, uncontrollable, and/or intense negative affect. Most often, the negative affect was anger or rage, but in some cases the affect was more depressed, moody, or irritable. Words or phrases such as "sudden" or "hot" temper, "uncontrollable anger," "rage," "snaps," "explodes," "loses it," and "ranting and raving" resulted in positive coding for this category. *Substance abuse* was defined as any household member described as abusing a drug or alcohol. The fourth category of life events was *loss through death,* defined as any loss in the immediate or extended family or individuals identified by the mother as important; the mother's miscarriages or loss of children through death was also coded, as well as the age of the subject at the time of any particular loss. These life events categories were coded in terms of presence/absence by two-person teams (four coders in all) who had no additional knowledge of the participants or the study hypotheses. Life event categories were defined a priori and refined with the assistance of the coders on a set of six training interviews. Inter-team reliability on events and age at which event occurred for a subsample of 19 interviews (agreements/agreements + disagreements) ranged from 87 to 100% across all categories.

Following life events coding, loss information was reduced to two categories that were intended to reflect expected difficulty to assimilate or resolve. One category was designated as *uncomplicated loss,* including the death of one or several grandparents, elderly relatives, or family friends in childhood or death of a single parent after age 18. The other category was designated as *complicated loss,* including the death before age 18 of a parent, sibling, or other young person living in the household; two or more deaths of significant figures (parents, siblings, and/or spouse) within 2 years of one another after age 18; accidental deaths of significant others at any age, loss of a child, and any loss of a family member within 2 years of the birth of the child who was a subject of the study or in the 2 years preceding participation in the study.

Protection-Related Ratings

The transcripts of mothers who had one or more positive indices of the "rage pattern" (n = 24) and four randomly selected cases without positive indices (total = 28) were rated on five 7-point rating scales designed to capture qualitative aspects of this experience. These scales were designed to parallel the helplessness indices used in coding and rating of the Caregiving Interview and derived both from attachment theory and our research regarding attachment in parental divorce (Solomon & George, 1999) and adult attachment (George & West, in press; George, West, & Pettem, 1999). Two scales captured failed protection. *Parent out of control* rated the intensity and persistence of parent behavior described as out of control, unpredictable, frightening, or frightened, including behavior referred to as "rage" (e.g., "enraged," "abusive," "ranting and raving," "screaming," "flipped out"). The score did not reflect the mother's recent revision of past events, when this was so noted by the mother. *Frightened/helpless* rated the intensity and persistence of feelings of fear, helplessness, and being unprotected in response to a household member who was perceived as out of control. Two scales measured successful protection. *Buffering* rated the promptness and effectiveness of attempts by one or more family members to protect the mother emotionally from harm or distress from the out-of-control individual. *Agency* rated the promptness and effectiveness of actions taken by the mother to protect herself from the out-of-control individual. Scores on all scales ranged from 1 to 7.

On all scales, scores between 1 and 7 reflected differences in the intensity and persistence of parent behavior. Scores for the parent out-of-control and frightened/helplessness scales were also higher when the mother was a direct recipient of this behavior rather than a bystander. For purposes of data reduction, the highest score on the parent out-of-control and frightened/helpless scales (pertaining either to mother or father or both) was used in statistical analyses. Due to the limited range of scores for buffering and agency and because relatively few mothers described themselves as showing agency, the highest score received by a mother on either of these scales was used in the analyses.

Rating on these scales was completed by an individual who had not participated in other coding and rating and who was blind to other information pertaining to the family. The correlation between independent scoring by this individual and the first author on six cases, randomly selected from the 28 cases described above, was .85 or higher on all scales.

RESULTS

Replication of Earlier Findings

The results of this study were expected to replicate our earlier findings (George & Solomon, 1989), which demonstrated correspondences among mothers' unresolved classification on the AAI, child disorganized–controlling attachment, and maternal caregiving helplessness. As shown in Table 2.1, there was statistically acceptable correspondence overall between the child and mother attachment measures (kappa = 65; $df = 1$, $p < .001$). This overall level of correspondence was comparable to our earlier study; however, the relation between mother unresolved status on the AAI and child disorganized/controlling classification was more limited in this study than in our previous study. Although three of the five unresolved mothers (60%) in the present sample had children classified as disorganized/controlling, these three cases represented only 20% of the D group in the sample. That is, of the 15 children judged to be disorganized/controlling in relation to mother, 12 (80%) had mothers who were not unresolved with respect to loss or

TABLE 2.1. Correspondence between Child and Maternal Attachment Classifications

Maternal classification	Child classification				
	Secure (B)	Avoidant (A)	Ambivalent (C)	Controlling (D)	Parent total
Autonomous (F)	14			1	15 (26%)
Dismissive (D)		14	1	3	18 (32%)
Preoccupied (E)			11	8	19 (33%)
Unresolved (U)	1		1	3	5 (9%)
Child total	15 (26%)	14 (25%)	13 (23%)	15 (26%)	

Note. Kappa = .65, $df = 1$, $p < .000$. Child classifications are based on child attachment behavior in reunion with the parent (Main & Cassidy, 1998); maternal attachment classifications are based on Adult Attachment Interview classifications (Main & Goldwyn, 1984).

abuse. The most common maternal AAI classification was preoccupied (E). In contrast, in our previous sample, 100% of unresolved mothers had children classified as disorganized/controlling and 67% of these children had mothers who were classified as unresolved.

The results concerning caregiving representational helplessness and child disorganized–controlling classification were consistent with our previous findings, however. These results are shown in Table 2.2. Univariate analysis of variance (ANOVA) showed a significant main effect of child classification on caregiving representational helplessness, $F(3, 46) = 41.98$, $p < .001$. Group comparisons using the conservative Bonferroni correction showed that mothers of disorganized/controlling children described themselves or their children as significantly more helpless than mothers of children in any of the other attachment groups.

Gender Differences

Preliminary analyses revealed an unpredicted but significant effect of gender on attachment classifications. This was most prominent in the D group, which comprised 11 boys (73%) and four girls (27%). Among children with organized classifications, 16 (38%) were boys and 26 (62%) were girls (likelihood ratio = 5.64, $df = 1$; $p = .018$). Given the limited sample size overall, it seemed that including gender as a factor in statistical analyses would reduce rather than increase the interpretability of the results. For this reason, we report below only differences between the organized and the disorganized

TABLE 2.2. Mean Caregiving Helplessness of Mothers for Each of the Child Attachment Classification Groups

	Caregiving helplessness ratings		
Child classification	Mean	SD	n^a
Secure (B)	2.85	1.07	13
Avoidant (A)	2.91	.77	11
Ambivalent (C)	2.83	.83	12
Controlling (D)	5.90	1.61	14

Note. Group D > than Groups B, A, and C, $p < .001$, with Bonferroni correction.
$^a n = 50$; cases in which either AAI or Caregiving Interviews that were missing were excluded from analysis.

classifications. The impact of this decision on the generalizability of results will be addressed in the discussion at the end of the chapter.

Maternal Rage Pattern Events and Protection

As shown in Table 2.3, the child disorganized/controlling classification was strongly and significantly related to maternal reports of rage and experiences of other unpredictably frightening or frightened behaviors on the part of family members. Mothers of all but two of the D children (13 of 15, 87%) reported the presence of one or more of the discrete rage pattern events (family violence, unpredictable anger/negative affect, substance abuse) in their families of origin. In comparison, only 26% ($n = 11$) of mothers whose children were classified into one of the organized attachment categories (A, B, C) reported one or more rage pattern events (likelihood ratio = 17.51, $df = 1$, $p = .000$). Considered separately, these three types of rage pattern events were likely to be reported more than twice as often by mothers of D children than by mothers of children whose attachments were organized. Substance abuse was particularly rare among mothers of organized children (2%; $n = 1$) as compared to mothers of disorganized/controlling children (53%; $n = 8$, likelihood ratio = 19.54, $df = 1$, $p = .000$).

Table 2.3 shows mean differences on the protection-related rating scales between mothers in the "rage sample" whose children were classified as controlling/D or organized. A multivariate ANOVA showed a significant overall effect for disorganization (Wilks's lambda = 4.32, $df = 3$, $p = .020$). Follow-up univariate tests showed significant between-group differences for all three variables. That is, mothers of D children described attachment fig-

TABLE 2.3. Frequency of Maternal Life Events Codes and Mean Protection Ratings for Children with Organized (A, B, C) or Controlling (D) Classifications

Attachment	Life events codes n (%)					Protection ratings mean (SD)		
	Any rage codes	Unpredictable	Violent	Substance Abuse	Complicated loss	Parent out of control	Child helpless	Buffer or agency
Controlling (D)	13*** (87%)	9** (60%)	8** (53%)	8*** (53%)	8* (53%)	5.31 (1.18)	3.50 (2.58)	1.77** (1.09)
Organized (A, B, C)	11 (26%)	9 (21%)	8 (21%)	1 (2%)	10 (24%)	4.55 (1.52)	3.27 (2.14)	3.50 (1.88)

Note. Total n = 57; controlling group n = 15; organized group n = 42.

*$p < .05$; **$p < .01$; ***$p < .001$.

ures as more out of control/frightening and themselves as more helpless/frightened with respect to those figures than mothers of organized children who also had rage experiences. Mothers of the organized children in this group, on the other hand, described attachment figures as more likely to provide protection and buffering or described themselves as higher in agency.

Maternal Loss Related to Rage Events and Child Disorganization

Eighteen mothers (32%) in the sample experienced "complicated losses." As predicted, this experience was significantly more common among mothers of D children than among other mothers. Over half of mothers in the D group (53%, n = 8) were coded as having complicated losses, compared to about one-quarter (24%, n = 10) of mothers in the organized group (chi-square = 4.46, df = 1; p = .040). It is noteworthy that all of the mothers who were classified as unresolved or CC (n = 2) on the AAI reported complicated losses; yet, clearly, not all of the mothers in the sample with complicated loss were classified as unresolved on the AAI.

Hierarchical loglinear analysis was used to test the hypotheses that early rage pattern experiences and complicated loss have additive effects on child disorganization, maternal lack of resolution, and caregiving helplessness. No significant interaction between the two event variables (presence vs. absence of any rage variable; complicated loss) on attachment organization versus disorganization was detected (change in chi-square after the two- and three-way interaction terms were deleted = 1.23, df = 2, p = .540). The effects of complicated loss and rage experiences (presence vs. absence) on caregiving helplessness and AAI lack of resolution scores were examined through two-factor univariate ANOVA. Early rage experience was significantly related to caregiving helplessness, F = 14.08, df = 49, p < .001), and marginally related to lack of resolution, F = 3.9, df = 40, p = .070, but neither complicated loss nor the interaction of rage experiences and complicated loss was predictive of caregiving helplessness or lack of resolution scores.

It was puzzling to find that mothers of D children were more likely than mothers of children with organized attachments to have experienced complicated loss and yet to find no effect of complicated loss and no interaction between loss and rage events on caregiving helplessness or lack of resolution scores. Moss and colleagues (Moss, Bureau, Cyr, Mongeau, & St-Laurent, 2004; Moss, Cyr, Bureau, Tarabulsy, & Dubois-Comtois, 2005; Moss, St-Laurent, Bureau, & Tarabulsy, Chapter 3, this volume) previously reported a link between recent maternal loss and child classification in the controlling–caregiving child attachment classification subgroup but not between maternal loss and the controlling–punitive classification subgroup. We had also noted in reading caregiving interviews that mothers of controlling–caregiving children were more likely than other disorganized/ controlling mothers to describe psychological merging and role-reversal and to "glorify" the child (i.e., describe the child in glowing, awe-struck terms). These representational features were sometimes reminiscent of the "eulogistic" speech sometimes associated with the AAI lack of resolution of mourning (Main & Goldwyn, 1984). We wondered if maternal complicated loss might be related only to the controlling–caregiving subgroup of mother–child attachments. Post-hoc examination of the data confirmed this view: the mothers of six out of seven children judged to be controlling–caregiving had experienced complicated loss, compared to two of the eight mothers of controlling–punitive children. This difference is significant (Fisher's exact test = .045).

DISCUSSION

This study advances our understanding of the intergenerational transmission of disorganized caregiving patterns in several important ways. As predicted, the results replicated our earlier finding (George & Solomon, 1996) of a link between maternal representational helplessness and child controlling and disorganized attachment classifications. In addition, we found that mothers of children with disorganized/controlling classifications were more likely than other mothers to describe their own attachment figures as out of control or unpredictable in the display of rage and other frightening behaviors. All but two of the 15 mothers of children with disorganized/controlling attachments described the behavior of a parent in these terms during the course of the AAI. In several families, both parents were frightening. For example, one participant described her experiences with her brutal stepfather. On occasion, her mother would violently restrain the stepfather, yet the mother was also a victim and tacitly colluded with beatings, humiliation, and fear at the hands of the stepfather. Another participant described her mother as having a breakdown after the loss of a baby and thereafter displaying wild swings in mood and behavior. Her father was a passive alcoholic.

Within the subsample comprised of the participants who described their parents as out of control, ratings for the intensity and chronic nature of the parent's behavior and the participant's own experience of fear and helplessness did not differentiate between mothers of organized and mothers of controlling children. Thus, these findings suggest that the common definition of trauma (i.e., as the overwhelming experience of life-threatening events) is not a necessary precursor to caregiving helplessness, a view that is consistent with the findings of Lyons-Ruth and colleagues' study of high-risk infants (Lyons-Ruth et al., 2003). Of greater significance was the presence or absence of protective factors. Mothers of disorganized and controlling children portrayed themselves as without protection or adequate adaptive strategies. In contrast, mothers in our sample who experienced comparable frightening parental behavior and fear but who also described a family figure or friend who served as a source of reassurance had children who were judged to be organized in attachment. Some of these protective figures intervened directly when the other caregiver was out of control, although this was not always the case. This result parallels well-known findings of the impact of novel and unpredictable events on the stress response of infants and young children and the ameliorative effects of a responsive attachment figure (Gunnar, Brodersen, Nachmias, Buss, & Rigatuso, 1996; Nachmias, Gunnar, Mangelsdorf, Parritz, & Buss, 1996). Other mothers of children with organized attachments described how they relied on their own resources to subdue, avoid, or outwit their frightening or maltreating parent or reached out to helpful persons from outside of the family. Whereas protection and coregulation of the child theoretically is inherent in the organization of the caregiving system (Bowlby, 1982; Polan & Hofer, 2008) mothers of controlling and disorganized children typically describe themselves as in need of protection *from* the child, as protected *by* the child, or both. Given mothers' representation of their attachment figures as threatening and failing to protect them, it is hardly surprising that they chronically or intermittently abdicate the position of the stronger and wiser member of the mother–child dyad (George & Solomon, 1989, 1996; Chapter 6, this volume; Solomon & George, 1996).

The results of this study are consistent with reports of previous investigators and clarify some of the ambiguities evident in their studies. Main and Hesse (1990), in attempting to formulate the etiology of disorganized attachment, have emphasized the connections between dissociative processes and both first- and second-generation experiences of fright, particularly fright related in some way to loss and physical abuse. Ainsworth and Eichberg (1991) had also noted that "insecurity" in general might potentiate a maladaptive response to loss, a view that we note is consistent with Bowlby's (1980) conceptualization of factors predisposing to incomplete mourning. Subsequent researchers have focused explicitly on maltreatment as a precursor to infant disorganization and "disrupted maternal communication" in high-risk or specially selected samples (Hughes et al., 2004; Hughes et al., 2006; Lyons-Ruth & Block, 1996).

Prior to the present study, a link between attachment disorganization and the mother's experience of maltreatment in childhood had not been established in a heterogeneous, nonclinical sample and it was not clear whether other aspects of insecurity might also be predictive. We expanded on previous approaches by attending to a broader but theoretically meaningful set of criteria, that is, negative parental behavior that was inherently frightening by virtue of its unpredictability. This permitted us to identify representational precursors to caregiving helplessness and disorganized caregiving in a normative, low-risk sample.

In contrast to our previous study, the mother's scores on the AAI for lack of resolution of loss or abuse explained little of the variance in child attachment organization. This finding is similar to what has been reported for a high-risk sample (Lyons-Ruth et al., 2003, 2005), but somewhat atypical for normative samples, at least when the focus is infant attachment organization (van IJzendoorn, 1995). However, in this study we focused on loss experiences with attention to the inherent psychological intensity or meaning of events by combining a variety of losses reported by mothers in the AAI into a single category, termed "complicated loss." It was through the lens of complicated loss, then, that we found a relation between maternal loss and disorganized/controlling attachment. This category included both early losses of significant members of the household and later losses of parents, children, and marital partners that were sudden or accidental, occurred in close proximity in time, occurred close to the time of birth of the child in the study, or were recent. The three mothers who were classified as unresolved/CC on the AAI reported complicated loss. Yet, contrary to predictions, the combination of complicated loss with the experience of an unpredictably frightening attachment figure did not predict mothers' lack of resolution scores on the AAI or caregiving helplessness.

This leads us to consider an intriguing but unanticipated finding of the study. Post-hoc analyses revealed that although parental frightening, out-of-control behavior was described by nearly all of the mothers of disorganized/controlling children, only the mothers of children in the controlling–caregiving subgroup also had experienced a complicated loss. All of the mothers who were classified as unresolved on the AAI had children who were in this subgroup. The Caregiving Interviews of mothers of caregiving–controlling children have several common features. Mothers describe themselves as quite constricted in the expression of anger and aggression toward the child. Occasionally they seem absent or dazed in the course of the interview. Finally, many of the mothers describe psychological merging between themselves and their precocious and highly sensitive child. We speculate that it is this subgroup that best conforms to Main's hypotheses (Hesse & Main, 2006; Main & Morgan, 1996) regarding the centrality of unresolved loss and dissociative processes in the behavior of mothers and their disorganized children and these processes may be especially relevant in predicting caregiving–controlling relationships.

To this point, we have framed the discussion in terms of the long-standing clinical theory that maternal representation and behavior in the present are in some way driven by the mother's experiences in the past. Although the Caregiving Interview and the AAI differ considerably in approach and content, it is possible that a mother's thinking about the current relationship with her child influenced her consideration of the past rather than the reverse (i.e., representational transcription of the past based on the present). If so, this would be more than a methodological confound; it might reveal important information about the development of the parent–child relationship and the corresponding representations that parent and child have of their mutual relationship. Spieker, Nelson, DeKlyen, Jolley, and Mennet (Chapter 4, this volume) examined AAI-Strange Situation prediction related to "intra-AAI stability" (stability of AAI discourse-based classifications over time) and "cross age/measurement stability" (concordance between infant Strange Situation and the AAI at a later time). Spieker et al. reported that the instability of mothers' lives in high risk samples may render experiences of loss or abuse as more or less a topic of importance when the mother is asked to respond to the questions in the AAI protocol *depending on her present life experiences*. Spieker et al.'s work centered on mothers at risk; but this thinking is certainly relevant for low-risk samples as well. Difficulties that the mother experiences with the child might constitute another kind of life experience that colors her current representation of the past; and this construction of the past, in turn, might reinforce her current perception of the child, making it more difficult for the dyad to overcome the negative spirals of interaction to which they are clearly subject.

The additional methodological limitations of the present study—both the limited sample size and the disproportionate gender distribution in the various attachment classification groups—constitute a second constraint on our ability to disentangle the effects of maternal history from child effects. Boys far outnumbered girls in the disorganized/controlling group and, given overall low power, we were not able to do analyses pertaining to gender. We are not aware of other samples with this kind of sex bias in the disorganized/controlling group.

Hazen, Jacobvitz, Higgens, Allen, and Jin (Chapter 7, this volume) have emphasized the difference in boys' and girls' responses to social stress as a source of phenotypic differences in the mother–child relationship (see also Taylor et al., 2000). There can be little doubt that a child's emotional reactivity, aggressiveness, or impulsiveness may resonate with troubling aspects of the mother's representation of herself and other attachment figures, biasing her toward interpreting such behavior according to her previous experience. On the basis of their behavioral tendencies, boys would seem to be at greater risk than girls to be the target of mothers' negative perceptions and maternal intrusiveness when boys are emotionally aroused or frustrated (Crockenberg, Leerkes, & Jo, 2008). Girls may also evoke representations of the past in their mothers, by virtue either of their challenging or accommodating behaviors. They have the additional protection, however, of being easier to identify with by their mothers. A mother who has some capacity to reflect on her own experiences, past and present, may find it easier to comprehend or at least attribute beneficent motives to her daughter than to her son. All of these processes, whether at the level of behavior or of representation, clearly merit further study.

We note that the unusual gender distribution in the study might be in some way linked to the unusual distribution of attachment classification groups in the sample as a whole (i.e., more insecure than secure attachments). Previously, we attributed this fact to a variety of self-selection biases believed to operate in the area from which the current sample is drawn (Solomon et al., 1995). The internal consistency that we have found in this sample among the major measures of attachment, caregiving, representation, and classroom behavior as well as the consistency between these data and those reported by other researchers (Lyons-Ruth & Jacobvitz, 2008; Moss, Bureau, et al., 2004; Moss, Cyr, & Dubois-Comtois, 2004; Moss, Parent, Gosselin, Rousseau, & St-Laurent, 1996; Moss et al., 2006) argues for the generalizability of the results from this sample.

The data from this study contribute an important element to our understanding of maternal helplessness and disorganized and disrupted caregiving, allowing us to extend our thinking about the proximate psychological mechanisms and development of these phenomena. Some time ago our child representational data led us to suggest that disorganized and controlling attachments reflect a form of rigid defensive exclusion that Bowlby (1980) termed a "segregated system." This was his attempt to integrate traditional notions of dissociation and repression with the cognitive science of his time (Solomon & George, 1999; Solomon et al., 1995). Segregated systems were described as compartmentalized but contradictory representations of relationships that could not be simultaneously integrated in awareness but might become activated and expressed in behavior at various times and somewhat unpredictably. Although one can question whether mothers in our normative sample actually dissociated when in interaction with the child, we have characterized the mothers' state as one of affective dysregulation and incompletely integrated states of mind (see also Lyons-Ruth et al., 2005).

Based on their descriptions of their upbringing, mothers in the disorganized–controlling group were subject as children to intense, unmodulated negative affect, both their own and their parents. In light of this, it would hardly be surprising if as adults these women were to lack flexible affect regulation strategies (Gunnar & Barr, 1998) and confidence that distress will be assuaged by loved ones. Without such experiences of their own, these mothers quite likely find it difficult to assist their children in similar circumstances. In addition, whether or not their experiences were traumatic in objective terms, the fact that mothers experienced their parents' moods and behaviors as unpredictable or inexplicable may well contribute to a failure to integrate these memories into coherent internal models of attachment and caregiving.

Many investigators use adult attachment measures to stand in for mothers' representation of themselves as caregivers and their likely caregiving behavior. However, the lack of correspondence between adult attachment and child classifications shown in the present study and in others (e.g., Bernier & Dozier, 2003; Dozier, Stovall, Albus, & Bates, 2001) indicates that these behavioral systems are to some degree independent. Developmentally, however, both systems draw to some degree on memories of the same interpersonal experiences, but from different perspectives. That is, children very likely learn both sides of the parent–child relationship, both passively (Gallese, Keysers, & Rizzolatti, 2004) and more actively, through processes of identification and symbolic play (Bretherton & Munholland, 2008)

We have argued that a woman's caregiving system cannot be fully consolidated until she takes over the care of a dependent individual, which is usually caring for her own child (George & Solomon, 2008; Solomon & George, 1996, 1999). She must make an internal shift in her sense of self, from an attachment *subject*, as it were, to herself as the child's attachment figure and protector in order for her caregiving to be appropriately and coherently organized around the welfare of that child. In the usual course of events, this inner shift will likely entail an integration of the (representational) perspective of her parents and memories of herself being cared for by them within her overall representation of herself. This shift in perspective is commonplace, described by many new parents as "finally understanding why my parents acted as they did." Maintaining a coherent sense of the self as both a caregiver and a care receiver is likely to be particularly challenging for the mother who has been raised by unpredictable, frightened, or frightening caregivers. Although she will necessarily have internalized her caregivers' behavior to some degree, memories related to her caregivers are likely to be extremely aversive, at least partially segregated, in Bowlby's terms, and inherently difficult to integrate in consciousness or to acknowledge as a part of one's self-as-a-caregiver. Thus, the woman's internal representation of her caregivers and of herself in relation to them may engender sharp discontinuities in perspective and sense of self in the course of interaction with her child. This unstable or incoherent sense of self plausibly may result in the "lapses in the monitoring" of maternal behavior that are observable as disrupted or contradictory communication (Lyons-Ruth et al., 1999; Lyons-Ruth et al., 2005) and frightened or dissociative behavior (Hesse & Main, 2006; Madigan et al., 2006; Out, Bakermans-Kranenburg, & van IJzendoorn, 2009), both of which have been found to be characteristic of some mothers of disorganized children. This view of disorganized caregiving is broadly consistent with the approaches of Liotti (Chapter 14, this volume) and Lyons-Ruth et al. (2005) to understanding the unintegrated states-of-mind of borderline and physically or sexually abused adults. The results of the present study demonstrate the applicability of these models to a nonclinical sample of mothers and their kindergarten-age children. Both researchers and clinicians may find that widening their focus to include experiences of unpredictable or inexplicable parental behavior, the capacity for self-agency, and parental failures to protect will improve prediction and deepen comprehension of the experiences of adults and children.

ACKNOWLEDGMENTS

We gratefully acknowledge the special contributions of Sabra Melamed, Paloma Hesemeyer, Bianca Hovda, Rebecca Jackly, and Megan McConnel, who assisted with the development of the Failed Protection Scales and the Life Events Coding system and spent long hours on coding and rating. Thanks are also due to the many Mills College students who donated their time and effort to this research.

REFERENCES

Ainsworth, M. D. S., & Eichberg, C. (1991). Effects on infant–mother attachment of mother's unresolved loss of an attachment figure, or other traumatic experience. In C. M. Parkes, J. Stevenson-Hinde, & P. Marris (Eds.), *Attachment across the life cycle* (pp. 160–183). New York: Tavistock/Routledge.

Bakermans-Kranenburg, M. J., Schuengel, C., & van IJzendoorn, M. H. (1999). Unresolved loss due to miscarriage: An addition to the Adult Attachment Interview. *Attachment and Human Development, 1*, 157–170.

Bernier, A., & Dozier, M. (2003). Bridging the attachment transmission gap: The role of maternal mind-mindedness. *International Journal of Behavioral Development, 27*, 355.

Bowlby, J. (1980). *Attachment and loss: Vol. 3. Loss: Sadness and depression.* New York: Basic Books.

Bowlby, J. (1982). *Attachment and loss: Vol. 1. Attachment.* New York: Basic Books. (Original work published 1969)

Bretherton, I., & Munholland, K. A. (2008). Internal working models in attachment relationships: Elaborating a central construct in attachment theory. In J. Cassidy & P. R. Shaver (Eds.), *Handbook of attachment: Theory, research, and clinical applications* (2nd ed., pp. 102–127). New York: Guilford Press.

Britner, P. A., Marvin, R. S., & Pianta, R. C. (2005). Development and preliminary validation of the Caregiving Behavior System: Association with child attachment classification in the preschool Strange Situation. *Attachment and Human Development, 7*, 83–102.

Cicchetti, D., & Barnett, D. (1991). Attachment organization in maltreated preschoolers. *Development and Psychopathology, 3*, 397–411.

Crockenberg, S. C., Leerkes, E. M., & Barrig Jo, P. (2008). Predicting aggressive behavior in the third year from infant reactivity and regulation as moderated by maternal behavior. *Development and Psychopathology, 20*, 37–54.

Dozier, M., Stoval, K. C., Albus, K. E., & Bates, B. (2001). Attachment for infants in foster care: The role of caregiver state of mind. *Child Development, 72,* 1467–1477.

Fraiberg, S., Adelson, E., & Shapiro, V. (1975). Ghosts in the nursery: A psychoanalytic approach to the problems of impaired mother–infant relationships. *Journal of the American Academy of Child and Adolescent Psychiatry, 14,* 387–422.

Gallese, V., Keysers, C., & Rizzolatti, G. (2004). A unifying view of the basis of social cognition. *Trends in Cognitive Science, 8,* 396–403.

George, C., Kaplan, N., & Main, M. (1984/1985/1996). *Adult Attachment Interview.* Unpublished manuscript. University of California at Berkeley.

George, C., & Solomon, J. (1989). Internal working models of caregiving and security of attachment at age six. *Infant Mental Health Journal, 10,* 222–237.

George, C., & Solomon, J. (1996). Representational models of relationships: Links between caregiving and attachment. *Infant Mental Health Journal, 17,* 18–36.

George, C., & Solomon, J. (1996/2002/2008). *Caregiving representation rating manual: Rating scales, and Caregiving Interview protocol.* Unpublished manuscript, Mills College, Oakland, CA.

George, C., & Solomon, J. (2008). The caregiving system: A behavioral systems approach to parenting. In J. Cassidy & P. R. Shaver (Eds.), *Handbook of attachment: Theory, research, and clinical applications* (2nd ed., pp. 833–856). New York: Guilford Press.

George, C., & West, M. (in press). *The Adult Attachment Projective Picture System.* New York: Guilford Press.

George, C., West, M., & Pettem, O. (1999). The Adult Attachment Projective: Disorganization of adult attachment at the level of representation. In J. Solomon & C. George (Eds.), *Attachment disorganization* (pp. 462–507). New York: Guilford Press.

Gunnar, M. R., & Barr, R. G. (1998). Stress, early brain development, and behavior. *Infants and Young Children, 11,* 1–14.

Gunnar, M. R., Brodersen, L., Nachmias, M., Buss, K., & Rigatuso, J. (1996). Stress reactivity and attachment security. *Developmental Psychobiology, 29,* 191–204.

Hesse, E. (2008). The Adult Attachment Interview: Protocol, method of analysis, and empirical studies. In J. Cassidy & P. R. Shaver (Eds.), *Handbook of attachment: Theory, research, and clinical applications* (2nd ed., pp. 552–598). New York: Guilford Press.

Hesse, E., & Main, M. (2006). Frightened, threatening, and dissociative parental behavior in low-risk samples: Description, discussion, and interpretations. *Development and Psychopathology, 18,* 309–343.

Hesse, E., & van IJzendoorn, M. H. (1998). Parental loss of close family members and propensities towards absorption in offspring. *Developmental Science, 1,* 299.

Hughes, P., Turton, P., Hopper, E., McGauley, G. A., & Fonagy, P. (2004). Factors associated with the unresolved classification of the Adult Attachment Interview in women who have suffered stillbirth. *Development and Psychopathology, 16,* 215–230.

Hughes, P., Turton, P., McGauley, G. A., & Fonagy, P. (2006). Factors that predict infant disorganization in mothers classified as U in pregnancy. *Attachment and Human Development, 8,* 113–122.

Lieberman, A. F. (2007). Ghosts and angels: Intergenerational patterns in the transmission and treatment of the traumatic sequelae of domestic violence. *Infant Mental Health Journal, 28,* 422–439.

Lieberman, A. F., & Van Horn, P. (2008). *Psychotherapy with infants and young children: Repairing the effects of stress and trauma on early attachment.* New York: Guilford Press.

Lyons-Ruth, K., & Block, D. (1996). The disturbed caregiving system: Relations among childhood trauma, maternal caregiving, and infant affect and attachment. *Infant Mental Health Journal, 17,* 257–275.

Lyons-Ruth, K., Bronfman, E., & Parsons, E. (1999). Maternal frightened, frightening, or atypical behavior and disorganized infant attachment patterns. *Monographs of the Society for Research in Child Development, 64,* 67–96.

Lyons-Ruth, K., Connell, D. B., Zoll, D., & Stahl, J. (1987). Infants at social risk: Relations among infant maltreatment, maternal behavior, and infant attachment behavior. *Developmental Psychology, 23,* 223–232.

Lyons-Ruth, K., & Jacobvitz, D. (2008). Attachment disorganization: Genetic factors, parenting contexts, and developmental transformation from infancy to adulthood. In J. Cassidy & P. R. Shaver (Eds.), *Handbook of attachment: Theory, research, and clinical applications* (2nd ed., pp. 666–697). New York: Guilford Press.

Lyons-Ruth, K., & Spielman, E. (2004). Disorganized infant attachment strategies and helpless–fearful profiles of parenting: Integrating attachment research with clinical intervention. *Infant Mental Health Journal, 25,* 318–335.

Lyons-Ruth, K., Yellin, C., Melnick, S., & Atwood, G. (2003). Childhood experiences of trauma and loss have different relations to maternal unresolved and hostile–helpless states of mind on the AAI. *Attachment and Human Development, 5,* 330–352.

Lyons-Ruth, K., Yellin, C., Melnick, S., & Atwood, G. (2005). Expanding the concept of unresolved mental states: Hostile/helpless states of mind on the Adult Attachment Interview are associated with disrupted mother–infant communication and infant disorganization. *Development and Psychopathology, 17,* 1–23.

Madigan, S., Bakermans-Kranenburg, M. J., van IJzendoorn, M. H., Moran, G., Pederson, D. R., & Benoit, D. (2006). Unresolved states of mind, anomalous parental behavior, and disorganized attachment: A review and meta-analysis of a transmission gap. *Attachment and Human Development, 8,* 89–111.

Madigan, S., Moran, G., Schuengel, C., Pederson, D. R., & Otten, R. (2007). Unresolved maternal attachment representations, disrupted maternal behavior and disorganized attachment in infancy: Links to toddler behavior problems. *Journal of Child Psychology and Psychiatry, 48,* 1042–1050.

Main, M., & Cassidy, J. (1988). Categories of response to reunion with the parent at age 6: Predictable from infant attachment classifications and stable over a 1-month period. *Developmental Psychology, 24,* 415–426.

Main, M., & Goldwyn, R. (1985). *Adult attachment scoring and classification system.* Unpublished manuscript, University of California at Berkeley.

Main, M., & Hesse, E. (1990). Parents' unresolved traumatic experiences are related to infant disorganized attachment status: Is frightened and/or frightening parental behavior the linking mechanism? In *Attachment in the preschool years: Theory, research, and intervention* (pp. 161–182). Chicago: University of Chicago Press.

Main, M., Kaplan, N., & Cassidy, J. (1985). Security in infancy, childhood, and adulthood: A move to the level of representation. *Monographs of the Society for Research in Child Development, 50,* 66–104.

Main, M., & Morgan, H. (1996). Disorganization and disorientation in infant Strange Situation behavior: Phenotypic resemblance to dissociative states. In L. K. Michel & W. J. Ray (Eds.), *Handbook of dissociation: Theoretical, empirical, and clinical perspectives* (pp. 107–138). New York: Plenum Press.

Main, M., & Solomon, J. (1986). Discovery of an insecure–disorganized/disoriented attachment pattern. In T. B. Brazelton & M. Yogman (Eds.), *Affective development in infancy* (pp. 95–124): Westport, CT: Ablex.

Main, M., & Solomon, J. (1990). Procedures for identifying infants as disorganized/disoriented during the Ainsworth Strange Situation. In M. T. Greenberg, D. Cicchetti, and E. M. Cummings (Eds.), *Attachment in the preschool years: Theory, research, and intervention* (pp. 121–160). Chicago: University of Chicago Press.

Marvin, R., Cooper, G., Hoffman, K., & Powell, B. (2002). The Circle of Security Project: Attachment-based intervention with caregiver–pre-school child dyads. *Attachment and Human Development, 4,* 107–124.

Moss, E., Bureau, J.-F., Béliveau, M.-J., Zdebik, M., & Lépine, S. (2009). Links between children's attachment behavior at early school-age, their attachment-related representations, and behavior problems in middle childhood. *International Journal of Behavioral Development, 33,* 155–166.

Moss, E., Bureau, J., Cyr, C., Mongeau, C., & St-Laurent, D. (2004). Correlates of attachment at age 3: Construct validity of the Preschool Attachment Classification System. *Developmental Psychology, 40,* 323–334.

Moss, E., Cyr, C., Bureau, J., Tarabulsy, G. M., & Dubois-Comtois, K. (2005). Stability of attachment during the preschool period. *Developmental Psychology, 41,* 773–783.

Moss, E., Cyr, C., & Dubois-Comtois, K. (2004). Attachment at early school age and developmental risk: Examining family contexts and behavior problems of controlling–caregiving, controlling–punitive, and behaviorally disorganized children. *Developmental Psychology, 40,* 519–532.

Moss, E., Parent, S., Gosselin, C., Rousseau, D., & St-Laurent, D. (1996). Attachment and teacher-reported behavior problems during the preschool and early school-age period. *Development and Psychopathology, 8,* 511–525.

Moss, E., Smolla, N., Cyr, C., Dubois-Comtois, K., Mazzarello, T., & Berthiaume, C. (2006). Attachment and behavior problems in middle childhood as reported by adult and child informants. *Development and Psychopathology, 18,* 425–444.

Nachmias, M., Gunnar, M., Mangelsdorf, S., Parritz, R. H., & Buss, K. (1996). Behavioral inhibition and stress reactivity: The moderating role of attachment security. *Child Development, 67,* 508–522.

Out, D., Bakermans-Kranenburg, M. J., & van IJzendoorn, M. (2009). The role of disconnected and extremely insensitive parenting in the development of disorganized attachment: Validation of a new measure. *Attachment and Human Development, 11*, 419–433.

Polan, H. J., & Hofer, M. A. (2008). Psychobiological origins of infant attachment and its role in development. In J. Cassidy & P. R. Shaver (Eds.), *Handbook of attachment: Theory, research, and clinical applications* (2nd ed., pp. 158–172). New York: Guilford Press.

Solomon, J., & George, C. (1996). Defining the caregiving systems: Toward a theory of caregiving. *Infant Mental Health Journal, 17*, 3–17.

Solomon, J., & George, C. (1999). The caregiving system in mothers of infants: A comparison of divorcing and married mothers. *Attachment and Human Development, 1*, 171–190.

Solomon, J., & George, C. (2000). Toward an integrated theory of maternal caregiving. In J. D. Osofsky & H. E. Fitzgerald (Eds.), *World Association of Infant Mental Health handbook of infant mental health* (Vol. 3, pp. 323–368). New York: Wiley.

Solomon, J., & George, C. (2006). Intergenerational transmission of dysregulated maternal caregiving: Mothers describe their upbringing and childrearing. In O. Mayseless (Ed.), *Parenting representations: Theory, research, and clinical implications* (pp. 265–295). New York: Cambridge University Press.

Solomon, J., George, C., & De Jong, A. (1995). Children classified as controlling at age six: Evidence of disorganized representational strategies and aggression at home and at school. *Development and Psychopathology, 7*, 447–463.

Tarabulsy, G. M., Pascuzzo, K., Moss, E., St-Laurent, D., Bernier, A., Cyr, C., et al. (2008). Attachment-based intervention for maltreating families. *American Journal of Orthopsychiatry, 78*, 322–332.

Taylor, S. E., Kein, L. C., Lewis, B. P., Gruenewald, T. L., Gurung, R. A. R., & Updegraff, J. A. (2000). Biobehavioral responses to stress in females: Tend-and-befriend, not fight-or-flight. *Psychological Review, 107*, 411–429.

van IJzendoorn, M. (1995). Adult attachment representations, parental responsiveness, and infant attachment: A meta-analysis on the predictive validity of the Adult Attachment Interview. *Psychological Bulletin, 117*, 387–403.

Van Zeijl, J., Mesman, J., van IJzendoorn, M. H., Bakermans-Kranenburg, M. J., Juffer, F., Stolk, M. N., et al. (2006). Attachment-based intervention for enhancing sensitive discipline in mothers of 1- to 3-year-old children at risk for externalizing behavior problems: A randomized controlled trial. *Journal of Consulting and Clinical Psychology, 74*, 994–1005.

West, M. L., & Sheldon-Keller, A. E. (1994). *Patterns of relating: An adult attachment perspective*. New York: Guilford Press.

Chapter 3

Understanding Disorganized Attachment at Preschool and School Age

Examining Divergent Pathways of Disorganized and Controlling Children

ELLEN MOSS, JEAN-FRANÇOIS BUREAU,
DIANE ST-LAURENT, and GEORGE M. TARABULSY

A mother and her 5-year-old son arrive at our laboratory playroom for their scheduled visit. We ask them to sit down. Two chairs are provided; one is a regular adult-sized chair and the other is a small chair, similar to those found in elementary school classrooms. The mother sits down in the large chair. Suddenly, the child becomes angry and says in a commanding voice, "Get up from that chair! It's for me. Go sit in the other one." The mother says nothing, looks sheepish, and quietly gets up and goes to sit in the small chair.

A second mother and her 5-year-old daughter enter the playroom. The mother sits down and the child immediately becomes involved in showing her mother a toy. The mother quickly loses interest and the child finds a second object which she brings to the mother's attention. The child appears to be quite animated and adopts a lively, happy voice when addressing her mother. By contrast, the mother appears deflated, unfocused, and expresses little emotion in voice or mannerisms. The play interaction continues with the child initiating most of the interactive exchanges and the mother sitting quite passively, sometimes in what appears to be a dissociated state.

In a third case, a 5-year-old boy is playing independently while his mother tries to draw his attention toward her. At one point, she asks the child to sing a song for her. He refuses, insisting that he wants to play on his own. The mother persists, saying that it will make her happy and that he is a good singer. The child continues to refuse to sing a song. As the tension escalates between them, the child breaks down, saying, "I will get beat up if I sing." The mother, surprised by his answer, asks him to explain himself. The child answers, "I'm ugly, like my father." The mother seems quite shocked and says, "You're not ugly and neither is Dad!" The child then seems very surprised as if he did not remember his previous statement, and asks, "What are you talking about?" Strikingly, during this whole interaction, the child's nonverbal behavior and posture remain neutral, and he keeps playing with his toys.

These three descriptions are typical of the observational notes that are used to classify disorganization at preschool and early school age. They represent the three patterns of child attachment to the caregiver that fall in the spectrum of controlling or disorganized behavior in children ages 3–7. The child in the first vignette presented was classified controlling–punitive, the second controlling–caregiver, and the third behaviorally disorganized using the Cassidy, Marvin, and McArthur Working Group on Attachment (1992) classification system. This coding system allows the classification of children based on their attachment behaviors into the secure category, the insecure–organized categories (insecure–avoidant and insecure–ambivalent), or one of the three insecure–disorganized categories described above. Previous studies have enabled us to better understand the individual and family processes that contribute to these different subtypes of disorganization which emerge by early school age, as well as their impact on child social–emotional and school adaptation. In this chapter, we attempt to broaden understanding of disorganization beyond infancy by discussing recent theoretical, methodological, and empirical findings that have substantially changed our conceptualization of this phenomenon. We begin by discussing changes in the behaviors associated with disorganization following the infancy period, and how developmental changes in the child, caregiving patterns, and traumatic family events contribute to these changes. We next discuss the impact of disorganized attachment on social–emotional and cognitive development during the school years. We believe that this chapter may be of interest to clinicians, as well as researchers, because it discusses the role of disrupted parenting, maternal psychosocial difficulties, and traumatic life events as factors playing a key role in the emergence of different forms of disrupted attachment at early school age.

CHANGES IN DISORGANIZED ATTACHMENT BEYOND INFANCY

As explained by Britner, Marvin, and Pianta (2005), the child attachment and parental caregiving systems are integrated in a manner that keeps the child organized and safe, while permitting exploration and the development of autonomy. During the preschool period, as the child's representational and communicative skills improve, caregiver–child interactions become increasingly focused on mutually affecting one another's plans (Marvin & Britner, 2008). The child, who is increasingly able to represent the attitudes, goals, and feelings that organize and regulate dyadic functioning, can play a greater role in maintaining an effective goal-corrected partnership (Bowlby, 1982) with the caregiver, which requires the ability to verbally negotiate shared plans that may conflict with individual motives. Balanced role structuring during the preschool period is also linked with the ability of the dyad to appropriately integrate affective experience. Research indicates that during the preschool period secure mother-child dyads evidence more reciprocity and greater interactive competence than insecure mother–child dyads (Barnett, Kidwell, & Leung, 1998; Moss, Rousseau, Parent, & Saintonge, 1998; Stevenson-Hinde & Shouldice, 1995). Mothers and their secure children show greater reciprocity in interactions, more freely explore emotional themes, and rely more on interpersonal experience to repair conflicts than do dyads with insecure children (Britner et al., 2005). Dyads with insecure–organized patterns of attachment are more likely to show interactive patterns that are less balanced and less mutually regulated in meeting the needs of both partners than do secure dyads. However, the unbalanced parent–child relationships that characterize dyads that involve a disorganized child reflect a relational structure in which one partner's initiatives are elaborated at the expense of the other partner's (Lyons-Ruth, Bronfman, & Atwood, 1999). In line with these ideas, our longitudinal data indicated that although reciprocity and balanced emotional expression improved for the sample over the course of the preschool period, the interactive quality of the disorganized subgroups either decreased or remained stable (Moss, Cyr, Bureau, Tarabulsy, & Dubois-Comtois, 2005).

Within the context of a greater child role in regulating the emotional content of the dyadic relationship, preschool and early school-age attachment profiles for secure, avoidant, and ambivalent children are thus qualitatively similar to those displayed in infancy. For these groups, some level of child dependency on the parent for dyadic regulation is maintained. However, a radical shift in role structuring within the mother–child dyad occurs for many children with disorganized attachment. Earlier follow-up studies of infants who had been classified as disorganized in infancy indicated that the majority developed a role-reversed controlling reunion pattern by age 6 (Main & Cassidy, 1988; Wartner, Grossman, Fremmer-Bombik, & Suess,

1994). Results of our more recent longitudinal study of a normative sample showed that the transition from disorganization to a controlling strategy occurs primarily between the ages of 3 and 5, and that a larger proportion of children than previously thought (7/23, or about one-third of the D group) remained behaviorally disorganized without developing a controlling strategy (Moss et al., 2005). This study also revealed that, despite a high rate of stability within the disorganized/controlling category, three distinct profiles of disorganization (controlling–punitive, controlling–caregiving, and behaviorally disorganized) had developed by age 5. How did these profiles emerge out of infant disorganization?

Disorganized/disoriented infants have been distinguished from those with more "organized" secure or insecure attachment strategies by their apparent failure to show a coherent behavioral strategy for dealing with separation and reunion with their mothers (Main & Solomon, 1990). These infants display bouts or sequences of behaviors that seemingly lack a goal and, in contrast to infants of other attachment classifications, appear to experience a "collapse of strategy" (Main, 1995). This collapse of strategy can be understood as the inability of the child to maintain an organized strategy for seeking proximity to the caregiver in stressful situations owing to overwhelming fear. Further expanding beyond Main's hypothesis, George and Solomon (2008) have suggested that maternal behavior (and internal working models) revealing helplessness and mother being out of control of herself, the child, or the situation leaves the child in momentary or prolonged states of feeling abandoned or unprotected. Thus, they suggested that it is not scary behavior per se, but the experience of abdicated care on the part of the attachment figure, that is frightening for the child. Children with a disorganized attachment pattern are therefore faced with a developmental paradox. The attachment figure is the only available caregiver in times of distress, but the child has already learned that to express distress in the presence of this parent is likely to evoke subtle or overt hostile or helpless parental behavior and thereby increase child distress.

Solomon, George, and De Jong (1995) suggested that the onset of controlling behavior in disorganized children may be linked to regulation of the child's own internal state and behavior, especially feelings of helplessness and being out of control. Mason (1968) noted that one of the psychological determinants of stress response is an individual's feeling that he or she does not have control over a situation. In this perspective, the development of parentified behavior over the preschool period may be the disorganized child's adaptive attempt to reduce stress levels, which cannot be regulated through child dependency on the caregiver (see also George & Solomon, 2008). Furthering this idea, a recent study also suggests that children's increase in controlling behavior with the caregiver during the preschool period may not only be linked to child self-regulation, but also with other-regulation by the child of the parent. Moss, Thibaudeau, Cyr, and Rousseau (2001) found that children's increase in controlling behaviors during the preschool period was associated with a reduction in parental anxiety and depression, suggesting that the controlling strategy may well function as a "pseudo"-mechanism for regulating parental emotional states. "Pseudo" refers to the fact that the underlying trauma or other parental problems related to their caregiving difficulties remain untreated. Results of this study also showed that, whereas there was a reduction in parental symptoms during the preschool period, there was a concomitant increase in child behavior problem symptoms during the same period. This supports the theory that the disorganized child's strategy of orienting away from seeking comfort, protection, and the meeting of his or her own needs and toward maintaining engagement with the parent on the parent's terms is likely to increase the likelihood of child psychopathology (Bowlby, 1982; Main & Cassidy, 1988). However, more recent findings (to be discussed below) suggest that particular events and conditions in the family contexts of disorganized children also influence the evolution of disorganization beyond infancy.

Longitudinal studies examining developmental precursors of the three different forms of disorganized/controlling groups that emerge by early school age are rare. Few studies contained sufficient numbers of disorganized and controlling children to do analyses by subgroup. We recently completed the first study of the preschool to school-age trajectories of the three disorganized subgroups. The objective of this study was to examine longitudinally the maternal caregiving and psychosocial patterns, the family characteristics, and the behavior problems of children classified as controlling–caregiving, controlling–punitive, and behaviorally disorganized at early school age. Owing to the large sample size of 242 families that we followed longitudinally between the ages of 3 and 8 years, we were able to split the 37 disorganized children by subgroup based on reunion patterns at 5 years of age (Moss, Cyr, & Dubois-Comtois, 2004). In this group, 13 children were evaluated as controlling–caregiving, 12 as controlling–punitive, and 12 retained a behaviorally disorganized classification.

Child attachment and stressful life events (the latter retrospectively: parental separation/divorce, hospitalization of a parent for a serious illness, and/or death of significant relatives) were measured at ages 5–7 years (Time 2), and mother–child interactive quality, parenting stress, marital satisfaction, and teacher-reported behavior problems were evaluated concurrently and 2 years earlier, when the children were ages 3–4 years (Time 1). We also recently conducted an age-8 follow-up of this sample, which included teacher reports of child behavior problems and school performance measures (Bureau, Moss, & St-Laurent, 2006). Attrition for the group of disorganized/controlling children as a whole between Time 1 and Time 2 and between Time 2 and Time 3 was comparable to that of the rest of the sample (roughly 15 %). Attrition rates for the disorganized subgroups (classified at age 5) were also comparable to one another (approximately 20%). Moreover, the attrition group did not differ from the rest of the sample on child gender, age and IQ, socioeconomic status, or child behavior problems. The only significant difference was that mothers from the attrition sample were more depressed than mothers who returned for follow-up $F(1, 239) = 5.27$, $p = .023$. However, the mothers of disorganized children in the attrition group ($n = 6$) were not more depressed than other mothers in the attrition sample ($n = 28$). An overview of the methodologies of the different studies conducted by our research group is presented in Table 3.1.

In undertaking this study, we expected that all the disorganized subgroups would experience a poorer caregiving environment, a greater number of traumatic family events, and more developmental risk related to socioemotional and academic functioning than secure children. Concerning maternal variables that have been found to influence parental caregiving, such as perceived stress and marital quality, we expected a higher level of maternal psychosocial difficulty for the disorganized subgroups, with different variables associated with different subtypes. In addition, on the basis of previous theoretical and empirical associations between disorganization of attachment relationships and the experience of potentially traumatic events in the family system, we expected that mothers of the disorganized subgroups might report higher levels of severe separation experiences, such as parental separation or divorce, parental hospitalization, or loss of significant family members. Finally, we hypothesized that the disorganized and the controlling groups would show different levels of externalizing and internalizing behavior problems. Although we had certain tentative hypotheses concerning comparisons among the controlling–caregiving, controlling–punitive, and insecure-other groups (which are discussed below), given the paucity of previous studies, we could not specify any further predictions concerning differences among the subgroups on study variables.

TRAJECTORIES OF CONTROLLING
AND BEHAVIORALLY DISORGANIZED CHILDREN

In this section, we summarize the current literature on disorganization in the preschool and school-age periods, integrating our own new findings on the separate trajectories of the three disorganized subgroups. We describe what is currently known about the role of caregiving, marital context, and traumatic life events in the development of disorganization. We then discuss sequelae of disorganization with respect to behavior problems and academic risk. Our emphasis in this section is on the postinfancy period, between preschool and early school age. Given that the bulk of the literature is com-

TABLE 3.1. Overview of the Methodology of the Recent Studies by Moss and Colleagues

Study	Sample	Study variables
Moss & St-Laurent (2001): Attachment, cognitive engagement, and academic achievement	108 dyads (Cohort 1), ages 6 and 8	Preschool child attachment; child cognitive engagement; quality of mother–child interaction; child mastery motivation; academic achievement
Moss, Bureau, et al. (2004): Validation of the preschool attachment system at 3 years of age	153 dyads (Cohort 2), age 3	Preschool child attachment; teachers' and mothers' report of behavior; maternal depression; maternal stress; stressful life events; maternal child-rearing practices
Moss, Cyr, & Dubois-Comtois (2004): Comparisons of controlling–disorganized subgroups	242 dyads (Cohorts 1 and 2), Ages 3 and 6	Preschool child attachment; quality of mother–child interaction; teachers' report of behavior; conjugal satisfaction; maternal depression; maternal stress; stressful life events
Moss et al. (2005): Stability of attachment during the preschool period (ages 3–5)	120 dyads (Cohort 2), ages 3 and 6	Preschool child attachment; quality of mother–child interaction; conjugal satisfaction; maternal depression; family risk index; stressful life events
Moss et al. (2006): Multiple informants of behavior problems	96 dyads (Cohort 1), ages 6 and 8	Preschool child attachment; self-, teachers', and mothers' reports of behavior

posed of studies that did not conduct analyses as a function of subgroup type (i.e., controlling–punitive, controlling–caregiving and behaviorally disorganized), we will first briefly summarize these studies and then describe in greater depth our results concerning subgroup differences. In order to illustrate certain points and also render this chapter more useful for clinical work, descriptions of observed interactive sequences will be included when relevant.

The Emergence of Different Forms of Disorganization at Early School Age: The Influence of Caregiving, the Marital Context, and Traumatic Life Events

An accumulating list of studies have indicated that infants identified as disorganized according to the Main and Solomon (1990) coding system experience the most dysfunctional caregiving when compared with other attachment groups (Carlson, 1998; Lyons-Ruth, Alpern, & Repacholi, 1993; Lyons-Ruth, Bronfman, & Parsons, 1999; van IJzendoorn, Schuengel, & Bakermans-Kranenburg, 1999). Additional research has associated infant disorganization with parental maltreatment, parental psychopathology, and disturbed parent–infant interactions (Madigan et al., 2006; van IJzendoorn et al., 1999), further suggesting that the child's inability to form comprehensible attachment behaviors may be influenced by parental characteristics related to unpredictable and aversive patterns of early care. The association between disorganization in infancy and frightened, frightening, or disrupted maternal behaviors has been confirmed in several independent samples (for a meta-analysis, see Madigan et al., 2006).

In a high-risk sample, mothers of infants classified disorganized using separation–reunion measures have been described as highly insensitive with repeated episodes of hostile intrusiveness and/or emotional detachment (Lyons-Ruth, Yellin, Melnick, & Atwood, 2005). Maternal internal working models revealing helplessness and hostility about their past experiences with attachment figures predicted both disrupted interaction and child disorganization (Lyons-Ruth et al., 1999, 2005). At preschool and school age, a similar profile has emerged for those classified as behaviorally disorganized or controlling (these two groups are generally combined in most studies) (Main, Kaplan, & Cassidy, 1985; Moss et al., 1998; NICHD Early Child Care Research Network, 2001; Stevenson-Hinde & Shouldice, 1995; Teti, 1999). Numerous studies indicate that both at preschool and at school age, mothers and disorganized/controlling children also evidence lower quality parent–child communication, affective attunement, reciprocity, and emotion regulation than insecure/organized dyads (Main et al., 1985; Moss, Bureau, Cyr, Mongeau, & St-Laurent, 2004; Moss, Cyr, & Dubois-Comtois, 2004; Moss, et al., 1998; Moss & St-Laurent, 2001; Moss, St-Laurent, & Parent, 1999; Stevenson-Hinde & Shouldice, 1990, 1995; Teti, 1999).

These studies have found less coordination and attunement for both the disorganized and the controlling groups when compared with children showing other attachment patterns. Our longitudinal data (Moss et al., 2005) indicated that, although reciprocity and balanced emotional expression improved for the sample over the course of the preschool period, the interactions of all the disorganized subgroups showed continued disrupted affective communication characterized by failed reciprocity, periods of very low engagement, or hostile, conflictual interaction.

Exploring the same longitudinal high-risk samples as Lyons-Ruth et al. (2005), Bureau, Easterbrooks, and Lyons-Ruth (2009) showed that maternal disrupted communication in infancy predicted child punitive and caregiving behavior 7 years later. More specifically, overall maternal disrupted communication predicted child punitive behavior, while maternal withdrawal in infancy predicted child caregiving behavior.

Moving beyond the parent–child dyad, a meta-analysis of combined infant, preschool, and school-age studies also indicate significant associations between disorganized attachment and unresolved loss or trauma and marital discord (van IJzendoorn et al., 1999). Bowlby (1953) discussed how severe and chronic parental illness, the death of important family members, and parental separation may raise child fears related to the lack of protection for the self or the caregiver. In several studies with preschool or school-age samples, mothers of disorganized children had higher levels of depression, dysfunctional marital relations, parenting stress, and difficulties in managing the caregiving role (George & Solomon, 1996; Moss, Bureau, et al., 2004; Solomon & George, 1999c; Stevenson-Hinde & Shouldice, 1995; Teti, Gelfand, Messinger, & Isabella, 1995). Not surprisingly, mothers of secure preschool children tend to report supportive romantic relationships and low levels of depression and stress; mothers of insecure children tend to report dysfunctional romantic relationships and high levels of maternal depression and parenting stress (Davies & Cummings, 1994; Mills-Koonce, Gariepy, Sutton, & Cox, 2008; Moss et al., 1998; Teti et al., 1995).

However, findings are not consistent from study to study, suggesting that discrepancies in the prevalence of different risk factors may be linked to differences between samples (e.g., higher or lower risk), which may also affect the proportion of children in each disorganized subgroup. For example, results from studies indicate that the ratio of behaviorally disorganized to controlling children may be considerably higher in psychiatrically at-risk (Speltz, Greenberg, & De Klyen, 1990) or maltreated samples (Cicchetti & Barnett, 1991).

The Controlling–Punitive Pattern: The Role of Maternal Stress and Caregiving

Children who are classified as controlling–punitive direct behaviors toward the caregiver that may include harsh commands, verbal threats, and occasional physical aggression toward the parent. In one sequence we observed, a 5-year-old boy became frustrated with a difficult toy during a separation episode. He called for the mother while angrily kicking the toy against the wall. When the mother returned for the reunion, the child displayed a mixture of crying and screaming as he went toward her, but before reaching her, abruptly turned around and headed in the opposite direction.[1] He then commanded the mother to leave the room, shouting, "Go outside, go outside!" After the third repetition, the mother sheepishly left the room to sit on a chair in the hallway. The child went out and ordered the mother to "move her chair farther away." The mother once again obeyed the child's order. Upon returning alone to the room, the child quickly calmed down and returned to normal play. Several minutes later the mother asked if she could come back in the room. The child refused; 5 minutes later when the mother asked again in a very submissive tone, "Can I come in now? It's getting lonely out there," the child acquiesced, the mother came in, and the dyad returned to normal interaction.

The most striking feature of this sequence is that the mother appears clearly intimidated by her child and helpless in the face of his punitive behavior, despite the fact that he is only a small 5-year-old boy in great distress. In fact, on a stress questionnaire completed by all mothers in our study, when their children were ages 5–7 years, mothers of controlling–punitive children reported the highest levels of child-related stress in the sample. They described their children as more hyperactive and less adaptable than did mothers of other attachment groups. Moreover, our longitudinal data showed that they viewed their children as increasingly difficult and out of control as they approached school age, despite the fact that most other parents perceive this period as increasingly easier from a child-rearing perspective, owing to a general child decrease in aggressive behavior. Interview data collected by George and Solomon (1996) also support these results in showing that mothers of controlling–punitive children described their relationships with their children as stressful, confrontational, and combative and experience themselves as helpless to control themselves or their children (see also George & Solomon, Chapter 6, this volume). Although we examined other family process measures such as maternal depression and experience of traumatic life events, we were unable to isolate any unique contextual factors that differentiated the controlling–punitive group from other attachment groups (both organized classifications and other disorganized subgroups). However, our measures did not include specific questions concerning maternal experience of maltreatment, of a past or present (e.g., spousal) nature.

It is possible that the maternal difficulties in responding appropriately to child distress that we have described here are related to the mother's own unresolved fearful experiences which may limit flexible attention to the child's current states and even lead to dissociative responses (Lyons-Ruth et al., 1999; Main & Hesse, 1990; Solomon & George, 2006; Chapter 2, this volume). Indeed, on an anecdotal level, in the case of several controlling–punitive dyads that we observed, mothers appeared to have little recollection of events occurring during episodes in which the child expressed distress or anger, suggesting temporary dissociation. For example, one 5-year-old boy asked his mother why she did not respond to his cries for help. The mother replied that the child had never asked for help. The videotaped segment in question clearly showed that the child had, in fact, asked for help, while simultaneously showing a mixture of whining, regressed behavior, and punitive anger directed at the mother. A second interesting example involved a clinical consultation in which the first author was involved. A teacher recounted the story of a 4-year-old boy who had attacked her in the presence of the child's mother, who showed no reaction immediately following the event. In an interview about this episode, the mother claimed that the attack had never occurred, although there were several witnesses, and the teacher in question required medical attention for injuries sustained during the attack. Further research on the maternal states of mind and antecedents in mother's own attachment history which are related to this attachment pattern are necessary.

The Controlling–Caregiving Pattern: The Impact of Loss

Although both interactions of controlling–punitive and controlling–caregiving dyads involve role-reversal and restricted emotional expression, so great are the qualitative differences in interactions of mothers and children in each subgroup that it is difficult to imagine that these dyads are part of the same disorganized spectrum. Children classified as controlling–caregiving direct the parent's activities and conversational exchanges by structuring interactions in a helpful and/or emotionally positive manner. Whereas the controlling–punitive child's interactions with the caregiver seem designed to humiliate her into submission through initiation of hostile and aggressive interactions, the controlling–caregiving child seems motivated to orient or protect the parent by being excessively cheery, polite, or helpful. It is notable, however, that, as is the case with the controlling–punitive group, there is a notable lack of reciprocity in these parent–child exchanges, and considerable affective disparity between the partners. For example, mothers often appear quite passive and disengaged, showing a neutral or negative affective expression. In contrast, the controlling–caregiving child appears lively and animated, and quite attentive to the needs of the mother.

For example, one child we observed was constructing a tower from a set of blocks. Mom was not at all actively involved in the game. When the tower fell, the child turned quickly to mother and said, "Don't worry, Mom, it'll be okay!" Another characteristic of children with the controlling–caregiving attachment pattern is that they seem not to show any signs of distress or related negative emotional expression in the presence of the mother. In the case of another child who was pretending to serve tea and cookies to her mother, when the latter harshly rejected the proffered items and attempted to redefine the game, the child, for an instant, became angry. However, abruptly, the child grabbed her own body in a strait-jacket mode, dropped her head, and became totally silent for about a minute. She then recovered with a bright smile and cheerily continued directing the game.

Despite the fact that both the controlling–punitive and the controlling–

caregiver subtypes are in a role-reversed relationship with the caregiver, there is evidence to suggest that the maternal experience is quite different. In contrast to mothers of controlling–punitive children who reported feeling increasingly more stressed and unable to cope with their children over the preschool period, mothers of controlling–caregiving children reported feeling increasingly better about their relationship with their children and described their children as more adaptable. Caregiving interviews conducted with mothers of controlling-caregiving children in a study by George and Solomon (1996) showed that mothers of controlling–caregiving children may paradoxically feel both disinvested (e.g., ceased to make an effort or take an interest in the relationship) in the mother–child relationship, and exceptionally close to their children, with an emphasis on the children's precociousness and, in some cases, the children's taking responsibility for maternal emotions.

One clue to the developmental trajectory of the caregiving group emerged when we compared attachment groups with respect to the incidence of traumatic separation-related experiences. Mothers of children who developed a controlling–caregiving pattern by early school age had a greater likelihood of loss of their own attachment figure than did any other attachment group (both organized attachment classifications and other disorganized subgroups). This association was also confirmed by Solomon and George (2006; Chapter 2, this volume) who described an unusually high rate of complicated bereavement reported by mothers of controlling–caregiving children.

The death of their attachment figure had occurred during *their child's* early childhood (birth to 5 years of age). Unresolved loss has been associated with infant disorganization in a number of studies (see van IJzendoorn, 1995, for a review). Lyons-Ruth and colleagues (1999) also reported that the mothers of disorganized/secure infants[2] (who, they suggest, may later become caregivers) had experienced a higher proportion of loss of *their own* parent through death, separation, or divorce during childhood than did infants who were classified as disorganized/insecure.

Bowlby (1980) suggested that parents experiencing difficulty coping with their own loss may seek comfort from their children, which leads to role-reversal. Although the mechanism by which mothers' loss experience is associated with the development of a controlling–caregiving strategy in her child is not yet understood, it is likely that a relational diathesis is implicated. As explained by Lyons-Ruth et al. (1999), if a caregiver has not experienced comforting in relation to her own past losses, the infant's own distress may evoke her own unresolved fearful affects, as well as her sense of helplessness in finding comfort. The caregiver must restrict her attention to the infant's stress cues in order to regulate her own negative arousal, leading to considerable imbalance in the parent–child relationship.

It is interesting that the reduction in stress over the course of the pre-school period that mothers of controlling–caregiving children report coincides with the emergence of caregiving behavior in their children. The emergence of punitive behavior over the same period is not similarly associated with maternal stress reduction, but in fact is related to increased stress. This suggests that the caregiving behavior of controlling–caregiving children may actually reduce parental negative arousal, but that controlling–punitive behavior does not. How and why this occurs is a topic for further research. Apart from loss experiences, we were unable to isolate any other family background factors that differentiated the families of controlling–caregiving children from other disorganized groups.

The Behaviorally Disorganized Group: The Impact of Marital Dysfunction and Parental Hospitalization

Although we found that the majority of children with preschool disorganized attachment patterns did change to a controlling pattern by early school age, one-third of this group remained behaviorally disorganized. These children resembled disorganized infants in displaying disordered, incomplete movements, confusion, and apprehension in the presence of the attachment figure and no coherent strategy for seeking proximity or in combining two insecure patterns (e.g., avoidant and ambivalent). It is important to note that postinfancy disorganized behaviors, such as contradictory sequencing, may be manifested in verbal as well as nonverbal exchange patterns. For example, during the reunion with mother described earlier, a 4-year-old child suddenly started to make bizarre, frightened, and self-depreciative comments. He then seemed to completely forget about this part of the conversation when his mother answered him back. The child also seemed to experience abrupt changes of state evidenced by a sudden shift of affect and disruption in his discourse.

Although affective disparity between the partners and in the dyad is common to both controlling and disorganized children at early school age, the abruptness of the changes seen in behaviorally disorganized children and their lack of an established communicative pattern, even if nonoptimal, such as in the caregiving or punitive patterns, make disorganized dyads appear more disrupted in their communication. Perhaps as Solomon et al. (1995) have suggested, behaviorally disorganized children, who lack a controlling strategy for regulating negative emotions and containing fear, act it out in a more obvious manner in their behavior.

However, why does this subgroup of children not develop a controlling strategy, as the majority of disorganized infants do? Our examination of family process variables for this group revealed that the behaviorally disorganized group was significantly higher than all other attachment groups (both organized classifications and other disorganized subgroups) on maternal reports of marital dissatisfaction. In fact, the mean score for marital problems reported by mothers of behaviorally disorganized children exceeded the clinical cutoff score for a dysfunctional couple relationship. This result is consistent with Bowlby's (1973) theorizing that marital conflict may lead to parental rejection, which in turn may lead to dysfunctions in the parent–child attachment system. This result is also in line with those by O'Connor, Bureau, McCartney, and Lyons-Ruth (2009) who obtained similar results in the National Institute of Child Health and Human Development (NICHD) sample with preschool-age children. Mothers of behaviorally disorganized children reported lower conjugal satisfaction than all other attachment groups, including controlling–punitive and controlling–caregiving. Whereas previous studies have found an association between high levels of marital discord and disorganized attachment (Moss, Cyr, et al., 2004; Owen & Cox, 1997; Solomon & George, 1999c; Teti & Gelfand, 1997; van IJzendoorn et al., 1999; Zeanah et al., 1999), no previous study had examined whether severe marital conflict was more likely to be associated with the development of a controlling or behaviorally disorganized strategy.

The unpredictability and overwhelming nature of the family environment, which is disrupted by severe marital conflict, may compromise the possibility of the child's forming an organized integrated model of attachment, even one of a role-reversed controlling nature. In order for the child to assume a controlling role in the family system, it is necessary for parents to allow, either complicitly or explicitly, such role-reversal. Secondly, for any organized attachment strategy to develop, there must be a predictable adaptive outcome for the child. In the families of controlling children, the child's involvement with the mother in a role-reversed fashion may be adaptive from a family systems perspective. In a family where a child has succeeded in taking control of one parent's behavior, there is an implicit disengagement on the part of both mother and father. A disengaged father might welcome child attempts to take responsibility for regulating his spouse's dysregulated emotional states and the child's overinvolvement may even play a functional role in regulation of marital tension.

However, in a family with high levels of marital tension, fathers have been shown to be more negative and intrusive with their children and patterns of child rearing to be more inconsistent (Belsky, Youngblade, Rovine, & Volling, 1991; Jacobvitz, Riggs, & Johnson, 1999). In such a context, child attempts to control maternal behavior are likely to increase paternal negativity toward the child and child feelings of rejection. In order to repair the relationship with the child's father, the child may form a temporary alliance with him against the mother, until resulting feelings of rejection lead him to change alliances once again. Thus, chronic marital conflict presents the child with both experiences of frightened or frightening parental behavior which may directly impact on feelings of insecurity, and diminished behavioral options to alleviate accompanying distress (Owen & Cox, 1997).

Apart from marital dysfunction, we also discovered that children classified as behaviorally disorganized had experienced a significantly higher proportion of parental hospitalization due to a serious illness or accident than secure children (see also George & Solomon, Chapter 6, this volume). In fact, half of this group had experiences of this kind. The serious disruption in the family that is occasioned by parental hospitalization may be associated with an increase in children's fears related to lack of protection for themselves or their caregivers, which in turn may lead to disorganization of attachment-related mental processes (Bowlby, 1980; Robertson, 1962). Parents experiencing their own or their spouse's hospitalization may adopt a helpless, rejecting, or even frightening stance in the face of their children's own attachment behavior. The poor communication patterns and greater marital conflict that also characterize the family environments of the behaviorally disorganized group would likely render any resolution of this trauma by family members even more difficult. The stressful life events questionnaire used in this study did not include reasons for parental hospitalizations, but further studies should examine whether parental hospitalization might be psychiatric in nature and thus embedded in a larger context of disrupted parental behavior. In addition, prevalence of other traumatic attachment-related events such as parental incarceration should be included in future studies.

DISORGANIZATION AT SCHOOL AGE: SOCIAL–EMOTIONAL DEVELOPMENT AND SCHOOL ADAPTATION

Disorganization and the Development of School-Age Behavior Problems

According to attachment theory, the quality of early relationships with caregivers has a continuing effect on patterns of interpersonal adaptation (Bowlby, 1982). As discussed above, insecurity and disorganization in particular may lead to unresolved anger, anxiety, and fear, and to related externalizing and internalizing problems. Given the disrupted caregiving and family patterns that characterize the disorganized/controlling groups, it is not surprising that disorganized attachment is associated with risk in a number of developmental domains. Several large-scale studies with both normative and higher risk samples have found externalizing behavior–problem associations for the disorganized/controlling group, when infant or preschool/school-age classifications are used as predictors (Bureau & Moss, 2010;

Greenberg, Speltz, DeKlyen, & Endriga, 1991; Lyons-Ruth, Easterbrooks, & Cibelli, 1997; Moss, Bureau, et al., 2004; Munson, McMahon, & Spieker, 2001; NICHD Early Child Care Research Network, 2001; Shaw, Owens, Vondra, Keenan, & Winslow, 1996). Studies have also noted increased risk for internalizing problems for this group during childhood and adolescence (Carlson, 1998; Moss, Cyr, et al., 2004; Moss, Bureau, et al., 2004).

Although at preschool and early school age, it is primarily an aggressive, disruptive behavior pattern that is associated with disorganization (George & Solomon, Chapter 6, this volume; Lyons-Ruth et al., 1997; Speltz et al., 1990), anxieties and fears related to performance, abilities, and self-worth become more pronounced in middle childhood (Cassidy, 1988; Jacobsen, Edelstein, & Hoffmann, 1994). In two recent studies, we found that children with disorganized patterns of attachment to the caregiver at 6 years of age were more likely than their peers to represent conflict themes and to depict chaotic and violent interpersonal relationships in their narratives 2 years later (Bureau & Moss, 2010; see also Solomon et al., 1995). Both the disorganized classification and the conflict narrative dimension predicted age-8 internalizing symptoms. In keeping with these ideas, several previous studies have noted increased risk for internalizing problems for the disorganized/controlling group at early school age, middle childhood, and adolescence (Carlson, 1998; Moss et al., 1998).

Disorganization and School Performance

These motivational and self-dimensions have important implications, not only for levels of behavior problems, but also for a wide range of competences related to academic performance. The considerable cognitive and attentional resources necessary to cope with a caregiver who induces fear or feelings of abandonment or threat in the child should considerably restrict the mental resources available for learning and exploration (Aber & Allen, 1987; Main, 1991). Secondly, as suggested by Main and Solomon (1990) and Solomon and George (1996), prolonged child exposure to a disorganized or frightening parent who does not assist the child in dealing with negative feelings may lead to problems in cognitive self-regulatory activity that influence both the processing of social–emotional information and tasks of an academic nature. Thirdly, lack of parental involvement in scaffolding children's emerging executive or metacognitive functions may hinder the development of child self-regulation in learning tasks (Moss, 1992; Moss, Gosselin, Parent, Rousseau, & Dumont, 1997; Zimmerman, 2002).

In support of these theoretical ideas, we found a number of important results related to the school performance of the disorganized/controlling group (all subgroups combined) at early school age and middle childhood in two studies that we conducted (Moss & St-Laurent, 2001; Moss et al., 1999). The clearest indicator of academic risk was the finding that controlling children, despite their similarity in IQ to other attachment groups, showed the poorest school performance of all attachment groups. In addition to low perceived competence, children displaying controlling attachment behavior showed metacognitive deficits at age 5, and poor math performance 2 years later. As hypothesized, disorganized children and their mothers were also the least likely of all attachment groups to display a collaborative pattern facilitative of joint problem solving. These results show continuity with studies indicating that mothers of disorganized infants and preschoolers were lowest on involvement, teaching skill, positive parent–infant mutuality, and conversational skill (Lyons-Ruth et al., 1997; Main et al., 1985; Moss, Bureau, et al., 2004; Solomon & George, 1999a; Stevenson-Hinde & Shouldice, 1995). We also tested the mediational role of self-esteem and mother–child interaction in explaining the demonstrated relation between controlling/noncontrolling attachment and academic performance. Our analyses revealed that both negative self-evaluations of children with a disorganized classification and their dis-synchronous mother–child interactive patterns mediated the relation between attachment and school performance. These findings are also supported by those of Jacobsen and her colleagues (Jacobsen et al., 1994; Jacobsen & Hoffmann, 1997), indicating that disorganization, as assessed by a representational measure of attachment at 7 years of age, predicted deficits in cognitive and metacognitive functioning during middle childhood and adolescence that were mediated by low self-confidence (Jacobsen et al., 1994). Together, these findings support the hypothesis that the cognitive self-regulatory activity of children and adolescents with disorganized representational strategies are not limited to the processing of socioemotional information but extend to tasks of an academic nature.

DISORGANIZED SUBGROUPS AND DEVELOPMENTAL RISK

These results, in conjunction with our previous findings concerning difficulties in social–affective components of interaction (Moss et al., 1998) support the idea that disrupted levels of cognitive as well as social engagement may characterize the interactive environment of disorganized children and their caregivers. However, owing to small sample sizes in these original studies, we were unable to examine the separate profiles of the three disorganized subgroups. In the following section, we discuss recent findings for each of these groups concerning behavior problem profiles and school adaptation.

Controlling–Punitive Children: Externalizing Behavior Problems and Underachievement

As described earlier, controlling–punitive children appear to use angry, contradictory patterns of avoidance and hostility to capture and maintain dyadic attention. The child's overt power assertion through attacking or humiliating the parent appears to increase maternal involvement (Jacobvitz & Hazen, 1999; Solomon & George, 1999b). In our recent study of the behavior problem profiles of the three disorganized attachment groups, we found that the controlling–punitive group was rated by their teachers as significantly higher than other attachment groups on the Externalizing problem scale. Even after controlling for child sex, IQ, and socioeconomic status, controlling-punitive attachment still was a significant predictor of children's externalizing behavior at ages 4, 5, and 8. Teti (1999) found that controlling–punitive preschoolers showed poorer functioning than secure children on measures of fussiness–difficultness and general emotional tone. Bureau et al. (2009) also found that punitive behaviors observed at age 8 were significantly associated with externalizing behaviors. Finally, O'Connor et al. (2009) reported that punitive preschoolers were more disruptive than other children.

Concerning the school performance of children with a controlling–punitive profile, we obtained results from a study examining scores for cognitive engagement during a joint problem-solving task at age 4 and academic performance at age 6 (Moss & St-Laurent, 2001). Our results showed that controlling–punitive children had lower scores than secure children on both variables. In a recent follow-up study of these children (Bureau et al., 2006) this earlier indication of academic risk was supported by our finding that controlling–punitive children were the only D subgroup to be evaluated by their teachers as having poorer academic performance than secure children in middle childhood. In a regression analyses that evaluated the contribution of different risk factors to the prediction of academic performance, we found that even after considering the role of child sex, IQ, and family socioeconomic status, controlling–punitive attachment was still a significant predictor of academic risk.

The adoption of a parentified role vis-à-vis the caregiver implies abdicated caregiving interactions (Solomon & George, 1996), which may be incompatible with the careful monitoring of and adjustment to the child's state required not only for adequate development of child affective-self functions, but also to facilitate the development of cognitive regulatory functions during the school-age period (Main, 1991; Vygotsky, 1978). Role-reversal in the caregiver–child dyad may interfere with the acquisition and consolidation of higher level cognitive skills important for school success. Alternatively, other cognitive or metacognitive deficits may underlie the academic underachievement of the controlling–punitive group. Although no deficits in overall IQ were evident for this subgroup, it is possible that more specific skills related to cognitive executive functioning underlie both the lack of aggressive inhibition and certain academic problems of the punitive group. Although a few studies have established links between metacognitive functioning and attachment disorganization (Moss & St-Laurent, 2001; Moss et al., 1999), no studies have yet examined whether these deficits are specific to one or more of the D subgroups.

Controlling–Caregiving Children: Higher Rates of Internalizing Problems and Lower Mastery Motivation Than Secure Children

Our earlier examples of the interactions between controlling–caregiver children and their mothers illustrate a style of emotion regulation that seems quite opposite to that of the controlling–punitive group. Controlling–caregiving children suppress their own negative affect and, at times, may attempt to animate or cheer up the mother. In line with these findings, our analyses of the behavior problem profiles of the controlling–caregiving group revealed no evidence of elevated risk for aggressive behavior problems, but rather significantly higher rates of internalizing behavior problems, when compared with secure children. It is not surprising that the child's strategy of containing distress should lead to elevated rates of anxiety, depression, and other internalizing symptoms. The discrepancy between keeping up the supercompetent self that the child is obliged to show to the mother and unsuccessfully trying to regulate the fearful, inner self may further the process of mental disorganization, leading to split, segregated, or confused models of self (Lynch & Cicchetti, 1991). The absence of externalizing problems is also consistent with the child's strategy of trying to appease maternal distress.

However, our examination of the academic profiles of controlling–caregiving children showed a lower level of academic risk in comparison with the controlling–punitive group. Their levels of cognitive engagement resembled that of the secure group at preschool age (Moss & St-Laurent, 2001). In our recent analyses, controlling–caregiving children also resembled secure children on academic performance based on school marks at early elementary level (Bureau et al., 2006). The only evidence of cognitive risk that emerged in our analyses was the finding that controlling–caregiving children had lower mastery motivation scores than secure children as assessed on the "goal orientation" questionnaire (Ames & Archer, 1988). Maintaining a caregiving profile implies focusing on maternal needs to the detriment of the child's own pursuits. Apart from the emotional burden of being unable to seek comfort from the caregiver in dealing with the child's own distress, the child may also neglect school tasks such as homework or other extracurricular activities that may draw the child away from home, rendering him or her less available to mother. Clinicians report cases in which children will not attend school on days that mother is feeling too depressed to function and the caregiver child is obliged to attend to the needs of younger children at home. It is easy to see how academic concerns will be of less importance to a child faced with such a situation. On a more positive note, the fact that controlling–caregiver children did not appear to show important deficits in academic performance suggests more positive outcomes in comparison with that of their punitive peers. It is likely that the differing social–emotional profiles of the two groups also have an influence on teachers' and peers' attitudes toward these groups in academic situations. On the one hand, their lack of aggressive behavior may render it easier for the controlling–caregiving child to receive academic assistance in the classroom. On the other hand, the controlling–punitive child's involvement in aggressive interactions in the school setting is likely to elicit negative attention from teachers and school authorities. The helpful, empathic attitude of the caregiver child, if extended to the school context, may elicit quite the opposite kind of attention.

Behaviorally Disorganized Children: Externalizing Problems and Underachievement

Our comparisons of the behavior problem profiles of the behaviorally disorganized group at ages 4 and 5 revealed that they, like controlling–punitive children, were marginally higher than their secure peers on the Externalizing scale. This result is supported by previous findings indicating a maladapted behavioral profile for this group at preschool age (Cichetti & Barnett, 1991; Teti, 1999). In our recent follow-up of this group at 8 years of age, we found a significant difference on the externalizing scale in comparison with the secure group (Moss et al., 2006). This result is not surprising given studies that have also associated high levels of marital conflict with the development of externalizing behavior problems. In their recent review, Cummings and Davies (2002) speculated that certain forms of children's internal regulation of exposure to interparental conflict may pose particularly substantial long-term risks for maladjustment. This result is also consistent with findings that suggest that those disorganized children who fail to develop even a compensatory controlling pattern by early school age may be at risk for more serious maladaptation (Speltz et al., 1990). Our findings suggest that there is a higher level of risk for these behaviorally disorganized children in comparison with those children who develop a controlling–caregiving strategy, but not in comparison with the controlling–punitive group. Similar results were also found in a study with school-age children (Bureau et al., 2009). That is, both the behaviorally disorganized and the controlling–punitive children developed higher levels of externalizing behavior problems as well as serious academic problems. It is important to note that these profiles apply to the middle childhood period and may change by adolescence.

CONCLUSION

In this chapter, we have presented theoretical ideas and empirical findings concerning disorganization in the preschool and school-age period, as well as new evidence clarifying the precursors and sequelae of different forms of disorganized behavior beyond infancy. We have provided descriptions and examples of each profile and what is currently known about each of these groups with respect to family background, child behavior problem profiles, and academic functioning in the preschool/school-age period. These findings support the importance of inadequate parenting, maternal psychosocial difficulties, and traumatic life events as factors playing a key role in the emergence of different forms of disorganized and controlling attachment at early school age. They also shed light on why disorganized children may adopt different strategies with their caregivers by school age and what the social–emotional cost to the child of these different strategies might be. The different pathways into middle childhood of the three disorganized subgroups appear to be mediated by different caregiving patterns, self processes, and family events that may seriously compromise both affective and cognitive development. Given the important role of family processes in explaining the types of difficulties, both social–emotional and academic, experienced by disorganized children at school age, interventions related to school underachievement that focus on the role of the child in the family context are likely to be more successful than those that focus only on individual child cognitive deficits.

One of the conclusions that we propose can be drawn from the current literature on disorganization is that the disorganized and controlling classifications no longer be considered to be a single group with similar family and child behavior problem profiles. In future studies, it will be important to attempt to study large enough samples that will enable separate analyses of these groups. In addition, researchers should focus attention on higher risk samples (e.g., maltreated children, children of adolescent mothers) that are likely to include higher numbers of disorganized and controlling children. Secondly, our findings concerning the important role of the marital relationship and of major separation events in the developmental trajectories of disorganized and controlling groups suggest that attachment theory needs to move beyond its focus on the mother–child dyad. Although this is not a new suggestion, researchers have been reluctant to incorporate family systems models within attachment theory. However, it is likely that further research into disorganization will benefit greatly from such efforts.

Finally, we would like to suggest ideas for future research into disorganization at school age. In attachment theory, behavioral patterns with caregivers and other social partners are believed to reflect internalized representations constructed on the basis of earlier attachment relationships and likely updated as a function of the ongoing quality of such relationships beyond infancy (Bowlby, 1973). During middle childhood, representations of specific relationships with caregivers are likely to become better integrated within higher order metarepresentational systems that influence children's overall view of themselves and relationships (Steele & Steele, 2005). We need to know more about the differences in child internal working models which characterize the disorganized subgroups and how experiences with different caregivers in the family system influence the development of these models. In addition, more in-depth examination of the histories of parents of the different disorganized subgroups, particularly concerning their experiences of abuse and neglect, might further our understanding of the intergenerational transmission of disorganization. Future studies are needed to examine these questions and to further trace the trajectories of disorganized and controlling children in the later school-age and adolescent period in order to verify whether the associations between particular attachment classifications and the problem profiles identified here are maintained.

It is also important to consider other possible pathways linking disorganization to academic problems. For example, given the importance of supportive peer relationships in determining school success (Epstein, 1992), it is likely that problems in peer social competence contribute to disorganized children's social–emotional and academic difficulties. Longitudinal studies, such as those conducted in Minnesota (Sroufe, Egeland, Carlson, & Collins, 2005) and Germany (Grossmann, Grossmann, & Waters, 2005), that further explore these processes and the school-age pathways discussed in this chapter are critical to linking the abundant literature on infancy with the accumulating evidence emphasizing the important metacognitive and affective differences associated with disorganization in adulthood.

ACKNOWLEDGMENTS

This research was supported by grants received from the Social Sciences and Humanities Research Council of Canada and the FQRSC (Fonds de recherche sur la société et la culture). We thank Chantal Cyr, Karine Comtois-Dubois, Katherine Pascuzzo, and Jean Begin for their invaluable support and contributions to this work.

NOTES

1. This is indicative of directly disorganized behavior.
2. When a child displays strong indices of disorganized or disoriented behavior, a primary disorganized (D) classification is given. A secondary classification of secure (B), avoidant (A), or ambivalent (C) or combined A-C is also given. Whereas the primary D classification refers to specific atypical child behaviors displayed in the presence of the caregiver, the secondary classification describes the overall strategy of child proximity seeking and parental response observed during reunion.

REFERENCES

Aber, J. L., & Allen, J. P. (1987). The effects of maltreatment on young children's socioemotional development: An attachment theory perspective. *Developmental Psychology, 23,* 406–414.

Ames, C., & Archer, J. (1988). Achievement goals in the classroom: Students' learning strategies and motivation processes. *Journal of Educational Psychology, 80,* 260–267.

Barnett, D., Kidwell, S. L., & Leung, K. H. (1998). Parenting and preschooler attachment among low-income urban African-American families. *Child Development, 69,* 1657–1671.

Belsky, J., Youngblade, L., Rovine, M., & Volling, B. (1991). Patterns of marital change and parent–child interaction. *Journal of Marriage and the Family, 53,* 487–498.

Bowlby, J. (1953). *Child care and the growth of love.* Harmondsworth, UK: Penguin Books.

Bowlby, J. (1973). *Attachment and loss: Vol. 2. Separation.* New York: Basic Books.

Bowlby, J. (1980). *Attachment and loss: Vol. 3. Loss.* New York: Basic Books.

Bowlby, J. (1982). *Attachment and loss: Vol. 1. Attachment* (2nd ed.). New York: Basic Books. (Original work published 1969)

Britner, P. A., Marvin, R. S., & Pianta, R. C. (2005). Development and preliminary validation of the caregiving behavior system: Association with child attachment classification in the preschool Strange Situation. *Attachment and Human Development, 7,* 83–102.

Bureau, J.-F., Easterbrooks, E. A., & Lyons-Ruth, K. (2009). Attachment disorganization and role-reversal in middle childhood: Maternal and child precursors and correlates. *Attachment and Human Development, 11,* 1–20.

Bureau, J.-F., & Moss. E. (2010). Behavioral precursors of attachment representations in middle childhood and links with child social adaptation. *British Journal of Developmental Psychology, 28,* 657–677.

Bureau, J.-F., Moss, E., & St-Laurent, D. (2006, June). The roles of attachment and individual and familial processes in the prediction of academic and cognitive functioning. In F. Lamb-Parker (Chair), *Attachment, adult–child relationships, and affect regulation: Contributions to children's later cognitive, social, and behavioral competence.* Symposium conducted at the Head Start's 8th National Research Conference, Washington DC.

Carlson, E. A. (1998). A prospective longitudinal study of disorganized/disoriented attachment. *Child Development, 69,* 1970–1979.

Cassidy, J. (1988). Child–mother attachment and the self in six-year-olds. *Child Development, 59,* 121–135.

Cassidy, J. & Marvin, R. S., with the McArthur Working Group on Attachment. (1992). *Attachment organization in 2½ to 4½ year olds: Coding manual.* Unpublished coding manual, University of Virginia, Charlottesville.

Cicchetti, D., & Barnett, D. (1991). Attachment organization in maltreated preschoolers. *Development and Psychopathology, 3,* 397–411.

Cummings, M. E., & Davies, P. (2002). Effects of marital conflict on children: Recent advances and emerging themes in process-oriented research. *Journal of Child Psychology and Psychiatry, 43,* 31–63.

Davies, P. T., & Cummings, E. M. (1994). Marital conflict and child adjustment: An emotional security hypothesis. *Psychological Bulletin, 116,* 387–411.

DeMulder, E. K., & Radke-Yarrow, M. (1991). Attachment with affectively ill and well mothers: Concurrent behavioral correlates. *Development and Psychopathology, 3,* 227–242.

Epstein, J. L. (1992). School and family partnerships. In M. Alkin (Ed.), *Encyclopedia of educational research* (6th ed., pp. 1139–1151). New York: Macmillan.

George, C., & Solomon, J. (1996). Representational models of relationships: Links between caregiving and attachment. *Infant Mental Health Journal, 17,* 198–216.

George, C., & Solomon, J. (2008). The caregiving system: A behavioral systems approach to parenting. In J. Cassidy & P. R. Shaver (Eds.), *Handbook of attachment: Theory, research, and clinical applications* (2nd ed., pp. 833–856). New York: Guilford Press.

Greenberg, M. A., Speltz, M. L., DeKlyen, M., & Endriga, M. C. (1991). Attachment security in preschoolers with and without externalizing problems: A replication. *Development and Psychopathology, 3,* 413–430.

Grossmann, K. E., Grossmann, K., & Waters, E. (2005). *Attachment from infancy to adulthood: The major longitudinal studies.* New York: Guilford Press.

Jacobsen, T., Edelstein, W., & Hoffmann, V. (1994). A longitudinal study of the relation between representations of attachment in childhood and cognitive functioning in childhood and adolescence. *Developmental Psychology, 30,* 112–124.

Jacobsen, T., & Hofmann, V. (1997). Children's attachment representations: Longitudinal relations to school behavior and academic competency in middle childhood and adolescence. *Developmental Psychology, 33,* 703–710.

Jacobvitz, D., & Hazen, N. (1999). Developmental pathways from infant disorganization to childhood peer relationships. In J. Solomon & C. George (Eds.), *Attachment disorganization* (pp. 127–159). New York: Guilford Press.

Jacobvitz, D., Riggs, S., & Johnson, E. M. (1999). Cross-sex and same-sex family alliances: Immediate and long-term effects on daughters and sons. In N. D. Chase (Ed.), *Parentified children: Theory, research and treatment* (pp. 34–55). Thousand Oaks, CA: Sage.

Lynch, M., & Cicchetti, D. (1991). Patterns of relatedness in maltreated and non-maltreated children: Connections among multiple representational models. *Development and Psychopathology, 3,* 207–226.

Lyons-Ruth, K., Alpern, L., & Repacholi, L. (1993). Disorganized infant attachment classification and maternal psychosocial problems as predictors of hostile–aggressive behavior in the preschool classroom. *Child Development, 64,* 572–585.

Lyons-Ruth, K., Bronfman, E., & Atwood, G. (1999). A relational diathesis model of hostile–helpless states of mind: Expressions in mother–infant interaction. In J. Solomon & C. George (Eds.), *Attachment Disorganization* (pp. 33–70). New York: Guilford Press.

Lyons-Ruth, K., Bronfman, E., & Parsons, E. (1999). Maternal frightened, frightening, or atypical behavior and disorganized infant attachment patterns. *Monographs of the Society for Research in Child Development, 64,* 67–96.

Lyons-Ruth, K., Easterbrooks, M. A., & Cibelli, C. D. (1997). Infant attachment strategies, infant mental lag, and maternal depressive symptoms: Predictors of internalizing and externalizing problems at age 7. *Developmental Psychology, 33,* 681–692.

Lyons-Ruth, K., Yellin, C., Melnick, S., & Atwood, G. (2005). Expanding the concept of unresolved mental states: Highly defended/helpless states of mind on the Adult Attachment Interview are associated with disrupted mother–infant communication and infant disorganization. *Development and Psychopathology, 17,* 1–23.

Madigan, S., Bakermans-Kranenburg, M. J., van IJzendoorn, M. H., Moran, G., Pederson, D. R., & Benoit, D. (2006). Unresolved states of mind, anomalous parental behavior, and disorganized attachment: A review and meta-analysis of a transmission gap. *Attachment and Human Development, 8,* 89–111.

Main, M. (1991). Metacognitive knowledge, metacognitive monitoring and singular (coherent) vs. multiple (incoherent) models of attachment: Findings and directions for future research. In C. Parkes, J. Stevenson-Hinde, & P. Marris (Eds.), *Attachment across the life cycle* (pp. 127–157). London: Routledge.

Main, M. (1995). Recent studies in attachment: Overview, with selected implications for clinical work. In S. Goldberg, R. Muir, & J. Kerr (Eds.), *Attachment theory: Social, developmental, and clinical perspectives* (pp. 407–474). Hillsdale, NJ: Analytic Press.

Main, M., & Cassidy, J. (1988). Categories of response to reunion with the parent at age six: Predictable from infant attachment classifications and stable over a 1-month period. *Developmental Psychology, 24,* 415–526.

Main, M., & Hesse, E. (1990). Parents' unresolved traumatic experiences are related to infant disorganized attachment status: Is frightened and/or frightening parental behavior the linking mechanism? In M. T. Greenberg, D. Cichetti, & M. Cummings (Eds.), *Attachment in the preschool years* (pp. 161–182). Chicago: University of Chicago Press.

Main, M., Kaplan, N., & Cassidy, J. (1985). Security of attachment in infancy, childhood, and adulthood: A move to the level of representation. In I. Bretherton & E. Waters (Eds.), Growing points in attachment theory and research. *Mono-*

graphs of the Society for Research in Child Development, 50(1–2, Serial No. 209), 66–104.

Main, M., & Solomon, J. (1990). Procedure for identifying infants as disorganized/ disoriented during the Ainsworth Strange Situation. In M. Greenberg, D. Cicchetti, & M. Cummings (Eds.), *Attachment in the preschool years: Theory, research, and intervention* (pp. 121–160). Chicago: University of Chicago Press.

Marvin, R. S. (1977). An ethological–cognitive model for the attenuation of mother–child attachment behavior. In T. M. Alloway, L. Krames, & P. Pliner (Eds.), *Advances in the study of communication and affect: Vol 3. Attachment behavior* (pp. 25–60). New York: Plenum Press.

Marvin, R. S., & Britner, P. A. (2008). Normative development: The ontogeny of attachment. In J. Cassidy & P. R. Shaver (Eds.), *Handbook of attachment: Theory, research, and clinical applications* (pp. 269–294). New York: Guilford Press.

Mason, J. W. (1968). A review of psychoendocrine research on the pituitary–adrenal cortical system. *Psychosomatic Medicine, 30,* 576–607.

Mills-Koonce, W. R., Gariepy, J.-L., Sutton, K., & Cox, M. (2008). Changes in maternal sensitivity across the first three years: Are mothers from different attachment dyads differentially influenced by depressive symptomatology? *Attachment and Human Development, 10,* 299–317.

Moss, E. (1992). The socioaffective context of joint cognitive activity. In L. T. Winegar & J. Valsiner (Eds.), *Children's development within social context: Vol. 2. Research and methodology* (pp. 117–154). Hillsdale, NJ: Erlbaum.

Moss, E., Bureau, J.-F., Cyr, C., Mongeau, C., & St-Laurent, D. (2004). Correlates of attachment at age 3: Construct validity of the preschool attachment classification system. *Developmental Psychology, 40,* 323–334.

Moss, E., Cyr, C., Bureau, J.-F., Tarabulsy, G., & Dubois-Comtois, K. (2005). Stability of attachment between preschool and early school-age and factors contributing to continuity/discontinuity. *Developmental Psychology, 41,* 773–783.

Moss, E., Cyr, C, & Dubois-Comtois, K. (2004). Attachment at early school age and developmental risk: Examining family contexts and behavior problems of controlling–caregiving, controlling–punitive, and behaviorally disorganized children. *Developmental Psychology, 40,* 519-532.

Moss, E., Gosselin, C., Parent, S., Rousseau, D., & Dumont, M. (1997). Attachment and joint problem-solving experiences during the preschool period. *Social Development, 6,* 1–17.

Moss, E., Rousseau, D., Parent, S., St-Laurent, D., & Saintonge, J. (1998). Correlates of attachment at school-age: Maternal-reported stress, mother–child interaction and behavior problems. *Child Development, 69,* 1390–1405.

Moss, E., Smolla, N., Cyr, C., Dubois-Comtois, K., Mazzarello, T., & Berthiaume, C. (2006). Attachment and behavior problems in middle childhood as reported by adult and child informants. *Development and Psychopathology, 18,* 425–444.

Moss, E., & St-Laurent, D. (2001). Attachment at school age and academic performance. *Developmental Psychology, 37,* 863–874.

Moss, E., St-Laurent, D., & Parent, S. (1999). Disorganized attachment and developmental risk at school age. In J. Solomon & C. George (Eds.), *Attachment disoganization* (pp. 160–187). New York: Guilford Press.

Moss, E., Thibaudeau, P., Cyr, C., & Rousseau, D. (2001, April). Controlling attachment and child management of parental emotion. In D. R. Pederson & C. A. DeOliviera (Chairs), *Attachment and the socialization of emotions.* Symposium conducted at the biennial meeting of the Society for Research in Child Development, Minneapolis, MN.

Munson, J. A., McMahon, R. J., & Spieker, S. J. (2001). Structure and variability in the developmental trajectory of children's externalizing problems: Impact of infant attachment, maternal depressive symptomatology, and child sex. *Development and Psychopathology, 13,* 277–296.

NICHD Early Child Care Research Network. (2001). Child-care and family predictors of preschool attachment and stability from infancy. *Developmental Psychology, 37,* 847–862.

O'Connor, E. E., Bureau, J.-F., McCartney, K. A., & Lyons-Ruth, K. (April, 2009). Maternal and child correlates of controlling and disorganized patterns of attachment at age three. In J.-F. Bureau & E. E. O'Connor (Chairs), *Disorganized and controlling attachment behaviors in childhood: Child and family correlates in low- and high-risk samples.* Symposium conducted at the Society for Research in Child Development biennial meeting, Denver, CO.

Owen, M. T., & Cox, M. J. (1997). Marital conflict and the development of infant–parent attachment relationships. *Journal of Family Psychology, 11,* 152–164.

Robertson, J. (1962). *Hospitals and children: A parents' eye view.* New York: Gollanz.

Shaw, D. S., Owens, E. B., Vondra, J. I., Keenan, K., & Winslow, E. B. (1996). Early risk factors and pathways in the development of early disruptive behavior problems. *Development and Psychopathology, 8,* 679–699.

Solomon, J., & George, C. (1996). Defining the caregiving system: Toward a theory of caregiving. *Infant Mental Health Journal, 17,* 183–197.

Solomon, J., & George, C. (1999a). The measurement of attachment security in infancy and childhood. In J. Cassidy & P. R. Shaver (Eds.), *Handbook of attachment: Theory, research, and clinical applications* (pp. 287–316). New York: Guilford Press.

Solomon, J., & George, C. (1999b). The caregiving system in mothers of infants: A comparison of divorcing and married mothers. *Attachment and Human Development, 1,* 171–190.

Solomon, J., & George, C. (1999c). The development of attachment in separated and divorced families: Effects of overnight visitation, parent and couple variables. *Attachment and Human Development, 1,* 2–33.

Solomon, J., & George, C. (2006). Intergenerational transmission of dysregulated maternal caregiving: Mothers describe their upbringing and childrearing. In O. Mayseless (Ed.), *Parenting representations: Theory, research, and clinical implications* (pp. 265–295). New York: Cambridge University Press.

Solomon, J., George, C., & De Jong, A. (1995). Children classified as controlling at age six: Evidence of disorganized representational strategies and aggression at home and at school. *Development and Psychopathology, 7,* 447–464.

Speltz, M. L., Greenberg, M. T., & DeKlyen, M. (1990). Attachment in preschoolers with disruptive behavior: A comparison of clinic-referred and non-problem children. *Development and Psychopathology, 2,* 31–46.

Sroufe, A. L., Egeland, B., Carlson, E., & Collins, A. W. (2005). Placing early attachment experiences in developmental context: The Minnesota Longitudinal Study. In K. E. Grossmann, K. Grossmann, & E. Waters (Eds.), *Attachment from infancy to adulthood: The major longitudinal studies* (pp. 48–70). New York: Guilford Press.

Steele, H., & Steele, M. (2005). The construct of coherence as an indicator of attachment security in middle childhood: The Friends and Family Interview. In K. A. Kerns & R. A. Richardson (Eds.), *Attachment in middle childhood* (pp. 137–160). New York: Guilford Press.

Stevenson-Hinde, J., & Shouldice, A. (1990). Fear and attachment in 2.5-years-olds. *British Journal of Developmental Psychology, 8,* 319–333.

Stevenson-Hinde, J., & Shouldice, A. (1995). Maternal interactions and self-reports related to attachment classifications at 4.5 years. *Child Development, 66,* 583–596.

Teti, D. M. (1999). Conceptualizations of disorganization in the preschool years: An integration. In J. Solomon & C. George (Eds.), *Attachment disorganization* (pp. 213–242). New York: Guilford Press.

Teti, D. M., & Gelfand, D. M. (1997). The Preschool Assessment of Attachment: Construct validity in a sample of depressed and nondepressed families. *Development and Psychopathology, 9,* 517–536.

Teti, D. M., Gelfand, D. M., Messinger, D. S., & Isabella, R. (1995). Maternal depression and the quality of early attachment: An examination of infants, preschoolers, and their mothers. *Developmental Psychology, 31,* 364–376.

van IJzendoorn, M. H. (1995). Adult attachment representations, parental responsiveness, and infant attachment: A meta-analysis on the predictive validity of the Adult Attachment Interview. *Psychological Bulletin, 117,* 387–403.

van IJzendoorn, M. H., Schuengel, C., & Bakermans-Kranenburg, M. J. (1999). Disorganized attachment in early childhood: Meta-analysis of precursors, concomitants, and sequelae. *Development and Psychopathology, 11,* 225–250.

Vygotsky, L. S. (1978). *Mind in society.* Cambridge, MA: Harvard University Press.

Wartner, U. G., Grossman, K., Fremmer-Bombik, E., & Suess, G. (1994). Attachment patterns at age six in South Germany: Predictability from infancy and implications for preschool behavior. *Child Development, 65,* 1014–1027.

Zeanah, C. H., Danis, B., Hirshberg, L., Benoit, D., Miller, D., & Heller, S. S. (1999). Disorganized attachment associated with partner violence: A research note. *Infant Mental Health Journal, 20,* 77–86.

Zimmerman, G. J. (2002). Achieving academic excellence: A self-regulatory perspective. In M. Ferrari (Ed.), *The pursuit of excellence through education* (pp. 85–110). Hillsdale, NJ: Erlbaum.

Chapter 4

Continuity and Change in Unresolved Classifications of Adult Attachment Interviews with Low-Income Mothers

SUSAN SPIEKER, ELIZABETH M. NELSON,
MICHELLE DEKLYEN, SANDRA N. JOLLEY,
and LISA MENNET

A frequently discussed finding in the developmental psychology literature has been the association between parental representations of attachment relationships, as measured by the Adult Attachment Interview (AAI;
George, Kaplan, & Main, 1984, 1985, 1996), and infant attachment patterns as measured by the Strange Situation (Ainsworth, Blehar, Waters, &
Wall, 1978). In an early meta-analysis, van IJzendoorn (1995) reported an
association for the three major adult classifications—dismissing (Ds), autonomous (F), and preoccupied (E)—with the corresponding three major infant
Strange Situation classifications—avoidant (A), r (108) = .42, secure (B),
r (274) = .48, and ambivalent (C), r (48) = .19. An association was also
found for the adult unresolved (U) classification and infant disorganized
classifications (D), r (118) = .31. A later meta-analysis of six studies, two
with high-risk subjects, found a somewhat smaller effect size, r (495) = .21,
$p < .01$ (Madigan, Bakermans-Kranenburg, et al., 2006). Of the two high-
risk studies in this sample, Madigan, Moran, and Pederson (2006) found
significant concordance, $r = .31$, and the other, Lyons-Ruth, Yellin, Melnick,
and Atwood (2003), did not, $r = .05$. All of these effect sizes, however, are
within the confidence interval (CI = .05–.36) reported by Madigan, Baker-

mans-Kranenburg, et al. (2006). Van IJzendoorn (1995) also reported no systematic differences between concurrent and retrospective (AAI administered some time after the Strange Situation) and prospective (AAI administered some time before the Strange Situation) designs. These findings suggest a degree of stability in AAI classifications over time, because if there were not some stability, then concurrent assessments would show stronger AAI–Strange Situation associations.

There are three kinds of continuity to consider. One is the stability of individual differences in infant attachment classification of Strange Situation behavior over varying time periods, which we call *intra-Strange Situation stability*. Another is the stability of AAI discourse classification over varying time periods in adulthood, or *intra-AAI* stability. A third is concordance between Strange Situation classification in infancy and AAI classification at a different time, which we call *cross-age/measurement stability*. Regarding intra-Strange Situation stability, Fraley (2002) conducted a meta-analysis on 15 published studies on continuity of Strange Situation dichotomous secure/insecure patterns within infancy. Fraley summarized the two-category test–retest effect as Pearson product–moment correlations (r, or phi correlations for 2 x 2 categorical data), as van IJzendoorn (1995) did in his meta-analysis. Fraley (2002) reported that the mean test-retest effect was modest, r (894) = .32, SD = .28, range = –.03 to .92. Both high- and low-risk samples contributed both high and low stability coefficients. In addition, Fraley conducted a meta-analysis of six studies (one unpublished) that examined cross-age/measurement stability from infant Strange Situation secure/insecure classification to late adolescent AAI secure/insecure classification. Again, the mean correlation was modest, r (216) = .27, SD = .29; range = .10 to .50, and both high- and low-risk studies contributed high and low stability coefficients.

Fraley's (2002) meta-analysis considered only the secure/insecure dichotomy, not continuity of the major Strange Situation classifications (A, B, C) to the major AAI classifications (Ds, F, E). Further, the published articles upon which it was based did not include the unresolved (U) AAI classification. Weinfield, Whaley, and Egeland (2004) partially addressed this issue when they reanalyzed the Waters, Merrick, Treboux, Crowell, and Albersheim (2000) data from a low-risk sample, using all of the participants (in the 2000 study participants with unstable classifications from 12 to 18 months had been excluded) and the D Strange Situation classifications, and found some cross-age/measurement stability. Security in infancy was associated with a lower incidence of unresolved status in adolescence, and disorganization in infancy was associated with a greater likelihood of insecurity in adolescence.

Three studies examined intra-AAI stability in low-risk samples using the four-way major classifications (Ds, F, E, U; Bakermans-Kranenburg & van IJzendoorn, 1993; Benoit & Parker, 1994; Crowell, Treboux, & Waters,

2002). Following Fraley's method, we computed phi *(r)* (Rosnow & Rosenthal, 1988) for stability of the F-not-F and U-not-U classification for all of these studies to make comparisons easier. Bakermans-Kranenburg and van IJzendoorn (1993) reported 71% concordance for 83 Dutch mothers over a 2-month period. All four Ds, F, E, and U categories showed significant stability when examined in a 4×4 table, phi (81) = .45 for dichotomous F-not-F and phi (81) = .37 for dichotomous U-not-U. Benoit and Parker (1994) collected AAI data during 84 women's last month of pregnancy and again when their infants were 11 months old. Concordance over this time period was 77%, and again there was significant stability for each of the major classifications, including F-not-F, phi (82) = .27, and U-not-U, phi (82) = .59. Finally, Crowell et al. (2002) studied 157 couples 3 months before marriage and again 18 months after marriage. The stability for F-not-F could not be computed because results were not reported for the four-way DFEU classifications. Stability for U-not-U was phi (210) = .42.

Only one of eight samples in van IJzendoorn's (1995) meta-analysis of four-way concordance included primarily low-income participants, and the association was *not* significant for this sample. Further, a "transmission gap" has been identified which applies to all groups. Van IJzendoorn's meta-analysis revealed that only 53% of disorganized infants had mothers whose AAI transcripts were judged to have evidence of lack of resolution. These finding leave us with two questions: What accounts for the lack of stability in unresolved attachment status among low-income, high-risk mothers, and why is there a transmission gap between unresolved mothers and disorganized infants? For many (e.g., Belsky, Campbell, Cohn, & Moore, 1996; Sroufe & Jacobvitz, 1989; van IJzendoorn, Juffer, & Duyvesteyn, 1995), the question of stability and change is important for attachment theory, which posits that working models endure by influencing the perception and interpretation of social and emotional information in interactions with others. On the other hand, these theorists note that working models can be revised in light of changing experience. Just how stable, how modifiable, and modifiable by what types of circumstances (therapeutic or otherwise) working models are has implications for our understanding of how parental working models of attachment influence outcomes—including children's attachment security—and the extent to which experiences and interventions can shift working models and behavior in both generations (see also Solomon & George, Chapter 2, this volume).

A growing body of literature suggests that conclusions about the nature of AAI classifications and their stability over time, largely derived from the study of middle-income samples, need to be adjusted to take into account findings from samples drawn from lower socioeconomic settings (e.g., Bailey, Moran, Pederson & Bento, 2007; Lyons-Ruth, Dutra, Schuder, & Bianchi, 2006; Lyons-Ruth, et al., 2003; Madigan, Moran, Schuengel, Pederson, &

Otten, 2007). These samples have higher rates of attachment-related losses and traumas.

It is the adult's unpredictable and unmonitored lapses in monitoring their discourse about experiences of loss or trauma that result in the U classification on the AAI. Coding for U relies on whether a small number of markers exceed a threshold. A U code depends on (1) whether the incident was discussed at all, and (2) whether it was discussed extensively and openly enough that lack of resolution markers had the opportunity to occur. Methodologically, coding for U may be more vulnerable to instability than other state of mind/discourse ratings that draw upon the interview as a whole in the assignment of Ds, F, or E classifications. Lack of resolution contributes to orthogonal attentional and cognitive processes that may temporarily or intermittently disrupt or disorganize an individual's primary dismissing, autonomous, or preoccupied stance (Bailey, Moran, Pederson, & Bento, 2007), thereby disrupting affective communication, which in turn contributes to insecure or disorganized infant attachment (Lyons-Ruth, Melnick, Bronfman, Sherry, & Llanas, 2004).

Given that low-income, high-risk mothers tend to have experienced significantly higher levels of trauma and loss, we speculated about the role these events might have played in their (shifting) attachment organization. Internal working models tend to endure if the life course remains fairly steady. Perhaps, in contrast, the traumatic losses and chaotic reversals that characterized the lives of many low-income, high-risk mothers leave them more vulnerable to events (positive and negative) that undermine established patterns of perceiving social and emotional information. In other words, these mothers' histories may have made them more susceptible to shifts in their internal organization, making it more likely that they would "move through" periods of lack of resolution over time. Might the birth of the child itself—particularly in light of a history of disruption and loss—have a profound impact on maternal mental organization? If so, this opens up the possibility that the timing of the mother's lack of resolution in the child's infancy could be one factor related to the "transmission gap."

The birth of a child can have profound effects on mothers and families. Parental caregiving behavior may become disregulated when certain characteristics of the infant trigger the effects of childhood traumatic experiences, as has been discussed in case studies in the infant mental health literature (e.g., Fraiberg, Adelson, & Shapiro, 1975; Pines et al., 2002; Cramer & Stern, 1988). Further, George and Solomon (2008; Solomon & George, 1996, Chapter 2, this volume) argued that the caregiving system is distinct from the adult attachment system. Infant characteristics (e.g., a medical problem or a resemblance to an abusing spouse) may elicit preoccupation with or intrusion from adverse experiences in the parent's past that create conditions for disorganized attachment in the infant but are distinct from the parent's lack of resolution of loss or trauma as measured by the AAI. Along the same line, though perhaps more rarely, a good parenting experience may also create conditions for the reorganization of attachment models in mothers who are more vulnerable to the impact of shifting life circumstances.

This chapter focuses on the stability across several years of AAI classifications in a high-risk sample of mostly young, highly stressed mothers and their children. We examine both intra-AAI stability and cross-generation agreement between adult AAI and infant attachment, with a particular emphasis on parental lack of resolution of loss and trauma and infant disorganization. We also consider the role of parental childhood trauma in cross-generation stability, and whether or not this trauma contributes to an unresolved state of mind.

METHOD

Overview of Study Design

The study reported here involved one of the 17 sites in the national Early Head Start (EHS) Research and Evaluation Project. The national study used an experimental design, with families randomly assigned at intake to either the EHS program group or to a comparison group that accessed services already available in the community. The study involved both common outcome measures and site-specific outcomes related to the focus of each program. Although analysis of the national EHS sample suggested numerous positive impacts (Office of Research and Evaluation & Head Start Bureau, 2001), at this site there were no differences between the program and comparison groups on parent or infant attachment security. Therefore, the program and comparison groups were combined.

Participants and Procedure

At this site, 179 low-income mothers who were pregnant or had a child less than 6 months of age were recruited in 1996 and 1997 from low-income, suburban neighborhoods. Eligible participants lived at or below the federal poverty level and, at this site, spoke English well enough to answer interview questions and were randomly assigned at intake to either the control condition or the EHS program. National and local evaluation data were collected at five face-to-face and three phone interviews during the child's first 3 years. Attrition was high across the years of the study. At each of the assessments, between 20 and 30% of the recruited sample could not be located or refused a data collection visit.

At baseline, 152 caregivers participated in the AAI interview. In the last year of the project, when children were between 4 and 5 years of age, limited funds were available to follow up a portion of the sample. During the follow-up, we administered the AAI a second time to 47 English-speaking birth mothers who had been the primary caregiver since the study child's birth and had completed the baseline assessment and most of the longitudinal assessments through 54 months. These 47 mothers and their children constitute the subsample in the current study. Analyses are based on the two AAI administrations (called Time 1 and Time 2) and the infant Strange Situation assessment at 19 months. On average, the interval between the two AAI assessments was 54.5 months ($SD = 3.0$).

In the subsample, 26 mothers (55%) enrolled in pregnancy and 21 (45%) enrolled within the first 6 months of the study child's birth; 66% were primiparous, 36% had not completed high school, 30% had a high school diploma or GED, and 34% had some postsecondary education. Mothers reported on the race and sex of the study child: 62% were white, 28% were African American, and the rest were multiracial; 47% of the children were male. Mothers' ages ranged from 15 to 40, with 43% being under 20 years at baseline. The sample for this study was compared with the larger recruited sample. Overall, participants in this sample were more likely to have been randomly assigned to the comparison group (67% vs. 50%) and to have somewhat higher vocabulary scores (Wechsler, 1981) ($M = 8.7$ vs. $M = 7.7$).

Measures

Adult Attachment/State of Mind with Respect to Attachment

Several variables related to caregiver representations of early attachment relationships were derived from the AAI (George et al., 1996). The AAI is a structured, hour-long, semiclinical interview during which the subject is queried about early experiences with caregivers. It was administered by interviewers who received extensive training from the third author. Early in the interview the subject is asked to list five adjectives that describe the relationship with each parent and then to describe specific memories that illustrate each adjective. There are questions about how the parents dealt with the subject's distress and sickness as a young child and whether the subject had been maltreated or experienced the loss of an important person. The intent of these questions is to "surprise the unconscious" of the subject and to direct attention to attachment-related events from childhood. The speaker must produce and reflect upon memories related to attachment, some of which may be highly charged with emotion, while at the same time maintaining a coherent discourse with the interviewer. The audiotaped interviews were transcribed verbatim and the third author, who was trained by M. Main and met criterion on a set of 30 reliability transcripts, coded the transcripts according to guidelines by Main, Goldwyn, and Hesse (2002).

Respondents were asked for memories of loss of attachment figures and significant others, experiences of early trauma (physical or sexual abuse), and loss of a child or prenatal losses due to miscarriage or elective termination. Individuals with high lack-of-resolution scores have discourse with indications of disorganization and disorientation in response to these questions or in other discussion about loss or trauma. Lack of resolution for loss of attachment figure, loss of another significant person, prenatal or child loss, and trauma were each rated on a 9-point lack-of-resolution scale. The highest rating involving lack of resolution of loss of attachment or significant person or child became the score for *highest unresolved loss* (U_L), which was separate from the rating for *unresolved prenatal loss* (U_p) and the rating for *highest unresolved trauma* (U_T). Finally, if multiple ratings of loss, prenatal loss, and trauma were present, the *highest lack-of-resolution score* (U_H) was recorded, regardless of type. When a particular U rating was not scored for any reason (e.g., loss or trauma did not occur, was not discussed, or was not discussed in sufficient detail to rate), a score of 0 was assigned.

In addition to lack of resolution, AAI transcripts were evaluated for state of mind with regard to attachment, which can be understood as varying across two dimensions: coherence and organization. In the AAI, coherent discourse occurs when the adult is able to both access and evaluate memories in response to specific questions and remain consistent, appropriate, and plausible as a discourse partner. These qualities were rated on the *coherence of mind* (CoM) 9-point scale. Organization is reflected in one of three classifications: secure–*freely autonomous (F)*, insecure–*dismissing (Ds)*, and insecure–*preoccupied (E)*. Transcripts are classified as F when they are internally consistent and reasonably clear, relevant, and succinct. They are classified as Ds when the discourse appears to minimize attachment-related experiences and as E when the discourse reveals a preoccupation with attachment figures and attachment experiences (Main et al., 2002).

Regardless of its organizational classification(Ds, F, E), a transcript with a U_H rating of 5 or higher also received a primary or secondary classification of *unresolved (U)* for lack of resolution of loss or trauma. According to convention, in our analyses we used the four-category Ds F E U classifications, three-category Ds F E classifications, and F-not-F and U-not-U dichotomies.

Life Events

AAI transcripts were also reviewed and coded using a modified, more limited version of the Life Events Coding Scale developed by Solomon and George (2006). The scale was used to summarize experiences of loss as well as potentially traumatic life circumstances, including physical abuse and family violence (capturing all forms of physical, emotional, and verbal harm in the respondent's family of origin), sexual abuse and molestation, caregiver mental illness, substance abuse by an attachment figure, neglect, and frequent changes in primary caregiver. Life event loss experiences included losing a caregiver to death; losing a caregiver due to abandonment, divorce, or separation (all before the age of 18); and pregnancy loss through miscarriage or elective termination at any age. In addition, a continuous variable ranging from 0 to 5 was included for the number of losses of other close individuals, excluding those listed above, an individual had experienced. Some experiences that may not have been discussed in enough depth on the AAI to warrant scoring for lack of resolution would still be considered significantly stressful life events on the Life Events Coding Scale. One goal of this coding was to determine whether specific life events or risk profiles were associated with a greater tendency toward unresolved or "U" responses, regardless of their contribution to a lack-of-resolution rating. A second goal was to relate these life events to infant attachment security and disorganization, independent of the mother's lack-of-resolution ratings on the AAI.

Different pairs of coders, trained to 75% agreement (agreements/agreements + disagreements) on a set of training transcripts coded Time 1 and Time 2 AAIs for these life events. A third coder rated 20% of the transcripts at each time point and agreement for categories reported in this study ranged from 75 to 100%.

Coding of life events also provided data used to assign a rating for both frequency of occurrence and severity of childhood maltreatment, based on the classification system developed by Barnett, Manley, and Cicchetti (1993). For example, a severity score of 3 would be assigned for physical or emotional force directed toward the individual that was beyond the boundaries of parental discipline, such as slapping, throwing, or hitting with objects, or frightening outbursts of anger directed toward the child. A frequency score of 3 indicated maltreatment that was ongoing. We computed a dichotomous maltreatment variable reflecting *ongoing, moderate to severe maltreatment* versus *none or lesser maltreatment*.

Infant–Parent Attachment Security

The Strange Situation (Ainsworth et al., 1978) assessed quality of attachment at 19 months. Videotapes of all Strange Situations were evaluated by a team of three experienced coders blind to other information about the child and family. All assessments were double-coded using the standard attachment classifications of secure (B), insecure–avoidant (A), insecure–resistant (C) (Ainsworth et al., 1978), insecure–disorganized (D), and insecure–unclassifiable (U) (Main & Solomon, 1990). The group and first author viewed disagreements at the major category level, and a code was assigned by consensus. For the current sample, across all coder pairs before conferencing, agreement with the 5-category classification system was 77% (kappa could not be computed because one coder assigned no C classifications). The dichotomous secure group consisted only of children classified in the B group, and the insecure group included all children in the A, C, D, and U groups. Agreement before conferencing for the B-not-B dichotomy was 81% (kappa = .62), and for the D-not-D dichotomy, 85% (kappa = .39). Coders also rated the 9-point security and disorganization scales. Interrater agreement (Pearson correlation) on these scales was .65 and .48, respectively. Although the correlation for disorganization was disappointingly low, 83% of the ratings were within 2 points.

RESULTS

AAI Classifications

The majority of AAI transcripts were classified as insecure at Time 1 (60%) and Time 2 (53%), and about one-third of these were U (defined as U_H of 5 or higher) at each time point (30% and 38%, respectively). All but three of the remaining insecure classifications were dismissing (Ds; 28% and 13%, respectively). As shown in Table 4.1, only 40% of the paired transcripts received the same Ds F E U classification at both time points, a level that was not better than chance, kappa = .11. There was also no evidence to suggest

TABLE 4.1. AAI Cross-Classifications at Time 1 and Time 2

AAI at Time 1	AAI at Time 2				
	Ds	F	E	U	Total
Ds					
Count	2	4	0	7	13
Expected	1.7	6.1	.3	4.7	
F					
Count	3	11	0	5	19
Expected	2.4	8.9	.8	6.9	
E					
Count	0	0	1	0	1
Expected	.1	.5	.0	.4	
U					
Count	1	7	1	5	14
Expected	1.8	6.6	.6	5.1	
Total count	6	22	2	17	47

Note. Kappa = .11, p > .10.

stability of the dichotomous classifications F-not-F, phi = .18, and U-not-U, phi = .06. This analysis was repeated using the three-way "forced" D F E classifications; results are presented in Table 4.2. These classifications were modestly stable, kappa = .29, p < .05, with 57% of paired transcripts classified in the same Ds F E classification at both time points.

Twenty-six mothers received the first AAI interview during pregnancy, and 21 were interviewed the first time within 6 months of the child's birth. Because parents in this sample had experienced considerable childhood sexual trauma that could be reactivated by experiences associated with childbirth (Born, Soares, Phillips, Jung, & Steiner, 2006), the stability of AAI U classifications was also analyzed separately by timing of the first AAI interview, before or after the child's birth. Stability of U-not-U classifications was significant only for the postnatal interviews, phi = .58, for which it was 76%, compared to 38% of interviews conducted before birth. Specifically, of the 21 mothers with both interviews after the child's birth, four of six mothers whose AAIs were classified as U were U at the second as well, and 12 of 15 whose AAIs were not-U at Time 1 were also not-U at Time 2. In contrast, for the 26 mothers for whom the birth of the study child occurred between the first and second AAI, only one of eight women whose AAIs were assigned U classifications at Time 1 had AAIs assigned U 4 years later, and one of 18 whose AAIs were not-U at Time 1 were assigned U at Time 2, a level of *instability* for U that was nearly significant (phi = −.35, p < .10).

Consistency of Life Event Reporting: Loss, Prenatal Loss, and Trauma

We examined the consistency with which respondents mentioned traumatic experiences and losses in the AAI. Eight (17%) reported the death of an attachment figure before the age of 18 at both interviews, and none reported this loss at one interview only. All were rated for lack of resolution of loss for both interviews. The majority of respondents reported other types of losses at Time 1 (81%) and Time 2 (66%). Regarding loss of other significant persons, eight respondents (17%) reported none in either interview, and nine (19%) reported losses inconsistently, at one interview only. Although 23 women (49%) at Time 1 and 17 (36%) at Time 2 reported prenatal loss through miscarriage or elective termination, only 12 (25%) made this report at both interviews. Of the 16 (34%) inconsistent reporters, only one had a loss that occurred in the interval between AAI interviews. Two of the 24 reporting loss at Time 1, and nine of the 17 reporting loss at Time 2, were not rated for lack of resolution of these losses, due to an insufficient response.

Consistencies of reports of maltreatment were analyzed in several ways. There were different patterns of inconsistency regarding physical abuse and

TABLE 4.2. Alternate Ds, F, and E Classifications, AAI at Time 1 by AAI at Time 2

AAI at Time 1	AAI at Time 2			
	Ds	F	E	Total
Ds				
Count	8	10	4	22
Expected	5.1	13.1	3.7	
F				
Count	3	17	2	22
Expected	5.1	13.1	3.7	
E				
Count	0	1	2	3
Expected	.9	2.5	.6	
Total count	11	28	8	47

Note. $X^2(4) = 10.6$, $p < .05$, kappa = .29, $p < .01$.

sexual abuse. Nineteen (40%) mothers reported at least one incident of childhood sexual abuse at both interviews, and five (11%) additional mothers reported sexual abuse at one interview only. The reports on physical abuse were less consistent. Seventeen (36%) mothers reported childhood physical abuse at both interviews; about the same number (34%) reported inconsistently across the two interviews. We also examined the cross-time consistency of reports of ongoing, moderate to severe maltreatment, a measure that reflects both frequency and severity of physical, sexual, and/or emotional abuse. Nineteen (40%) mothers reported that they had experienced ongoing moderate-to-severe maltreatment in childhood at both interviews; nine (19%) others reported this experience at one time only. As with prenatal loss, 13 of 35 women reporting at least one childhood maltreatment trauma at Time 1, and 11 of 34 at Time 2 gave insufficient detail for a rating of lack of resolution of trauma.

There were few associations among reports of these life events. The various types of losses did not tend to co-occur with each other or with reports of ongoing, moderate-to-severe maltreatment. Reports of physical and sexual abuse were also unrelated, but both were correlated with ongoing abuse that was moderate to severe. At Time 2 only, reports of childhood sexual abuse and prenatal loss were associated, $r(47) = .36$, $p < .05$.

Consistency of Resolution and CoM Ratings

The four lack-of-resolution ratings: prenatal loss (U_P), loss (U_L), trauma (U_T), and the highest of the three (U_H), and the overall CoM rating, were correlated with each other within time points. At Time 1, U_p, U_L, and U_T were unrelated, r's (47) = –.22 to .21. U_H was significantly associated with all of the individual U scores, r's (47) = .32 to .52, and marginally associated with CoM, r (47) = –.26, p < .10. At Time 2 again U_p, U_L, and U_T were unrelated, r's (47) = –.16 to .20. U_H was associated with both U_L and U_T, r's (47) = .65 and .66, but not U_p. CoM was unrelated to U_p or U_L, and significantly related to U_T, r (47) = –.34, p < .05, and U_H, r (47) = –.46, p < .001.

All of the lack of resolution ratings but U_L showed significant stability over time, r's (47) = .30 to .64. It is noteworthy that there were only modest correlations across time for each lack-of-resolution rating, and that they were not correlated with each other. These correlations include the whole sample by assigning a score of "0" when no rating was applied; this would inflate the correlations for variables with relatively more "0" ratings, so comparisons should be made cautiously. The findings from the within- and across-time correlations seem to highlight the specificity of each type of lack of resolution rating, and suggest that lack of resolution of trauma contributes more to the overall coherence ratings at both time points than lack of resolution of loss. For this reason we explore the events of loss, trauma, and prenatal loss separately in analyses to follow.

Life Events and AAI

Table 4.3 summarizes analyses with which we examine the associations of the various U ratings and CoM with life events mentioned in the AAI narrative at Time 1 and Time 2 separately. As we reviewed above, inconsistent reporting was not rare and for any life event; between 10 and 35% of the sample reported an event at one time only. Methodological and psychological reasons why events might not be discussed consistently across interviews will be explored in the discussion.

One salient finding is that the fact of a death of an attachment figure before the age of 18 was not related to any U rating at either time point. Having at least one loss other than an attachment figure was related to U_L at Time 1 but not at Time 2, whereas a prenatal loss was related to U_L at Time 2 but not at Time 1. Reporting a prenatal loss was associated with U_p at Time 1 and Time 2. Incidence of physical abuse was not related to U_T, but incidence of sexual abuse was related to U_T at both time points, as was maltreatment that was moderate to severe and ongoing (which may include physical, emotional, and/or sexual abuse). Finally, there were no associations of any life event with CoM at Time 1. At Time 2 only the ongoing moderate-to-severe maltreatment had a modest association with CoM, r (47) = –.32, p < .05.

TABLE 4.3. Correlations between Lack of Resolution Ratings and Coherence Rating at Time 1 and Time 2 and Selected Life Events Reported at Either Time ($n = 47$)

AAI life event	Lack of resolution ratings				
	U_P	U_L	U_T	U_H	CoM
			Time 1		
Maltreatment, ongoing	.03	−.20	.60***	.26+	−.16
Sexual abuse	.06	−.10	.54***	.29*	−.08
Physical abuse	−.17	.09	.23	.24+	−.13
Prenatal loss	.74***	−.16	.13	.15	.11
Death of attachment figure	−.17	.04	−.18	−.20	−.05
Multiple losses	.02	.46***	−.10	.29*	−.00
			Time 2		
Maltreatment, ongoing	.04	.14	.63***	.42**	−.32*
Sexual abuse	.04	.06	.41**	.22	−.22
Physical abuse	.13	−.01	.05	−.01	−.00
Prenatal loss	.51***	.30*	.01	.32*	−.22
Death of attachment figure	−.04	.23	−.17	.03	.18
Multiple losses	.12	.24	.10	.25+	.03

Note. U_P, lack of resolution of prenatal loss; U_L, lack of resolution of loss; U_T, lack of resolution of trauma; U_H, highest lack of resolution score; CoM, coherence of mind.

+$p < .10$; *$p < .05$; **$p < .01$; ***$p < .001$.

AAI and Infant Attachment

We examined the correlation of the child's 9-point Strange Situation security rating at 19 months with the lack of resolution ratings, U_P, L_P, U_L, and U_H, and CoM from the AAI interviews at both time points. At both time points U_H was negatively related to infant security, r's (47) = −.36 and −.51, and U_P was positively related to infant disorganization, r's (47) = .31 and .36. Also at Time 2, U_T was negatively associated with infant security, r (47) = −.33, $p < .05$, and CoM was marginally related to infant security, r (47) = .27, $p < .10$.

To compare our results with the existing meta-analyses, we calculated phi using dichotomous AAI F-not-F and U-not-U, and Strange Situation B-not-B, and D-not-D classifications. Intergenerational congruence for F-not-F and B-not-B was nonexistent for the Time 1 AAI, phi = 0.0, and modestly (65%) significant at Time 2, phi = .30, $p < .05$. Intergenerational congruity for U-not-U and D-not-D was not evident at Time 1, phi = .07, but was marginal at Time 2, phi = .21, $p = .10$.

Life Events and Infant Attachment

Finally, we examined the association between selected dichotomous indicators of the occurrence of life events reported at Time 1 and Time 2 and the child's security and disorganization ratings at 19 months. As presented earlier, these life events included ongoing moderate-to-severe maltreatment (a measure that reflects both frequency and severity of any abuse type), sexual and physical abuse (which may or may not also qualify as severe maltreatment), death of an attachment figure, and deaths of other significant persons, all before the age of 18, and prenatal loss occurring at any age. At Time 1, there were no associations between any life event reported in the interview and infant attachment outcomes. At Time 2, there were several associations. Ongoing moderate-to-severe maltreatment was associated with both security r (46) = $-.37$, $p < .05$, and disorganization, r (46) = .28, $p < .10$. The correlations with sexual abuse and security, r (46) = $-.26$, $p < .10$, and disorganization, r (46) = .33, $p < .05$, were small to moderate. Whether or not the mother mentioned a prenatal loss at Time 2 was also strongly correlated with infant security, r (46) = $-.44$, $p < .01$, and disorganization, r (46) = .54, $p < .001$. These analyses were performed controlling for the U_p rating. At Time 2, the associations between reporting a prenatal loss and infant security, r (43) = $-.37$, $p < .05$, and disorganization, r (43) = .44, $p < .001$, respectively, were only slightly attenuated, suggesting that mentioning the prenatal loss at Time 2 was associated with disorganization, even after the effect of lack of resolution of prenatal loss, the only Time 2 lack-of-resolution rating that had a significant association with disorganization, was taken into account.

Summary of Cases That Were Ever Unresolved

Table 4.4 summarizes all 26 cases that had a primary or secondary U classification (U_H score of 5 or higher) at one or both time points. Of the five cases in the first group, considered U at both time points, all were scored for lack of resolution of both loss and trauma at Time 1. Four of the five were also rated for lack of resolution of prenatal loss at Time 1, and three were rated high enough to be U_p; two of these three continued to have high U_p ratings at Time 2 and the other did not mention a prenatal loss at the second interview. In all but one instance of prenatal loss (case 14 at Time 2), respondents also reported other losses or traumas that were sufficient to assign U. All of the five had the first AAI after the study child's birth. Of the nine cases U at Time 1 only, all were rated for U_L at both time points, but each had a lower U_L rating at Time 2, some considerably lower. Four of the women were cases of simple' U_L with no other rated trauma or prenatal loss (except that case 16 received a U_p rating of 1 at Time 2). All four were

TABLE 4.4. Summary of Study Participants Ever Having an AAI Transcript Rated as Unresolved (Highest U rating ≥ 5)

	Time 1					Time 2				
ID—Age	AAI	U_T	U_L	U_P	CoM	AAI	U_T	U_L	U_P	CoM
	U score 5 or higher at Time 1 and Time 2 ($n = 5$)									
01–19 ny	E/U_T	5.5	5.0	0.0	1.5	U_T/E	5.5	5.0	0.0	3.5
34– 17 ny	U_T/Ds	5.0	4.0	1.0_m	2.0	U_L/E	4.0	5.0	0.0	2.0
42– 29 yn	U_{TL}/E	5.0	0.0	5.0_a	3.0	U_T/E	5.0	0.0	0.0	4.5
44–18 nn	U_L/Ds	5.0	7.0	5.5_m	2.0	U_L/Ds	1.0	7.0	4.0_a	3.0
46–28nn	U_L/Ds	1.0	5.5	5.5_a	4.0	F/U_L	0.0	0.0	5.0_a	5.0
	U score 5 or higher at Time 1 only ($n = 9$)									
05–16 yy	U_L/Ds	0.0	5.5	0.0	2.0	F	0.0	3.0	0.0	5.5
09–25 ny	U_{LT}/Ds	6.5	5.5	4.0_a	2.0	E	4.0	4.0	0.0	2.5
16–15 yy	U_L/E	0.0	5.0	0.0	4.0	F	0.0	1.0	1.0_a	6.5
22–17 yy	Ds/U_L	0.0	5.0	0.0	4.0	F	0.0	3.5	0.0	8.5
23–31 yy	U_T/F	5.5	1.0	5.0_m	4.5	F	0.0	1.0	0.0	6.0
24–22 yy	F/U_T	5.0	3.0	0.0	4.5	F	0.0	2.0	0.0	7.0
25–16 yy	U_L/Ds	0.0	6.0	0.0	3.0	Ds	0.0	4.0	0.0	2.0
33– 35 yn	F/U_T	5.0	4.0	1.0_a	6.0	F	2.0	2.0	0.0	8.0
36–20 ny	U_L/Ds	4.0	5.5	0.0	4.5	F	0.0	1.0	0.0	5.5
	U score 5 or higher at Time 2 only ($n = 12$)									
02–26 yn	Ds	0.0	4.0	0.0	2.5	Ds/U_T	5.0	3.0	0.0	4.0
04–16 yy	Ds	0.0	1.0	0.0	4.0	F/U_L	0.0	5.0	0.0	6.0
06–31 yn	Ds	2.0	4.5	2.5_a	2.0	Ds/U_L	0.0	5.0	0.0	3.0
07–24 yy	F	4.5	3.0	0.0	4.5	U_T/E	5.0	2.0	0.0	4.0
10–24 ny	Ds	4.0	1.0	0.0	3.0	U_T/Ds	6.0	1.0	0.0	2.5
14–20 yy	F	2.0	4.5	$5.5_{c/r}$	7.0	U_L/E	0.0	3.0	5.0_a	2.0
20–24 yn	Ds	0.0	4.0	0.0	3.5	U_T/E	6.0	4.0	0.0	3.5
26–21 yy	Ds	0.0	4.5	0.0	5.0	U_L/F	4.5	5.5	0.0	5.0
27–21 yy	F	3.0	3.0	1.0_m	5.0	F/U_T	5.0	2.0	0.0	6.0
32–18 ny	F	4.0	2.0	1.0_a	5.0	F/U_L	1.0	5.0	0.0	8.0
35–22 nn	F	3.0	4.0	0.0	8.0	U_L/ F	5.0	5.5	0.0	5.0
37–19 yy	Ds	3.0	1.0	0.0	2.5	U_T/Ds	5.0	1.0	0.0	3.0

Note. Letters next to maternal age report whether the first AAI was a prenatal interview (y = yes, n = no) and whether the target child was a first birth (y = yes, n = no). Lack of resolution ratings of 0 indicated that the transcript was not scored for that state of mind; a score of 1 indicates that it was scored, and no evidence of lack of resolution was discerned. U_T, lack of resolution of trauma; U_L, lack of resolution of loss; U_P, lack of resolution of prenatal loss; CoM, coherence of Mind; T, trauma; L, loss; a, abortion; m, miscarriage; c/r, can't rate/not discussed or denied at Time 2.

adolescents at Time 1 (ages 15–17), and all had had their first AAI interview during pregnancy. Not only were these four mothers not rated U_L at Time 2, three of them moved from D or E insecure classifications to F, autonomous–secure. This change raises the question of whether they could be considered to have become "resolved" with regard to the earlier loss. Of the remaining five cases in this group, four were U_T at Time 1 and the fifth had a U_T score of 4. However, four of the five were classified as F at Time 2; three of these were not even rated for lack of resolution of trauma at Time 2. These scenarios raise the question if these three have become "resolved" or are more defended with regard to earlier trauma. For all but one of these mothers the study child was their firstborn child, and most were interviewed in pregnancy ($n = 6$) or soon after the birth ($n = 2$), facts that indicate that they were both young and new to motherhood at Time 1, with the arc of their adult trajectory still before them, with great potential for change.

The largest group in Table 4.4 consists of those 12 that were U at Time 2 only. Four of these cases involved "simple" loss at Time 1: cases 02, 04, 20, and 26. For case 04, interviewed at Time 1 in pregnancy at age 16, lack of resolution of this loss increased, even as her overall state of mind changed from Ds to F. The other three cases of "simple" loss did not remain simple, as all revealed early trauma at Time 2 that had not been revealed at Time 1. With the exception of case 14, the eight remaining cases showed more subtle differences in the values of the various ratings that increased enough to "qualify" for U classification. The story of case 14 is elaborated in the section below. In summary, differences in maternal life course between the group with U scores 5 or higher at both time points and the group with U scores of 5 or higher only at Time 1 are possible, with the former being more experienced mothers at both interviews, and the latter for the most part making the transition to motherhood between the first and second interviews.

CASE STUDIES OF INSTABILITY
IN THE AAI UNRESOLVED CLASSIFICATION

In order to understand more fully the dynamics of change in U classifications, we selected some specific examples based on examination of the scoring sheets for the two interviews. In some cases with unstable U classifications the differences between one time point's U classification and the other time point's primary classifications of F, Ds, or E were small, while in others the differences were rather dramatic. This variability was not captured well in the quantitative analyses, nor did we collect detailed biographical information about respondents' activities and events between the two assessments. We studied the AAI interviews themselves for clues. The second and third authors reviewed both of the transcripts for all respondents with an interview classified as U at either time point to determine if some instability might have been due to coding error. Despite the passage of several years, they agreed with the original classifications in all cases. The final step was to compare the two narratives for both content and quality to learn what was similar and different about them. Results of this approach are summarized in the next sections.

AAI Unresolved to Dismissing

Case 25 was 16 years old and pregnant with her first child at the initial AAI interview. Her story is typical of young mothers in this sample, with early losses but no reported childhood traumas. She lived with her parents in a neighborhood with many relatives from her extended family. At Time 1 her transcript was classified as U_LDs. She consistently insisted on lack of recall and moderately idealized her mother. She insisted she had no relationship with her father. She was unresolved regarding the loss of her mother's aunt, who had been ill and had died rather suddenly on New Year's Day 5 years earlier. Ever since she would wake up on that date at just the hour they had received the call of her great aunt's death. She had passed out at the funeral. Even now, she says: "It feels weird when I go to their house—she's not there—to make me smile."

Almost 5 years later, at the second AAI interview, only the participant, her mother, and her son were in the household, and her father was not mentioned. Many relatives in her extended family had passed away in the previous year. However, the discussion of these losses was brief. In explaining how these losses had affected her, she said "Nobody's gonna be with me forever.... I mean, you gotta enjoy them while they here, you know." The great aunt whose loss had not been resolved 5 years earlier was not even mentioned in the second interview. Overall, the transcript of the second AAI was Ds, with similar experience and state-of-mind scales as reported for the first interview. At 19 months, her infant was classified as disorganized.

AAI Unresolved to Secure

Case 23 was 31 years old, living alone, and pregnant with her first child at the time of the first AAI interview. Her case was representative of women who reported quite different childhood trauma content in the two AAI interviews. She was classified as U_TF at Time 1 and F at Time 2. She and her three biological siblings had been adopted. At Time 1 she reported that her parents voluntarily sent her to a group home for a year when she was an adolescent because she talked back to them and assaulted her mother once. She also described almost daily emotional and physical abuse from her mother. But at the second interview there was no mention of the abuse or of living in the group home, and her adjectives describing her mother were positive: supportive, involved, giving. She saw her parents regularly and celebrated holidays with them. She was now married and planning to go back to school. Her infant was classified as avoidant at 19 months.

AAI Secure to Unresolved

Case 14 was 20 years old, pregnant with her first child, and living with her boyfriend at the time of her first interview. Her primary classification at Time 1 was F. She earned high enough lack-of-resolution scores at both times to qualify for U categorization related to elective termination of a pregnancy. Because this had occurred within a year of the first interview it did not qualify her for a U classification at Time 1, according to the AAI coding manual. It was the reason she was classified U at Time 2.

In the first interview, this participant reported minimal evidence of idealization, derogation, anger, lack of memory, or passivity. Her narrative gave little support for an organized–insecure classification. She described a number of events qualifying for some lack-of-resolution score including several deaths, and sexual molestation by an uncle at age 4, in addition to the pregnancy termination. She also had a lengthy discussion of pets dying or getting hurt, suggestive of mental disorganization probably detailed and unusual enough to qualify for a lack of resolution score if the subject matter had qualified. When she was probed about the molestation episode, she said, "I don't really talk about that." Case 14 did describe a close and positive relationship with her mother and with her grandmother who provided some caregiving. Although she reported being "afraid" of her demanding and yelling father, she also expressed admiration of him; their relationship was not portrayed as excessively difficult.

At her second interview, the subject and her child lived alone. The primary classification of the second interview was U_L/E. Case 14 indicated that her feelings about the elective termination were "getting worse" and she blamed the decision to abort on her father, who "made me do it." She expressed considerable anger toward him, and when asked about her current relationship with her parents said, "I can't stand them" and "They make me ill," and described her "whole life" as traumatic. Thus it was her elective termination that provided a sufficiently high lack-of-resolution score to qualify for a U classification. Only two other losses were noted this time, but again she wept as she described the death of her dog as traumatic. The sexual molestation was again noted, but she said "I've drawn a blank in my memory" regarding it, and the episode was not further probed. This is similar to the first AAI interview in which she was not willing to discuss that trauma, suggesting possible traumatic memory loss. In addition, this interview warranted moderately high scores for idealization, anger, and lack of recall, and the alternate classification was clearly insecure–preoccupied with anger. Her infant was classified as disorganized at 19 months, which seems congruent with the spirit if not the letter of the coding system.

Case 35 was 22 and living with her husband, new infant, and two young children at the time of the first interview. She is an example of an individual with a probable secure childhood whose AAI classification changed from F to U_L/F at Time 2. She reported the death of her cousin in both interviews. In the first interview she described it as a clearly distressing event indicating it did affect her relation with her own children, but her narrative did not display sufficient disorganization to warrant a high lack-of-resolution rating. In this interview she also noted additional losses as well as other abusive episodes, none of which evoked sufficient disorganization for high U scores. Case 35's responses to queries about each loss and about the abuse were quite brief, and she did not indicate either as having an influence on her relationships with her own children. However, traumatic memory loss is a possibility because she said she had blocked out memories of the molestation by a neighbor when she was 6 or 7 years old. Throughout this interview, case 35 provided authentic episodic memories that portrayed a loving family and a generally objective, autonomous state of mind.

At the second interview, case 35 was divorced from her husband and living with her three children and her fiancé. In her second interview, categorized as U_L/F, she again described the death of her cousin, the sexual abuse incidents, and the death of one of the relatives mentioned in the first interview, as well as a miscarriage and an elective termination. This time she described the events in considerable detail. She noted that her cousin's death had a significant effect on her and that she had blamed herself for a long time. Only after being in counseling was she able to "forgive" herself. She also discussed both abuse events at length, with apparent emotion, and described how it affected her and how it influenced her behavior with her own children. Consequently, her U_L score for lack of resolution for loss of her cousin and U_T score for sexual abuse by nonattachment figures both appear to warrant primary categorization as U. She reported that she had previously blocked memories of the early abuse "until I'd gone to some serious therapy" but did not seem to have continuing traumatic memory loss. Perhaps of significance, she reported a physically and psychologically abusive relationship with her former husband and hesitation about getting married again.

This mother's representations of her parents in the second interview were consistently positive and although many of the specific memories were different, they also appeared genuine. Her responses were longer and seemed more confiding in this interview. Given low scores for state of mind related to idealization, anger, derogation, lack of recall, and passivity, and her positive evaluation of attachment relationships (all similar to the first interview), her alternate classification was F. Her child was classified as avoidant with a disorganization rating of 5 at 19 months.

AAI Dismissing to Unresolved

Three separate instances of a shift from Ds to U will be summarized. The first has similar ratings from Time 1 to Time 2, and the second two quite different ratings. All the respondents whose interviews are presented here showed greater willingness to discuss specific traumas or losses in the second interview compared with the first, which allowed more opportunities to reveal narrative incoherence. This was so even though often the same traumas or losses were described in both interviews.

Case 37 was 19, married, and pregnant with her first child at the time of the first interview. At the second interview she was single with three children. The transcript of the first interview was rated high for insistence in lack of recall and idealization of her mother, and was classified as Ds. Her mother's boyfriend had physically abused her and her mother and siblings for about 5 years, until she went to live with her father at age 12. The U_T rating was 3. She only briefly and narrowly described the abuse. "After my mom was divorced, then um—she had this boyfriend that used to hit us, I mean all of us.... " When asked if the experience affected her now, she replied: "Yeah because sometimes I start to think you know—'cuz he, he had a lot of anger, you know, now that I think about it, but it's just you know, I hope that—that it doesn't reflect on me. But you know, ha—I don't think I'm, I hope I'm not gonna be like that."

When the abuse was described in the second interview, the interviewer asked the participant to name five words to describe her relationship with her mother's boyfriend. This had not been done for the first interview. She could only think of one word, "mean." But when the interviewer probed for a story about it, she said, "My sister and I were talking about it not too long ago—about this one time, she asked me if I remembered—he, she said he used to tie my hands to something an' then hit me or somethin', but I—don't remember it, so I can't—really, you know. I know I blocked out a lot of things." The subject then went on to give several specific examples of severe beatings to her and her siblings. The U_T rating was 5. Overall, the transcript was classified U_T/D_S. Her child was classified as avoidant at 19 months.

Case 20 was married, 24, and pregnant with her third child at the time of her first AAI interview, and pregnant with her fifth child at the time of the follow-up AAI. She was in contact with her mother, but not her father. She had not seen either of them, however, since leaving home at age 17. At Time 1 her transcript was judged to be Ds. She had lost her grandfather only weeks before, and the U_L score, though the loss was too recent to record it, had been rated 4.

In the second interview this participant was clearly preoccupied with events in her childhood that, although alluded to at Time 1, had not been accompanied by much detail or emotional content. Within a year after the Time 1 interview she had begun counseling and was treated for depression. She was prescribed medication for her depression and had taken it until she learned of her current pregnancy. She reported that both the counseling and the medication had made a great difference in her life. What became very clear in the transcript of the second interview was the extent to which she and her siblings had endured years of physical abuse from their mother. In the first interview, the participant described her mother as being "pretty physical" with the kids over minor transgressions. When asked about it, she described her mother's behavior briefly, "hitting, pinching, throwing things … we got spanked quite a bit." In the second interview, in response to the same question and probes, the subject specifically labels her mother's behavior as physical abuse, and the descriptions of the behavior were detailed and mentioned frequently throughout the interview. It was clear in this interview how frightened of their mother's violence she and her siblings had been.

At Time 2 case 20's transcript was judged to be U_T/E. The U_L score for the loss of her grandfather was still judged to be 4, but the U_T score, which was not rated at Time 1, was now 6. Her child was classified as avoidant at 19 months.

At the time of the first AAI interview, case 26 was 21, married, pregnant with her first child, and living with her husband in her mother's house, the home she had grown up in. This transcript was rated Ds. At the second interview, the participant's living status was unchanged, except that now her preschool-age child was also in the household. The transcript of the second interview was judged to be U_L/F. Her story is an example of the idea that the incoherence that accompanies exploration of loss or trauma may be an intermediate step between a dismissing and an autonomous state of mind.

In the first interview case 26 could think of no adjectives to describe her early relationship with her mother, but in the second, she listed five, and told a story about each. She lost her father from a sudden heart attack when she was 9. In the first interview, this was her only memory of her father. In the second, she was also able to share a memory of crawling up into his lap when he had his morning coffee and a cigarette. In terms of her resolution of his loss, in the first interview she simply related the story of the day of his death, with minimal reflection on how the loss had affected her, saying, "I didn't really have a male role model that was positive." In the second interview she seemed to be able to acknowledge that she had still not resolved the loss of her father. She said, "I just go wild that's why I'm still, it still makes me very numb. At the same time I can be very casual. People say, ask me about my dad, 'Oh he died when I was little.' " She acknowledged that the loss "definitely had a lasting effect on who I am." The shift in lack of resolution of trauma scores reflected how she described being raped when she was 17. She discussed the incident in both interviews, but in the first interview the discussion was so brief that there was no evidence of lack of resolution. When asked if the rape affected her now, she replied, "No. I—it did for a while—I can't say for a long time," whereas in the second interview she described the event, her feelings at the time, and how it still affected her now: "I didn't realize it would hurt until afterward but it does, even though I was there ... [3 seconds] pretty, very.... " The outlines of her life story were essentially the same in both interviews. The differences in the narrative, however, support the conclusion that she was moving toward a more autonomous perspective (U_L/F) from her dismissing one, and that she is on the way to resolving the loss of her father. Her child was classified as secure at 19 months.

DISCUSSION

We began this chapter with a review of the commonly acknowledged association between parental representations of attachment relationships as measured by the AAI and infant attachment behavior in the Strange Situation. We noted that high-risk samples were underrepresented in van IJzendoorn's (1995) meta-analyses and suggested that both intra-AAI stability and intergenerational congruity may be weaker in families with young, low-income mothers with a history of childhood loss and trauma. Our results were consistent with this idea. In this mostly young, high-risk sample, the distribution of the AAI classifications, Ds F E U, was not significantly different at either time point from that reported by van IJzendoorn and Bakermans-Kranenburg (1996) for five samples ($n = 350$) of low socioeconomic status mothers. However, because of the risk factors experienced by this sample and the 4 years between assessments, it is not surprising that we found low stability in AAI secure–autonomous classification (phi = .18), compared to the stability reported in low-risk samples by Bakermans-Kranenburg and van IJzendoorn (1993), phi = .45, over 2 months, and Benoit and Parker (1994) over 12 months, phi = .27. Stability coefficients for the unresolved classification in the range of .37 to .59 would have been predicted by the three published low-risk studies that reported such stability, compared to our finding of phi = .06. In contrast, when the forced or best-fitting D F E classifications were used, there was modest F-not-F stability, phi = .33, $p <$ .05, suggesting more cross-time consistency in the qualities of overall state of mind and more variability in the indices of lack of resolution of loss or trauma for individuals from low socioeconomic status samples.

Similarly, the results on intergenerational congruence of AAI and Strange Situation classifications were at odds with van IJzendoorn's (1995) meta-analysis. Concordance between parent and infant security for the two AAI interviews was phi = .00 and .30, respectively, compared with the meta-analysis phi = .48. The concordance between parental "U" and infant "D" was phi = .07 and .21 for the two AAI interviews, respectively. The Time 2 statistic compares favorably with both van IJzendoorn's (1995) meta-analysis effect size of .31, and Madigan, Bakermans-Kranenburg, et al's. (2006) meta-analysis effect size of .21. Time 1 AAIs were administered at a time of rapid change and many pregnancy stresses; by the time infant attachment was assessed and the second AAI interview administered, there may have been more stability in the family's situation, and hence more concordance of mother and child attachment.

The pattern of correlations between various negative life events and AAI ratings of lack of resolution of loss and trauma had some consistency from Time 1 to Time 2. However, at both time points, a third to a half of respondents' reports of potentially traumatic maltreatment or prenatal losses were not reported in sufficient detail to be rated for lack of resolution. These differences may reflect both methodological limitations and individual psychological processes. We noted cases in which a respondent had a dismissing, minimizing stance toward an abuse experience during one interview, resulting in an event that could not be rated for lack of resolution, and a somewhat preoccupied, disorganized stance toward it in the other. One example is case 20, whose experience in therapy between the first and second AAI interviews clearly contributed to her state of mind shift form Ds to U_T/E. On the other hand, interviewers who elicit more content also create more opportunities for the respondent to reveal disorganized thought processes. A good example is case 37. The interviewer at Time 2 asked for adjectives about the respondent's relationship with her mother's boyfriend and we learned about abuse that was not reported in much detail to the earlier interviewer who had not asked for five adjectives to describe her relationship with her mother's boyfriend. Her rating for lack of resolution of trauma changed from 3 to 5; it was enough to shift her classification from Ds to U_T/Ds.

Respondents' growth-promoting life experiences in the 4 years between the two interviews also served to increase their ability to discuss a painful childhood. As these (mostly) young people matured, they talked with friends, sisters, and counselors and began to confront and reinterpret their earlier lives. It was our impression that for at least some respondents, indices of lack of resolution at Time 2 were expressed because they were moving from a predominantly dismissing attitude to one of more understanding and compassion for their younger selves.

In addition to lack-of-resolution ratings, we examined associations of mothers' reports of childhood life events at both AAI interviews with infant attachment security and disorganization, as assessed in the Strange Situation at 19 months, about midway between the two assessments. There were weak but consistent associations at both time points between reports of early ongoing, moderate-to-severe maltreatment, in particular sexual abuse, and infant insecurity and disorganization. The strongest associations, however, were for maternal reports of prenatal loss at Time 2, including both elective termination and miscarriage. In this small sample, more respondents (51%) reported prenatal loss in the first AAI assessment compared to the second (36%) 4 years later. Overall, 60% of the sample reported experiencing prenatal loss at some time in their lives. Reporting a prenatal loss at Time 2 was moderately related to infant D-not-D classification, phi = .35, $p < .01$. At Time 1, there was no association between reporting fetal loss and infant D-not-D classification, phi = .09, $p > .10$.

Most women who reported a prenatal loss did not receive a U_P rating of 5 or higher for that loss. At Time 1, 17% of those reporting a prenatal loss qualified for U on that basis, and at Time 2, only 4% did. Nevertheless, the association of prenatal loss at Time 2 with infant D remained, even when controlling for U_P. In accord with what would be predicted by Hughes, Turton, Hopper, McGauley, and Fonagy (2004), we found that 50% of infants classified as D at 19 months had mothers who later reported both prenatal loss and ongoing moderate-to-severe childhood maltreatment, compared to 16% of infants who were not classified as D. Similar proportions held for mothers being classified as U at Time 2: 41% of women with U_H scores of 5 or higher reported both, compared to 13% of those who were not U.

Having a U_H rating of 5 or higher was marginally related to infant D classification, phi = .21, $p = .10$, as would be predicted, but only at Time 2. Sixty-three percent of infants classified as D had mothers with U_H scores of 5 or higher at Time 2, compared with 32% of infants who were not D. Time 2 reports of sexual abuse, phi = .20, $p < .10$, and most of all prenatal loss, phi = .35, were both associated with the D classification as well. There seem to be associations between prenatal loss, unresolved status, and infant disorganized attachment for women already vulnerable from early child maltreatment. The experience of other early loss, however, was not a contributing factor. Lyons-Ruth et al. (2003), following a high-risk sample, also found that early losses did not predict to infant D beyond 1 year.

Finally, the fact that ongoing, moderate-to-severe maltreatment is associated with infant disorganization, but the lack of resolution of trauma rating U_T is not, suggests several issues. Interviewers may fail to probe sufficiently when this painful material is touched on in the interview, and respondents can defensively minimize or choose not to discuss a painful topic in the interview that still has a disorganizing effect on state of mind and/or the caregiving system, resulting in infant disorganization. Some respondents appeared to take the latter path in the second interview, perhaps because they had some memory of the first and chose "not to go there." A more rigorous standardization of follow-up prompts could mitigate, though not eliminate, the variability in response patterns we observed. Alternatively, childhood trauma may be related to hostile–helpless states of mind, which in turn predict infant disorganization (Lyons-Ruth et al., 2003). Finally, some women, especially perhaps those who were adolescents at the first interview and experienced early loss but no trauma, truly seemed to have become more resolved over the 4 years since the first AAI interview.

Overall, we found more expected associations with infant attachment for the second AAI interview, compared to the first. These findings may be due to the combined factors of life experience, the transition to adulthood, and the developing child's presence as an elicitor of "ghosts" from the past. Research focusing on the parent's "working model of the child" (e.g., Benoit, Parker, & Zeanah, 1997) or the parent's representation of her relationship with the child (e.g., Slade, Belsky, Aber, & Phelps, 1999) may address this process more directly.

Similarly, the timing of the first AAI, before or after the birth of the study child (which was usually the mother's first child as well), affected the stability of the AAI U-not-U classification across a span of over 4 years, with significant stability found only when both interviews occurred after the birth of the child. Future research attempting to replicate and understand this intriguing finding might focus on the role of the attention and memory systems. It is likely that the mother's interactions with her child, centered as they are on the child's initially presymbolic affective regulation and engagement behaviors, activates her implicit (procedural) memory system. This system, which stores models of predictable sequences of interpersonal interactions (Siegel, 1999), may hold information about "ways of being with" important attachment figures that is outside of explicit, autobiographical memory—the memory system that is tapped by the AAI. The baby, but not the AAI, might trigger a mother's experience of a childhood trauma because the trauma experience, perhaps because it occurred very early in life, was never fully represented symbolically (semantically). Before the child's birth (at the time of some of our initial AAIs), perhaps memories of the trauma were processed in a defensive way—as in the dismissing person's tendency to fail to remember details from the past and not attend to heightened interpersonal cues in the present (Fraley, Davis, & Shaver, 1998; Fraley, Garner, & Shaver, 2000; Mikulincer & Orbach, 1995). This defensive stance may be difficult to maintain following the birth of the baby, however, because the activated implicit memory system has brought attachment-related material closer to the surface, where it is then more available for symbolization by the explicit memory system, and can be captured by the postnatal AAI. Even autonomous (at Time 1) individuals could have unevenness in the degree to which trauma is integrated across memory systems, so that a discussion, in the prenatal AAI, of past trauma would only activate semantically processed memories, while the infant's pain cry activates an associative network of implicit memories having to do with vulnerability, fear, and lack of protection. The repeated activation of these painful, previously disavowed feelings might account for the shift from an F classification before the infant's birth to a U classification after birth for some of our mothers.

However, we also found significant movement away from U for the subsample of women interviewed for the first time before birth of the child. Perhaps for some of these mothers, the experience of parenting opened up their implicit memory system, enabling them to access body memories of being soothed and cared for prior to later loss and abuse experiences. It may have been the case that the process of parenting was ultimately integrating for those new mothers who were young, had family support, and reported childhood loss but no trauma.

CONCLUSION

Our sample of young, high-risk mothers experienced significantly greater early trauma and loss than is typical for middle-class samples. It is our impression that these experiences created both more opportunity for lack of resolution (and thus a U code) and for greater instability of U status across time. A history of traumatic upheavals creates "opportunities" for lack of resolution around any number of individual events. But it may also create a complex and fragmented mental landscape where both an individual's ability and inclination to make meaning of a particular traumatic event *and* the meaning made change over time, often in response to newer disruptions and reversals. When the developmental reorganization of adolescence and early adulthood is factored in, it is perhaps unsurprising that many of these young mothers passed through periods of lack of resolution as reflected in their shifting personal narratives.

Though our sample was characterized by low stability of attachment classifications overall, our results suggest that the presence of the child, and the experience of parenting, may have had a crystallizing effect on maternal attachment-related representations. We found greater concordance between adult and child attachment status when the AAI was administered several years after the birth of the study child, which suggests that the experience of the mother–infant relationship itself—wherein each partner shapes interactions in a mutually influencing, recursive process—brought attachment representations and expectations closer into alignment for many of our subject dyads.

We also found greater stability in adult attachment classifications across

4 years when the initial interview was conducted after the birth of the child. We speculate that the experience of parenting the new infant unlocks access to previously warded-off implicit relational information, making it more available for explicit semantic processing from that point forward. This thinking fits well with George and Solomon's (2008) proposed model of the development of the caregiving system.

It appears that use of the AAI alone at multiple time points does not allow for making distinctions between the mother whose accounts across time differ because of increased access to implicit models of interaction (leading to increased or decreased defensiveness) and the mother for whom a previously painful and unresolved event has since become integrated and resolved. Future longitudinal research on stability of attachment would benefit from the use of additional measures, such as one that notes the quality of a therapeutic alliance, an independent trauma interview (e.g., Bailey, Moran, & Pederson, 2007) for a history of traumatic life events, and a measure that taps into implicit forms of dyadic communication, such as Lyons-Ruth's AMBIANCE scale (Lyons-Ruth et al., 2003), for use in combination with the AAI. It is also possible that a semiprojective technique may be better able to detect the influence of traumatic loss and abuse than an autobiographical interview that is likely to raise defenses in some individuals (see Buchheim & George, Chapter 13, this volume).

ACKNOWLEDGMENTS

This work was supported by the United States Department of Health and Human Services (Administration on Children, Youth, and Families) Local Research Partnerships of Early Head Start Programs, Grant Nos. 90YF0013/01 (5/96–4/01) and 90-YF-0024 (5/01–4/05).

REFERENCES

Ainsworth, M. S., Blehar, M. C., Waters, E., & Wall, S. (1978). *Patterns of attachment: A psychological study of the Strange Situation*. Hillsdale, NJ: Erlbaum.

Bailey, H. N., Moran, G., & Pederson, D. R. (2007). Childhood maltreatment, complex trauma symptoms, and unresolved attachment in an at-risk sample of adolescent mothers. *Attachment and Human Development, 9*, 139–161.

Bailey, H. N., Moran, G., Pederson, D. R., & Bento, S. (2007). Understanding the transmission of attachment using variable- and relationship-centered approaches. *Developmental Psychopathology, 19*, 313–343.

Bakermans-Kranenburg, M. J., & van IJzendoorn, M. H. (1993). A psychometric study of the Adult Attachment Interview: Reliability and discriminant validity. *Developmental Psychology, 29*, 870–879.

Barnett, D., Manly, J. T., & Cicchetti, D. (1993). Defining child maltreatment: The interface between policy and research. In D. Cicchetti & S. L. Toth (Eds.), *Child abuse, child development, and social policy* (pp. 7–74) Norwood, NJ: Ablex.

Belsky, J., Campbell, S. B., Cohn, J. F., & Moore, G. (1996). Instability of infant–parent attachment security. *Developmental Psychology, 32,* 921–924.

Benoit, D., & Parker, K. C. (1994). Stability and transmission of attachment across three generations. *Child Development, 65,* 1444–1456.

Benoit, D., Parker, K. C., & Zeanah, C. H. (1997). Mothers' representations of their infants assessed prenatally: Stability and association with infants' attachment classifications. *Journal of Child Psychology and Psychiatry, 38,* 307–313.

Born, L., Soares, C. N., Phillips, S. D., Jung, M., & Steiner, M. (2006). Women and reproductive-related trauma. *Annals of the New York Academy of Science, 1071,* 491–494.

Cramer, B., & Stern, D. N. (1988). Evaluation of changes in mother–infant brief psychology: A single case study. *Infant Mental Health Journal, 9,* 20–45.

Crowell, J. A., Treboux, D., & Waters, E. (2002). Stability of attachment representations: The transition to marriage. *Developmental Psychology, 38,* 467–479.

Fraiberg, S., Adelson, E., & Shapiro, V. (1975). Ghosts in the nursery: A psychoanalytic approach to the problems of impaired infant–mother relationships. *Journal of the American Academy of Child Psychiatry, 14,* 387–421.

Fraley, R. C. (2002). Attachment stability from infancy to adulthood: Meta-analysis and dynamic modeling of developmental mechanisms. *Personality and Social Psychology Review, 6,* 123–151.

Fraley, R.C., Davis, K. E., & Shaver, P. R. (1998). Dismissing-avoidance and the defensive organization of emotion, cognition, and behavior. In J. A. Simpson & W. S. Rholes (Eds.), *Attachment theory and close relationships* (pp. 249–279). New York: Guilford Press.

Fraley, R.C., Garner, J.P., & Shaver, P. R. (2000). Adult attachment and the defensive regulations of attention and memory: Examining the role of preemptive and post-emptive defensive processes. *Journal of Personality and Social Psychology, 79,* 816–826.

George, C., Kaplan, N., & Main, M. (1984). *The Adult Attachment Interview.* Unpublished manuscript, University of California at Berkeley.

George, C., Kaplan, N., & Main, M. (1985). *The Adult Attachment Interview.* Unpublished manuscript, University of California at Berkeley.

George, C., Kaplan, N., & Main, M. (1996). *The Adult Attachment Interview.* Unpublished manuscript, University of California at Berkeley.

George, C., & Solomon, J. (2008). The caregiving system: A behavioral systems approach to parenting. In J. Cassidy & P. R. Shaver (Eds.), *Handbook of attachment: Theory, research, and clinical applications* (2nd ed., pp. 833–856). New York: Guilford Press.

Hughes, P., Turton, P., Hopper, E., McGauley, G. A., & Fonagy, P. (2004). Factors associated with the unresolved classification of the Adult Attachment Interview in women who have suffered stillbirth. *Development and Psychopathology, 16,* 215–230.

Lyons-Ruth, K., Dutra, L., Schuder, M. R., & Bianchi, I. (2006). From infant attachment disorganization to adult dissociation: Relational adaptations or traumatic experiences? *Psychiatric Clinics of North America, 29,* 63–86.

Lyons-Ruth, K., Melnick, S., Bronfman, E., Sherry, S., & Llanas, L. (2004). Hostile–helpless relational models and disorganized attachment patterns between parents and their young children: Review of research and implications for clinical work. In L. Atkinson & S. Goldberg (Eds.), *Attachment issues in psychopathology and intervention* (pp. 65–94). Mahwah, NJ: Erlbaum.

Lyons-Ruth, K., Yellin, C., Melnick, S., & Atwood, G. (2003). Childhood experiences of trauma and loss have different relations to maternal Unresolved and Hostile–Helpless states of mind on the AAI. *Attachment and Human Development, 5,* 330–352.

Madigan, S., Bakermans-Kranenburg, M. J., van IJzendoorn, M. H., Moran, G., Pederson, D. R., & Benoit, D. (2006). Unresolved states of mind, anomalous parental behavior, and disorganized attachment: A review and meta-analysis of a transmission gap. *Attachment and Human Development, 8,* 89–111.

Madigan, S., Moran, G., & Pederson, D. R. (2006). Unresolved states of mind, disorganized attachment relationships, and disrupted interactions of adolescent mothers and their infants. *Developmental Psychology, 42,* 293–304.

Madigan, S., Moran, G., Schuengel, C., Pederson, D. R., & Otten, R. (2007). Unresolved maternal attachment representations, disrupted maternal behavior and disorganized attachment in infancy: Links to toddler behavior problems. *Journal of Child Psychology and Psychiatry, 48,* 1042–1050.

Main, M., Goldwyn, R., & Hesse, E. (2002). *Adult attachment scoring and classification systems.* Unpublished manuscript, University of California at Berkeley.

Main, M., & Solomon, J. (1990). Procedures for identifying infants as disorganized/disoriented during the Ainsworth Strange Situation. In M. T. Greenberg (Ed.), *Attachment in the preschool years: Theory, research, and intervention* (pp. 121–160). Chicago: University of Chicago Press.

Mikulincer, M., & Orbach, I. (1995). Attachment styles and repressive defensiveness: The accessibility and architecture of affective memories. *Journal of Personality and Social Psychology, 68,* 917–925.

Office of Research and Evaluation and Head Start Bureau. (2001). *Building their futures: How Early Head Start programs are enhancing the lives of infants and toddlers in low-income families, summary report.* Washington, DC: Department of Health and Human Services, Administration on Children, Youth and Families.

Pines, R. J., Bleiberg, E., Fonagy, P., Lebovici, S., McDonough, S., & Ware, L. (2002). A 3-year-old "monster." In J. M. Maldonado-Duran (Ed.), *Infant and toddler mental health* (pp. 345–360). Washington, DC: American Psychiatric Publishing.

Rosnow, R. L., & Rosenthal, R. (1988). Focused tests of significance and effect size estimation in counseling psychology. *Journal of Counseling Psychology, 35,* 203–208.

Siegel, D. J. (1999). *The developing mind.* New York: Guilford Press.

Slade, A., Belsky, J., Aber, J. L., & Phelps, J. L. (1999). Mothers' representations of their relationships with their toddlers: Links to adult attachment and observed mothering. *Developmental Psychology, 35,* 611–619.

Solomon, J., & George, C. (1996). Defining the caregiving system: Toward a theory of caregiving. *Infant Mental Health Journal, 17,* 183–197.

Solomon, J., & George, C. (2006). Intergenerational transmission of dysregulated maternal caregiving: Mothers describe their upbringing and childrearing. In O. Mayseless (Ed.), *Parenting representations: Theory, research, and clinical implications* (pp. 265–295). New York: Cambridge University Press.

Sroufe, L. A., & Jacobvitz, D. (1989). Diverging pathways, developmental transformations, multiple etiologies and the problem of continuity in development. *Human Development, 32,* 196–203.

van IJzendoorn, M. H. (1995). Adult attachment representations, parental responsiveness, and infant attachment: A meta-analysis on the predictive validity of the Adult Attachment Interview. *Psychological Bulletin, 117,* 387–403.

van IJzendoorn, M. H., & Bakermans-Kranenburg, M. J. (1996). Attachment representations in mothers, fathers, adolescents, and clinical groups: A meta-analytic search for normative data. *Journal of Consulting and Clinical Psychology, 64,* 8–21.

van IJzendoorn, M. H., Juffer, F., & Duyvesteyn, M. G. (1995). Breaking the intergenerational cycle of insecure attachment: A review of the effects of attachment-based interventions on maternal sensitivity and infant security. *Journal of Child Psychology and Psychiatry, 36,* 225–248.

Waters, E., Merrick, S., Treboux, D., Crowell, J., & Albersheim, L. (2000). Attachment security in infancy and early adulthood: A twenty-year longitudinal study. *Child Development, 71,* 684–689.

Wechsler, D. (1981). *Manual for the Wechsler Adult Intelligence Scale—Revised.* San Antonio, TX: Psychological Corporation.

Weinfield, N. S., Whaley, G. J., & Egeland, B. (2004). Continuity, discontinuity, and coherence in attachment from infancy to late adolescence: Sequelae of organization and disorganization. *Attachment and Human Development, 6,* 73–97.

Chapter 5

Genetic and Environmental Determinants of Attachment Disorganization

GOTTFRIED SPANGLER

Attachment is a central developmental issue that becomes salient in infancy and remains a critical contributor to the child's adaptation (Bowlby, 1982; Sroufe, 1979). The development of attachment requires adaptation to the caregiving environment, including organizing, coordinating, and integrating perceptions, emotions, and behaviors with those of the caregiver (Ainsworth, 1973). This process of attachment formation is facilitated by species-specific adaptations, individual differences in infant social responsiveness, and individual differences in the readiness of the caretaker to perceive and to respond to the infants needs. By the end of the first year, different patterns of infant attachment can be observed in Ainsworth's Strange Situation, a laboratory assessment (Ainsworth, Blehar, Waters, & Wall, 1978) that is designed to activate the attachment system by confronting the child with a strange person and short separations from the caregiver followed by reunions with the caregiver. According to Ainsworth's traditional classification, the infant's attachment strategies in the Strange Situation are categorized into three groups: secure, insecure–avoidant, or insecure–ambivalent.

In addition to the traditional groups, Main and Solomon (1986) described an additional attachment group conceptualized as disorganized/disoriented. The essential characteristic of infants in this group is behavior that demonstrates a striking absence of a coherent behavioral strategy upon reunion in coping with the emotional challenge caused by the separation from the caregiver (Main & Solomon, 1990). These infants seem to lack a readily observable goal, intention, or explanation. Their behavior is marked by temporal disorder, by functional contradictions such as proximity seeking with avoiding gaze, incompleteness or interruptions of movements, breaks, stereotypies, confusion, and apprehension. According to Main and Solomon, disorganized/disoriented behaviors are coded separately from the traditional secure and insecure patterns of attachment. Thus, the quality of infant–parent attachment can be described with respect to two conceptually different behavioral dimensions, the security of the attachment relationship as well as the coherence or organization of a specific attachment pattern, although it is not always easy to discern the underlying organized pattern when infants are disorganized.

The focus of this chapter is on the biological foundation of attachment disorganization, including both the psychobiological processes underlying the organization of the attachment system and the genetic characteristics of infants who are classified as disorganized. First, I review empirical findings that support the view of disorganized attachment status as indicating a dysfunctional behavioral pattern for managing emotionally stressful situations. Second, I review empirical evidence for a strong genetic component to infant disorganized attachment status, including interesting new findings that demonstrate an interaction between genetic characteristics of the infant and specific experiences with the caregiver in the development of attachment disorganization. This review of recent empirical studies serves as a basis for a discussion of theoretical and unresolved questions in understanding the biological basis for disorganized attachment.

BIOLOGICAL PROCESSES ASSOCIATED WITH REGULATION IN DISORGANIZED INFANTS

Main and Hesse (1990) suggested that disorganization reflects an intense alarm response on the part of an infant. They argued that, in the presence or upon return of the mother, the disorganized infant seems to experience a strong conflict between approach (activated by separation) and withdrawal (presumably activated by fear of the parent), with the consequence that the activation of attachment behavior cannot be systematically controlled by an organized, goal-oriented behavioral strategy. This conflict is revealed in the more-or-less subtle or intense behaviors of infants indicative of disorientation or disorganization or, in later developmental periods, strong attempts to control the behavior of the caregiver in either a caregiving or a punitive way (Main & Cassidy, 1988). The interpretation of these behaviors as signs of disorganization is supported by findings indicating the involvement of biological systems in the regulation of disorganized infants, in particular biological systems that indicate defensive responses to or inappropriate coping with attachment-related emotional stress.

Changes in cardiac activity have been used as indicators of the way in which the individual evaluates the current context. An increase in heart rate may be part of a defensive response (Graham & Clifton, 1966), may be interpreted as an index of emotional and behavioral activation (Fowles, 1980), or may indicate a fast-acting and short-lasting activation to cope with aversive situations (Ursin, Baade, & Levine, 1978). If disorganized behaviors in infants are indicative of alarm and the infant's evaluation of the situation as threatening, we would expect cardiac responses, in particular, a phasic heart rate acceleration, immediately upon the occurrence of these behaviors, such as when the parent approaches upon reunion in the Strange Situation. Furthermore, if the notion of alarm is correct, we would also expect a higher overall cardiac activation in disorganized infants as compared to nondisorganized ones, especially during separation. Thus, phasic responses accompanying specific infant behaviors labeled disorganized may support the validity of those behaviors as indications of alarm, while a tonic activation during separation may indicate an extreme emotional activation such as that assumed to be experienced by disorganized infants.

In our investigations, we found both types of cardiac activation associated with infant attachment disorganization. First, disorganized infants, as compared to infants with an organized attachment pattern, showed a heightened tonic heart rate during separation. This indicated a particularly high emotional activation, suggesting that disorganized infants experienced more intense alarm during separation than organized infants (Spangler & Grossmann, 1993). Second, infant behaviors defined as indicative of attachment disorganization in the presence of the attachment figure were found to be accompanied by phasic heart rate accelerations (Spangler & Grossmann, 1999). Following Graham and Clifton (1966), this pattern indicates defensive responses to the behavior of the caregiver. Moreover, both types of cardiac responses may reflect the greater effort needed by disorganized infants than organized infants to produce an effective coping response (Lundberg & Frankenhaeuser, 1980).

While, according to a stress arousal model (Selye, 1952), the cardiac system may mirror negative emotional reactivity in response to activation of the attachment system or to threatening stimuli, the function of the hypothalamic–pituitary–adrenal (HPA) system, which controls adrenocortical activity, has been related to the availability and efficacy of behavioral or psychological coping strategies (e.g., Levine, Wiener, Coe, Bayart, & Hayashi, 1987; von Holst, 1986). Accordingly, adrenocortical responses can be used to evaluate the quality of coping strategies. In the specific context of the Strange Situation (or any situation that activates the attachment system), adrenocortical responses may be indicators of the appropriateness of specific attachment strategies used for emotional regulation. This parallels Bowlby's (1973) conception of different rings of homeostasis, in which a failure of emotional regulation on the behavioral level ("outer ring" of homeostasis) leads to a physiological activation ("inner ring"). In the present case, this inner ring would be expressed as adrenocortical activation.

Empirical evidence from different studies confirms Main and Solomon's notion (1990) that disorganized status reflects an ineffective response to separation and/or reunion. In our first study on this topic (Spangler & Grossmann, 1993), securely attached infants showed no adrenocortical activation during the Strange Situation. There were significant increases in cortisol levels in infants with insecure attachment patterns, particularly in infants with disorganized attachment. A similar finding was reported by Hertsgaard, Gunnar, Erickson, and Nachmias (1995). In a replication study, however, Spangler and Schieche (1998) did not find heightened cortisol responses in disorganized infants, but they did find that expression of negative emotion was associated with adrenocortical activation in disorganized infants (as well as in avoidant and ambivalent ones), but not in secure ones. Thus, the use of emotional expression for an efficient dyadic emotional regulation within the attachment relationship, which would be expressed in a downregulation of the adrenocortical system, seems to be impaired in disorganized infants.

These findings provide evidence on a biological level for the validity of the concept of infant disorganization as a failure to organize or achieve effective attachment behavioral strategies in the Strange Situation. Although the classification of disorganized attachment is based on a great variety of behaviors, these behaviors in infants seem to be symptomatic of poor psychobiological organization. Thus, the hypothesis that disorganized infants experience more intense alarm and negative emotional arousal than organized infants, irrespective of their underlying attachment category, seems to be additionally supported by heightened activity of different biological systems (cardiac and adrenocortical) during the Strange Situation.

SOCIAL AND INDIVIDUAL DETERMINANTS
OF DISORGANIZED ATTACHMENT

About 15% of 1-year-old infants in low-risk and up to 86% in high-risk populations showed disorganized attachment behavior in the Strange Situation (Barnett, Ganiban, & Cicchetti, 1999; Main & Solomon, 1990; van IJzendoorn, Schuengel, & Bakermans-Kranenburg, 1999). There were for a long time in the field only assumptions regarding the determinants of attachment disorganization with little or no emprirical evidence. Main and Hesse (1990) suggested that, in an otherwise adequate caregiving relationship, there may sometimes be elements of fear in the interactions arising from frightening or frightened behavior of the parent and they assumed that such parental behavior may have a disorganizing effect on the infant's attachment behavior. When this occurred, infants were frightened but did not have an attachment solution to address their fear (Main & Solomon, 1990). Empirical support for this explanation was provided only later when research findings showed that maternal frightened or frightening behavior indeed was observed more often, although not exclusively, in mothers of infants with disorganized attachment (Goldberg, Benoit, Blokland, & Madigan, 2003; Hesse & Main, 2006; Schuengel, Bakermans-Kranenburg, & van IJzendoorn, 1999).

Additional support for the view that frightening or frightened maternal behaviors might be central in the etiology of attachment disorganization came from studies reporting high rates of disorganization in maltreated infants (Barnett et al., 1999; Lyons-Ruth & Jacobvitz, 1999). Empirical studies of high-risk samples have shown that mothers of infants with attachment disorganization show higher rates of atypical maternal behavior, such as hostile–intrusive behaviors, extreme withdrawal, and communication errors (Lyons-Ruth, Repacholi, McLeod, & Silva, 1991; Lyons-Ruth, Bronfman, & Parsons, 1999; Madigan, Moran, & Pederson, 2006).

Forbes, Evans, Moran, and Pederson (2007) conducted a study with adolescent mothers that potentially allows for causal interpretation of the relation between atypical maternal behavior and attachment disorganization. They found that a decrease of maternal disrupted communication during the second year of infant life was accompanied by a decrease in the proportion of infants with disorganized attachments.

In all of these studies, little or no information was provided about the infants' individuality independent of the interactions with the caretaker. Although temperament by itself rarely predicts quality of infant attachment (Vaughn, Bost, & van IJzendoorn, 2008), the prevalence of infants with disorganized attachments in high-risk populations is noteworthy and research on determinants of child abuse points to child contributors as well as parental factors (Starr, 1988). It is also noteworthy that child-related factors such as neurological impairment or autism seem to contribute to the same behavior charateristics as attachment disorganization (Capps, Sigman, & Mundy, 1994; Pipp-Siegel, Siegel, & Dean, 1999). Nevertheless, with only a few exceptions, there has been little interest in a systematic investigation of the effects of child characteristics on infant attachment disorganization until recently.

Several studies of infants have examined the contributions of mother and child characteristics to attachment. Spangler, Fremmer-Bombik, and Grossmann (1996) found that infants in a low-risk sample classified as disorganized during the Strange Situation at 12 months, as compared to nondisorganized infants, were characterized as newborns by low levels of behavioral organization (low orientation and low emotional regulation). At the same time, these authors found no significant differences between mothers of disorganized and nondisorganized infants for maternal sensitivity. Fish (2001), studying attachment in a low socioeconomic status sample, investigated the maternal and child contributions to attachment differences assessed in the Strange Situation at 15 months. While contextual factors and maternal interaction during the first year predicted attachment security, disorganized infants were best distinguished by infant characteristics, including a greater likelihood of being male and being wary without using the mother as a secure base at 9 months. Finally, Goldberg and colleagues (2003) found that a substantial proportion of the mothers of infants with attachment disorganization were not coded as disruptive in their parenting, and that there were no significant differences in maternal fearful or intrusive behaviors between the disorganized and the nondisorganized groups. The authors concluded that both infant factors and contextual factors might contribute to the development of attachment disorganization.

Based on these findings, it seems that the development of attachment disorganization might be influenced by an infant's individual dispositions. The behavioral indices of disorganization during the Strange Situation could indicate a more general deficit in behavioral regulation that can be observed as early as in the newborn period. Thus, attachment disorganization might also be conceived as an, at least partly, individual construct, in contrast to attachment security being perceived as a relationship characteristic.

GENETIC CORRELATES OF DISORGANIZED ATTACHMENT

The conception of disorganization as also including individual characteristics (see Spangler et al., 1996; Spangler & Grossmann, 1999) has been regarded somewhat skeptically by most attachment reserachers for a long time. This view changed when a Hungarian research group published a pioneering molecular-genetic study at the millenium that suggested a genetic contribution to attachment disorganization (Lakatos et al., 2000). In order to assess the molecular-genetic foundations of psychological processes, association studies are often used to test whether individuals with a specific behavioral or psychological characteristic are more frequently carriers of a variant of a specific gene candidate than those without this characteristic. Candidate genes used in psychological research are genes contributing to the regulation of important neurotransmitters like dopamine or serotonin or to the efficiency of signal transmission.

Lakatos and colleagues (2000) were the first to show in an emprical study that differences in attachment disorganization were associated with specific genetic markers of the dopaminergic system which is involved in attentional, motivational, and reward mechanisms and associated with negative emotionality and stress reactivity (Diamond, 2001). They found that the 7-repeat allele of the dopamine receptor D4 (*DRD4*) gene was more frequent in infants classified as disorganized with respect to quality of infant–mother attachment. It should be noted that this association is probabilistic rather than deterministic, because a significant proportion of infants with the 7-repeat allele was not disorganized (about one-third), while disorganization was also found among those without a 7-repeat allele (also about one-third). In further publications, the Hungarian group presented additional evidence for genetic contributions to infant attachment disorganization. Lakatos et al. (2002) indicated that a second polimorphism, the *-521 C/T* single nucleotide polymorphism in the regulatory region of the DRD4 gene, was involved in the development of attachment disorganization. Their study showed that the previous association with the 7-repeat allele was significant solely in the presence of the *-521 T* allele. Moreover, by applying family-based analyses (transmission equilibrium test), Gervai et al. (2005) found a preferential transmission of the 7-repeat allele from parents to disorganized infants, and thus could exclude population stratification in their sample. This means that the findings could be interpreted in terms of an association between genes and disorganization rather than in terms of a priori differences in allele frequencies of the subsamples of disorganized and nondisorganized infants. These studies can be regarded as a turning point leading to a more differentiated view of the possible origins of attachment disorganization.

A first attempt to replicate the findings of the Hungarian group in a Dutch twin study was not successful. Bakermans-Kranenburg and van IJzendoorn (2004) failed to identify an association between infant attachment disorganization and the presence of the 7-repeat allele of the *DRD4* gene. In addition, a study reporting on the behavioral genetic analyses using this same twin sample did not yield major genetic effects on the explained variance of attachment disorganization (Bokhorst et al., 2003). Rather, attachment differences were mostly explained by shared environment variance, that is, differences in environmental experiences shared by the twins. There are two further behavioral genetic studies with equivocal findings. Finkel and Matheny (2000) in a twin study found that 25% of the variance of attachment security was attributable to genetic influences, but most of the variance was explained by nonshared environment, the specific experiences of each of the twins. O'Connor and Croft (2001), however, could not identify a significant proportion of genetic variance. Unfortunately, neither of these studies included analyses for attachment disorganization.

A further indication of the role of the *-521 C/T* gene polymorphism in the regulatory region of the *DRD4* gene was found in a recent study, however. Frigerio and colleagues (2009) investigated the relation between quality of attachment, including disorganization, and several different gene markers (*SERT, DRD4, -521 CT,* and *GABRA* 6). These researchers did not find relations to *DRD4, SERT,* and *GABRA,* but they did find an effect regarding the distribution of the *-521 C/T* gene. While a high proportion of the ambivalent infants had two C-alleles, almost all (12 of 13) of the avoidant infants had at least one T-allele. There was no significant effect for the disorganized infants. However, it has to be noted that 17 of 20 disorganized infants also had at least one T-allele.

Following this wave of initial studies, there was a second wave of studies that have adopted a broader approach that includes gene–environment interactions. The questions now asked were whether infants with specific genetic characteristics *were more susceptible to environmental influences* than those with other characteristics and whether the influence of genetic characteristics was moderated by the infant's experiences with the caregiver. In a study by van IJzendoorn and Bakermans-Kranenburg (2006), both infant genetic characteristics and characteristics of the attachment figure known to be related to infant attachment disorganization were included in the analysis as predictors of attachment disorganization. Among the maternal predictors, they included unresolved loss or trauma as a distal risk factor and frightened/frightening behavior as a proximal risk factor. The findings indicated that infants with a 7-repeat polymorphism on the *DRD4* gene were more vulnerable to the environmental risk presented by maternal unresolved loss or trauma, that is, they were more likely to be classified as disorganized, when the mother was also unresolved.

It is noteworthy, however, that a comparable interaction was not found between allelic variation and maternal frightened or frightening behavior. Gervai and colleagues (2007) found evidence for the second type of gene–environment interaction, the moderating role of genetic factors in response to challenging maternal behavior. This study investigated the interplay between *DRD4* gene polymorphism and atypical behavior in a combined low-risk and high-risk sample from Hungary and the United States, respectively. As expected, attachment disorganization was significantly greater in high-risk families and in infants of mothers showing atypical behavior. However, the prediction of attachment disorganization from atypical maternal behavior was moderated by infant *DRD4* genotype. Disorganization was not associated with atypical maternal behavior in infants carrying a 7-repeat *DRD4* allele, but was predictable from maternal behavior in infants who lacked the 7-repeat allele. The authors speculated that functional variations in the *DRD4* gene expressed preferentially in brain regions of the reward circuit might modulate sensitivity to differences in maternal caregiving behavior.

Obviously, the results of these two studies are not unequivocal. Although both studies provide evidence for *DRD4* gene polymorphism moderation of caregiver influences on attachment disorganization, they found different susceptibility in different groups of infants. Infants carrying a 7-repeat allele were *more* sensitive to maternal influences in the van IJzendoorn and Bakermans-Kranenburg (2006) study and *less* sensitive in the Gervai et al. (2007) study.

Molecular-genetic research in the field of attachment has not been restricted to genes underlying the dopamine regulation system. While the study of Frigerio et al. (2009) included a variety of gene markers, a second more frequently used gene polymorphism is the serotonin transporter gene *5HTT-LPR (SERT)*, which was found to be related to emotional reactivity and regulation, specifically with respect to fear and anxiety and impulsiveness and aggressivity (e.g., Carver & Miller, 2006; Caspi et al., 2003; Greenberg et al., 2000; Hariri & Holmes, 2006; Lesch & Bengel, 1996). Regarding attachment disorganization, this polymorphism had already been included in the studies of Lakatos et al. (2000) and Frigerio et al. (2009), but was not found to be associated with quality of attachment in these studies. However, two further studies provided evidence that the *SERT* gene polymorphism is also involved in the development of attachment differences in infancy.

Barry, Kochanska, and Philibert (2008) investigated the predictability of attachment insecurity from low maternal responsiveness depending on the *SERT* polymorphisms. They found that an insecure infant–mother attachment relationship was only predicted by low maternal responsiveness in infants carrying a short version of the *SERT* gene, but not for those with a long allele. They interpreted these findings in terms of a higher genetic vulnerability of infants with a short *5HTT-LPR* allele. Unfortunately, insecurely attached and disorganized infants were combined into one group in this study and the authors did not conduct separate analyses for the disorganized infants. It is obvious from close study of their data, however, that all disorganized infants were carriers of the short allele of the *SERT* gene. In a follow-up assessment of the same sample an interaction between genetic risk and quality of infant–mother attachment was found to predict further development (Kochanska, Philibert, & Barry, 2009). Children with an insecure attachment who were carrying a short *SERT* allele developed poor regulatory capacities during preschool, while there was no effect of attachment security for children carrying two long alleles. The authors interpreted their findings as showing that secure attachment may a protective factor in the presence of risk conferred by a genotype. Again, no separate analyses were done regarding attachment disorganization.

Clear evidence for the role of the *SERT* gene for the development of attachment disorganization has been found in our research using the Regensburg Longitudinal Sample IV (Spangler, Johann, Ronai, & Zimmermann, 2009). First, we found an association between the *SERT* gene and attachment disorganization. Infants carrying a short allele had a higher probability to be classified as disorganized than infants carrying two long alleles. This effect was moderated by differences in maternal behavior. The effect was evident in infants whose mother showed a low responsiveness to the infant's signals, but was not found in infants with highly responsive mothers. We interpreted this finding in terms of the protective function of parental behavior. Perceiving the short allele of the *SERT* gene as a genetic risk for infant attachment disorganization, responsive parental behavior would provide a protection for the child against this risk as it externally contributes to the child's emotional regulation.

In sum, molecular-genetic association studies provide substantial evidence that there is a genetic foundation of attachment disorganization in addition to and in interaction with influences brought about by the behavior of the caregiver. The overall pattern of findings, however, is far from being clear.

DISCUSSION

Attachment theory essentially is a theory about the development of emotional regulation. Depending on the quality of experiences with the caregiver, infants use specific attachment strategies for emotional regulation. While securely attached infants are able to regulate their emotions by seeking proximity to or contact with the caregiver, insecure–avoidant infants, driven by fear of rejection, "down-regulate" their emotional expression and avoid contact with the caregiver. Insecure–ambivalent infants anxiously try to keep close contact and seek proximity, but have an inefficient strategy for regulating their emotions. The typical characteristic of disorganized infants as opposed to each of the other groups is the lack of any coherent strategy. Caught by the conflict between seeking proximity to and fear of the caregiver (Main & Hesse, 1990), they are not able to organize their behavior to make use of the attachment figure to regulate their emotional arousal. Thus, drawing from Bowlby's model of homeostasis, we would particularly expect biological or physiological responses to be indicators of the activation of the inner ring of homeostasis in disorganized infants. The empirical evidence supports this prediction. Disorganized infants show a high sympathetic arousal when the attachment system is activated during separation and disorganized behavior is accompanied by heart rate responses that indicate a defensive evaluation in presence of the mother. Finally, the ineffectiveness of the disorganized behavioral pattern is expressed by the endocrine responses of the HPA system, which is usually activated when behavioral coping is not working.

In sum, the empirical evidence shows that behavioral and biological systems participate in the emotional regulation process of disorganized infants, and that they interact in terms of biobehavioral function. The involvement of biological processes poses the question whether genetic dispositions also contribute to the development of attachment disorganization.

Genes and Attachment Disorganization

Although the molecular-genetic studies clearly demonstrate that there is some genetic foundation of attachment disorganization, the studies provide a somewhat equivocal picture regarding the specific gene marker. While some of the studies show attachment disorganization to be related to dopamine receptor polymorphisms (DRD4) and do not find relations to the serotonin transporter gene (SERT), the reverse pattern is reported in other studies. Different explanations may be offered based on the functional interpretation of the two genes.

According to Diamond (2001), the prefrontal cortex and the dopamine pathways are engaged in attentional, motivational, and reward mechanisms, as well as negative emotionality, social withdrawal, and sensitivity to stressful situations. Polymorphisms of the DRD4 differ in the quality of dopamine-based signal transmission, especially in the prefrontal cortex. The signal transmission is weaker for subjects carrying a 7-repeat polymorphism. In contrast, the SERT gene (5HTT-LPR) is related to emotional reactivity and regulation, specifically with respect to fear and anxiety and impulsiveness and aggressivity (e.g., Carver & Miller, 2006; Caspi et al., 2003; Greenberg et al., 2000; Hariri & Holmes, 2006; Lesch & Bengel, 1996). Polimorphisms of the SERT gene differ in transcription activity of serotonin. Transcription activity is higher in subjects carrying a long polimorphism as compared to those with a short polimorphism. Thus, in general, both genes are related to psychological regulation processes. However, while the SERT gene seems to be particularly involved in processes of emotional reactivity, the DRD4 gene may be more involved in regulation of attention and learning processes.

The association of attachment disorganization with the SERT gene supports the hypothesis that individual dispositions in regulatory capacities contribute to the development of attachment disorganization, as has been indicated by research using behavioral assessment (Spangler et al., 1996). A possible developmental pathway could lead from individual difficulties in emotional and behavioral regulation already detectable in the newborn period to later attachment disorganization in a stressful situation such as the Strange Situation by the end of the first year. The poor orientation and high negative emotionality of the newborns in the Spangler et al. (1996) study who were later classified as disorganized and also found in studies of infants carrying two short 5-HTTLPR alleles (Auerbach et al., 1999; Ebstein et al., 1998) are consistent with this perspective. Regarding the DRD4 genes (the 7-repeat allele of the dopamine receptor D4 and the -521 C/T gene), the findings of the Gervai et al. study (2005) highlight the developmental changes in dopamine levels and the density of dopamine receptors in the prefrontal cortex in the second half of the first year of life, when the first attachment relationships emerge. They proposed that the DRD4 genotype influences learning processes during this period; depending on the polymorphism, infants may differ in the perception of and the responses to stressful situations and the behavior of the caregiver. Thus, both the *DRD4* and the *SERT* genes may be involved in the development of individual differences regarding attachment disorganization. As a consequence, discrepancies in the findings of different studies may not be contradictory; rather they may be regarded as complementary.

An alternative explanation for the different genetic associations regarding attachment disorganization might be that the associations depend on specific characteristics of the samples in these studies; that is, the findings could be sample-specific. The classification of attachment disorganization is based on a great variety of behaviors. For example, some infants are classified as disorganized mainly due to their emotional responses (e.g., fear or apprehension), while others are classified due to their contradictory attempts to organize or regulate their behavior. These processes may be controlled by different regulation systems and thus may be associated with different gene markers. A detailed comparison of the disorganized infants of the different samples would be necessary to clarify this assumption.

Social and Individual Determinants of Attachment Disorganization

Based on findings about prediction of attachment disorganization by newborn behavioral organization, Spangler et al. (1996) addressed the possibility of conceiving of attachment disorganization as an individual construct (see also Spangler & Grossmann, 1999). While there was not much attention to these findings and conclusions for a long time, the recent genetic findings providing repeated evidence regarding associations between genetic characteristics and attachment disorganization provide clear evidence for the notion that individual dispositions are likely to contribute to individual differences in disorganization. Infant disorganization has been linked to maternal characteristics in several ways including unresolved traumatic attachment experiences of the mother (Ainsworth & Eichberg, 1991), maternal postnatal depression (Murray, 1992), maternal frightening behavior (Schuengel et al., 1999), hostile and neglectful behavior of mothers in high-risk samples (Carlson, Cicchetti, Barnett, & Braunwald, 1989; Lyons-Ruth et al., 1991), and cultural conditions of communally approved nocturnal separation of infants from their parents (Sagi, van IJzendoorn, Aviezer, Donnell, & Mayseless, 1994). Social influences on attachment disorganization are not in opposition to the proposed pathway related to individual disposition (see Spangler & Grossmann, 1999). Regarding genetic and social influences on attachment disorganization as independent factors, there may be different pathways to the development of attachment disorganization. Disorganization may be biased toward individual origin in some cases and biased toward social origin in other cases. Thus, some infants may be disorganized in their attachment strategy because they have general restrictions in their ability to regulate and organize their behavior. This may be brought about by inappropriate prenatal experiences due to chronic stress or may be due to genetic dispositions. For example, Schneider and Coe (1993) suggested that stress during pregnancy may lead to restricted behavioral and physiological organization in the newborn. Thus, infants later categorized as disorganized might be exposed to more chronic prenatal stress; their mothers, eventually due to their own traumatic attachment experiences, may experience their pregnancy and pending new attachment relationship as more stressful than mothers with gratifying childhood attachment histories. In these cases, we would expect indications of disorganization not only in the domain of attachment but also in other behavioral domains. Consequently, disorganization would be conceived as an individual construct. Alternatively, other infants may develop attachment disorganization because they are confronted with inappropriate behavior of the caregiver. This may be frightening or frightened behavior according to Main and Hesse (1990), atypical intrusive interactive behavior according to Lyons-Ruth et al. (1999), or maternal helplessness and role reversal according to George and Solomon (2008; Chapter 6, this volume). In these cases, we would expect that disorganization should only be observed in the domain of attachment behavior, or more specifically, in attachment behavior directed to a specific caregiver. This does not preclude behavioral consequences in other domains which may emerge later as a consequence of dysfunctional caregiving behavior.

Determinants of Attachment Disorganization: Heredity, Environment, and the Question of Mechanisms

In her seminal 1958 article, Anna Anastasi pleaded for overcoming asking questions whether, at that time, intelligence is of hereditary *or* environmental origin. Instead she argued for the need to investigate the *processes of how* genes and environment work together to foster development. Attachment researchers for a long time excluded hereditary processes or individual dispositions as potential sources of individual differences. Probably, thinking in terms of "genes *or* environment," they were afraid of challenging the concept of attachment as a dyadic construct by acknowledging individual contributions to attachment differences. Now, half a century after Anastasi's plea, the findings of the recent molecular-genetic studies regarding attachment disorganization provide a platform for discussing the interplay of genetic and environmental processes even in the field of attachment development. Thus, in addition to the different "separate" developmental paths to attachment disorganization described above, developmental paths can be described that include both genetic dispositions and individual experiences with the caregiver interacting with each other.

Taken together the gene–environment effects indicate that some of the gene variants contribute to the development of attachment disorganization, but not as determinants, rather as risk factors the influence of which only becomes obvious when there are restrictions in the quality of the (maternal) caregiving environment. Thus, the short version of the serotonin transporter seems to be a genetic risk for the development of attachment disorganization, but this is only the case when the infants' mothers behave in an unresponsive manner toward the child (Spangler et al., 2009; see also Barry et al., 2008). High maternal responsiveness seems to work as a protective factor, as the genetic effect seems not to be expressed in infants of highly responsive mothers. From this perspective, supportive caregiving can be regarded as a social buffer against genetic risk.

But one can also take a different perspective. Low parental responsiveness may be a social risk factor for attachment disorganization, yet the presence of two long alleles of the serotonin gene may be interpreted as a protective factor, at least when exposed to low responsive mothers. Such a protective effect associated with two long 5-HTTLPR alleles has also been reported by Caspi and colleagues (2003) with respect to the influence of stressful life events on the development of depression. Additionally, in a comparative study, Barr and colleagues (2003) found that the behavioral and emotional regulation was restricted compared to mother-reared primates in peer-reared rhesus macaques carrying the short serotonin transporter allele. A similar type of gene–environment interactions was reported by Gervai et al. (2007) regarding the DRD4 gene polymorphism. They found that maternal disruptive behavior predicted infant attachment disorganization, but only for those infants without a DRD4 7-repeat allele. Thus, the DRD4 7-repeat polymorphism turned out to be a protective factor. As noted earlier, however, gene–environment interactions regarding the DRD4 gene are not unequivocal. Van IJzendoorn and Bakermans-Kranenburg (2006), using a similar design, found that the 7-repeat gene heightened the risk of disorganization in infants.

An important difference between these two studies concerns the measures used. In the Gervai et al. (2007) study, maternal behavior was used as a proximal measure. In the van IJzendoorn and Bakermans-Kranenburg (2006) study, a distal variable (maternal unresolved loss or trauma) was responsible for the positive associations between gene markers and disorganized attachment. Further studies should focus on the three-way interaction between genetic markers, unresolved trauma or loss, and atypical behavior. Specifically, it would be interesting to see the gene-specific transmission in infants of mothers with high or low values. In a very recent study on genetic associations with attachment representation (Reiner & Spangler, 2010), adult ratings of parents as unloving in the Adult Attachment Interview were positively related to an insecure adult attachment *representation* only in subjects without a 7-repeat *DRD4* polymorphism. Comparable to the Gervai et al. (2007) study, the 7-repeat allele seems to be a protective factor regarding the development of a secure attachment representation.

Belsky, Bakermans-Kranenburg, and van IJzendoorn (2007) discussed different explanation models regarding gene–environment interaction effects on development. According to the dual-risk model, a negative developmental outcome would be expected in the case of co-occurrence of child and parent risk, while normal development would be expected otherwise. According to the differential susceptibility model, a child characteristic would predict a negative outcome in the case of negative parenting behavior, and a positive outcome in the case of positive parenting behavior, and thus would indicate a higher sensitivity to both positive and negative environmental influences rather than a risk. Related to attachment disorganization, the question is whether infants with a certain gene variant have a higher risk for attachment disorganization, or whether they are more sensitive to social influences and get more often disorganized in the case of problematic maternal behavior, but less often in the case of sensitive and supporting maternal behavior. Although known phenotypical behavior associated with specific gene variants could indicate a risk status (e.g., association of the short allele or the *SERT* with fear and anxiety; e.g., Lesch et al., 1996), we cannot exclude the possibility that such associations are based on broader characteristic like sensitivity, which may provide positive learning experiences to the child, and thus is indicating susceptibility rather than risk.

Most of the studies reporting gene–environment interactions for attachment disorganization explicitly or implicitly interpreted their findings in terms of a genetic vulnerability. This interpretation may have been facilitated as the genes identified as risky genes had been identified as risky genes already in other studies. The studies of Gervai et al. (2007) and of van IJzendorrn and Bakermans-Kranenburg (2006), however, demonstrate that a clear classification of a gene variant as risky or protective is not always possible (see also Reiner & Spangler, 2010). Also, although van IJzendoorn and Bakermans-Kranenburg (2006) initially interpreted their findings in terms of genetic vulnerability, they argued for an alternative interpretation based on the same data 1 year later, now in terms of a differential susceptibility (Bakermans-Kranenburg & van IJzendoorn, 2007).

FINAL REMARKS

Taken together, the studies reporting gene–environment interactions contribute to an integration of different theoretical assumptions and empirical findings regarding the determinants of attachment disorganization. According to Anastasi (1958), it is obvious that we should not ask the questions whether attachment disorganization is caused either by inappropriate parenting or by individual dispositions. Rather, these studies show that both dimensions are involved in the development of attachment disorganization and that identifying an individual or genetic predictor does not mean that social experiences are not important for attachment development. These statistical interactions may mirror interaction processes between the infant and the mother on the behavioral level underlying the development of attachment disorganization. Of course, such interactions are influenced by maternal behavioral characteristics as well as by individual dispositions of the infant.

The focus of this chapter was on the psychobiology of attachment disorganization in infancy. Molecular-genetic research in the field of attachment is not restricted to this area. Recent research themes focus, for example, on the genetic associations of attachment research in adults (e.g., Caspers et al., 2009; Reiner & Spangler, 2010) or on the role of a secure attachment relationship as a protective factor in the development of emotional regulation in children with genetic risks (Zimmermann, Mohr, & Spangler, 2009). I am sure that the inclusion of genetic information into the study of the development and sequelae of individual differences in attachment patterns will contribute essentially to our knowledge in the field of attachment research.

ACKNOWLEDGMENTS

My research projects underlying this chapter were supported in part by the German Research Foundation and by the Köhlerstiftung (Munich). I am very indebted to Klaus and Karin Grossmann for their supportive encouragement to adopt a psychobiological approach in the study of attachment; to Judit Gervai, Kriszta Lakatos and Ildiko Toth, who led me the way to and guided me on the genetic path; and to Peter Zimmermann, my colleague and friend, who would accompany many of my research ideas and projects as a stimulating discussant and/or supportive collaborator. Last, but not least, I want to thank my coworkers and students for their tremendous input of ideas, knowledge, motivation, and workload for translating our plans and ideas into action.

REFERENCES

Ainsworth, M. D. S. (1973). The development of infant–mother attachment. In B. M. Caldwell & H. N. Riciutti (Eds.), *Review of child development research* (Vol. 3, pp. 31–96). Chicago: University of Chicago Press.

Ainsworth, M. D. S., Blehar, M. C., Waters, E., & Wall, S. (1978). *Patterns of attachment: A psychological study of the Strange Situation.* Hillsdale, NJ: Erlbaum.

Ainsworth, M. D. S., & Eichberg, C. G. (1991). Effects on infant–mother attachment of mother's unresolved loss of an attachment figure, or other traumatic experience. In C. M. Parkes, J. Stevenson-Hinde, & P. Marris (Eds.), *Attachment across the life cycle* (pp. 160–183). New York: Routledge.

Anastasi, A. (1958). Heredity, environment and the question "how. " *Psychological Review, 65,* 197–208.

Auerbach, J., Geller, V., Lezer, S., Shinwell, E., Belmaker, R. H., Levine, J., et al. (1999). Dopamine D4 receptor (D4DR) and serotonin transporter promoter (5–HTTLPR) polymorphisms in the determination of temperament in 2–month-old infants. *Molecular Psychiatry, 4,* 369–373.

Bakermans-Kranenburg, M. J., & van IJzendoorn, M. H. (2004). No association of the dopamine D4 receptor (DRD4) and -521 C/T promoter polymorphisms with infant attachment disorganization. *Attachment and Human Development, 6,* 211–218.

Bakermans-Kranenburg, M. J., & van IJzendoorn, M. H. (2007). Genetic vulnerability or differential susceptibility in child development: The case of attachment. *Journal of Child Psychology and Psychiatry, 48,* 1160–1173.

Bakermans-Kranenburg, M. J., van IJzendoorn, M. H., & Juffer, F. (2005). Disorganized infant attachment and preventive interventions: A review and meta-analysis. *Infant Mental Health Journal, 26,* 191–216.

Barnett, D., Ganiban, J., & Cicchetti, D. (1999). Atypical attachment in infancy and early childhood among children at developmental risk: V. Maltreatment, negative expressivity, and the development of type D attachments from 12 to 24 months of age. *Monographs of the Society of Research in Child Development, 64,* 97–118.

Barr, C. S., Newman, T. K., Becker, M. L., Parker, C. C., Champoux, M., Lesch, K. P., et al. (2003). The utility of the non-human primate model for studying gene by environment interactions in behavioral research. *Genes, Brain and Behavior, 2,* 336–340.

Barry, R. A., Kochanska, G., & Philibert, R. A. (2008). G · E interaction in the organization of attachment: Mothers' responsiveness as a moderator of children's genotypes. *Journal of Child Psychology and Psychiatry, 49,* 1313–1320.

Belsky, J., Bakermans-Kranenburg, M. J., & van IJzendoorn, M. H. (2007). For better and for worse: Differential susceptibility to environmental influences. *Current Directions in Psychological Science, 16,* 300–304.

Bokhorst, C. L., Bakermans-Kranenburg, M. J., Fearon, R. M. P., van IJzendoorn, M. H., Fonagy, P., & Schuengel, C. (2003). The importance of shared environment in mother–infant attachment security: A behavioral genetic study. *Child Development, 74,* 1769–1782.

Bowlby, J. (1973). *Attachment and loss, Vol. 2: Separation: Anxiety and anger.* New York: Basic Books.

Bowlby, J. (1982). *Attachment and loss, Vol. 1: Attachment.* New York: Basic Books. (Original work published 1969)

Capps, L., Sigman, M., & Mundy, P. (1994). Attachment security in children with autism. *Development and Psychopathology, 6,* 249–261.

Carlson, V., Cicchetti, D., Barnett, D., & Braunwald, K. (1989). Disorganized/disoriented attachment relationships in maltreated infants. *Developmental Psychology, 25,* 525–531.

Carver, C. S., & Miller, C. J. (2006). Relations of serotonin function to personality: Current views and a key methodological issue. *Psychiatry Research, 144,* 1–15.

Caspers, K. M., Paradiso, S., Yucuis, R., Troutman, B., Arndt, S., & Philibert, R. (2009). Association between the serotonin transporter promoter polymorphism (5-HTTLPR) and adult unresolved attachment. *Developmental Psychology, 45,* 64–76.

Caspi, A., Sugden, K., Moffitt, T. E., Taylor, A., Craig, I. W., Harrington, H. et al. (2003). Influence of life stress on depression: Moderation by a polymorphism in the 5-HTT gene. *Science, 301,* 386–389.

Diamond, A. (2001). A model system for studying the role of dopamine in the prefrontal cortex during early development in humans: Early and continuously treated phenylketonuria. In C. A. Nelson & M. Luciana (Eds.), *Handbook of developmental cognitive neuroscience* (pp. 433–472). Cambridge, MA: MIT Press.

Ebstein, R. P., Levine, J., Geller, V., Auerbach, J., Gritsenko, I., & Belmaker, R. H. (1998). Dopamine D4 receptor and serotonin transporter promoter in the determination of neonatal temperament. *Molecular Psychiatry, 3,* 238–246.

Finkel, D., & Matheny, A. P. Jr. (2000). Genetic and environmental influences on a measure of infant attachment security. *Twin Research, 3,* 242–250.

Fish, M. (2001). Attachment in low-SES rural Appalachian infants: Contextual, infant, and maternal interaction risk and protective factors. *Infant Mental Health Journal, 22,* 641–664.

Forbes, L. M., Evans, E. M., Moran, G., & Pederson, D. R. (2007). Change in atypical maternal behavior predicts change in attachment disorganization from 12 to 24 months in a high-risk sample. *Child Development, 78,* 955–971.

Fowles, D. C. (1980). The three arousal model: Implications of Gray's two-factor learning theory for heart rate, electrodermal activity, and psychopathy. *Psychophysiology, 17,* 87–103.

Frigerio, A., Ceppi, E., Rusconi, M., Giorda, R., Raggi, M. E., & Fearon, P. (2009). The role played by the interaction between genetic factors and attachment in the stress response in infancy. *Journal of Child Psychology and Psychiatry, 50,* 1513–1522.

George, C., & Solomon, J. (1996). Representational models of relationships: Links between caregiving and attachment. *Infant Mental Health Journal, 17,* 198–216.

George, C., & Solomon, J. (2008). The caregiving system: A behavioral systems approach to parenting. In J. Cassidy & P. R. Shaver (Eds.), *Handbook of attachment: Theory, research, and clinical applications* (2nd ed., pp. 833–856). New York: Guilford Press.

Gervai, J., Nemoda, Z., Lakatos, K., Ronai, Z., Toth, I., Ney, K., et al. (2005). Transmission disequilibrium tests confirm the link between DRD4 gene polymorphism and infant attachment. *American Journal of Medical Genetics, Part B (Neuropsychiatric Genetics), 132B,* 126–130.

Gervai, J., Novak, A., Lakatos, K., Toth, I., Danis, I., Ronai, Z., et al. (2007). Infant genotype may moderate sensitivity to maternal affective communications:

Attachment disorganization, quality of care, and the DRD4 polymorphism. *Social Neuroscience, 2,* 307–319.

Goldberg, S., Benoit, D., Blokland, K., & Madigan, S. (2003). Atypical maternal behavior, maternal representations and infant disorganized attachment. *Development and Psychopathology, 15,* 239–257.

Graham, F. K., & Clifton, R. K. (1966). Heart-rate change as a component of the orienting response. *Psychological Bulletin, 65,* 305–320.

Greenberg, B. D., Li, Q., Lucas, F. R., Hu, S., Sirota, L. A., Benjamin, J., et al. (2000). Association between the serotonin transporter promoter polymorphism and personality traits in a primarily female population sample. *American Journal of Medical Genetics, 96,* 202–216.

Hariri, A. R., & Holmes, A. (2006). Genetics of emotional regulation: The role of the serotonin transporter in neural function. *Trends in Cognitive Science, 10,* 182–191.

Hertsgaard, L., Gunnar, M., Erickson, M. F., & Nachmias, M. (1995). Adrenocortical responses to the Strange Situation in infants with disorganized/disoriented attachment relationships. *Child Development, 66,* 1100–1106.

Hesse, E., & Main, M. (2006). Frightened, threatening, and dissociative parental behavior in low-risk-samples: Description, discussion, and interpretations. *Development and Psychopathology, 18,* 309–343.

Kochanska, G., Philibert, R. A., & Barry, R. A. (2009). Interplay of genes and early mother–child relationship in the development of self-regulation from toddler to preschool age. *Journal of Child Psychology and Psychiatry, 50,* 1331–1338.

Lakatos, K., Nemoda, Z., Toth, I., Ronai, Z., Ney, K., Sasvari-Szekely, M., et al. (2002). Further evidence for the role of the dopamine D4 receptor gene (DRD4) in attachment disorganization: Interaction of the III exon 48 bp repeat and the -521 C/T promoter polymorphisms. *Molecular Psychiatry, 7,* 27–31.

Lakatos, K., Toth, I., Nemoda, Z., Ney, K., Sasvari-Szekely, M., & Gervai, J. (2000). Dopamine D4 receptor (DRD4) gene polymorphism is associated with attachment disorganization in infants. *Molecular Psychiatry, 5,* 633–637.

Lesch, K. -P., & Bengel, D. (1996). Association of anxiety-related traits with a polymorphism in the serotonin transporter gene regulatory region. *Science, 274,* 1527–1531.

Levine, S., Wiener, S. G., Coe, C. L., Bayart, F. E. S., & Hayashi, K. T. (1987). Primate vocalization: A psychobiological approach. *Child Development, 58,* 1408–1419.

Lundberg, U., & Frankenhaeuser, M. (1980). Pituitary–adrenal and sympathetic–adrenal correlates of distress and effort. *Journal of Psychosomatic Research, 24,* 125–130.

Lyons-Ruth, K., Bronfman, E., & Parsons, E. (1999). Maternal frightened, frightening, or atypical behavior and disorganized infant attachment patterns: Atypical attachment in infancy and early childhood among children at developmental risk. *Monographs of the Society for Research in Child Development, 64,* 67–96.

Lyons-Ruth, K., & Jacobvitz, D. (1999). Attachment disorganization: Unresolved loss, relational violence, and lapses in behavioral and attentional strategies. In J. Cassidy & P. R. Shaver (Eds.), *Handbook of attachment: Theory, research, and clinical applications* (pp. 520–554). New York: Guilford Press.

Lyons-Ruth, K., Repacholi, B., McLeod, S., & Silva, E. (1991). Disorganized attachment behavior in infancy: Short-term stability, maternal and infant correlates, and risk-related subtypes. *Development and Psychopathology, 3,* 377–396.

Madigan, S., Moran, G., & Pederson, D. R. (2006). Unresolved states of mind, disorganized attachment relationships, and disrupted mother–infant interactions of adolescent mothers and their infants. *Developmental Psychology, 42,* 293–304.

Main, M., & Cassidy, J. (1988). Categories of response to reunion with the parent at age 6: Predictable from infant attachment classifications and stable over a 1–month period. *Developmental Psychology, 24,* 1–12.

Main, M., & Hesse, E. (1990). Parents' unresolved traumatic experiences are related to infant disorganized attachment status: Is frightened and/or frightening parental behavior the linking mechanism? In M. T. Greenberg, D. Cicchetti, & E. M. Cummings (Eds.), *Attachment in the preschool years* (pp. 161–184). Chicago: University of Chicago Press.

Main, M., & Solomon, J. (1986). Discovery of an insecure disorganized/disoriented attachment pattern: Procedures, findings and implications for the classification of behavior. In T. B. Brazelton & M. Yogman (Eds.), *Affective development in infancy* (pp. 95–124). Norwood, NJ: Ablex.

Main, M., & Solomon, J. (1990). Procedures for identifying infants as disorganized/disoriented during the Ainsworth Strange Situation. In M. T. Greenberg, D. Cicchetti, & E. M. Cummings (Eds.), *Attachment in the preschool years* (pp. 121–160). Chicago: University of Chicago Press.

Murray, L. (1992). The impact of postnatal depression on infant development. *Journal of Child Psychology and Psychiatry, 33,* 543–561.

O'Connor, T. G., & Croft, C. M. (2001). A twin study of attachment in preschool children. *Child Development, 72,* 1501–1511.

Pipp-Siegel, S., Siegel, C. H., & Dean, J. (1999). Neurological aspects of the disorganized/disoriented attachment classification system: Differentiating quality of the attachment relationship from neurological impairment. In J. I. Vondra & D. Barnett (Eds.), *Atypical attachment in infancy and early childhood among children at developmental risk. Monographs of the Society for Research in Child Development, 64,* 25–44.

Reiner, I., & Spangler, G. (2010). Adult attachment and gene polymorphisms of the dopamine D4 receptor and serotonin transporter (5-HTT). *Attachment and Human Development, 12,* 209–229.

Sagi, A., van IJzendoorn, M. H., Aviezer, O., Donnell, F., & Mayseless, O. (1994). Sleeping out of home in a kibbutz communal arrangement: It makes a difference for infant–mother attachment. *Child Development, 65,* 902–1004.

Schneider, M. L., & Coe, C. L. (1993). Repeated social stress during pregnancy impairs neuromotor development on the primate infant. *Developmental and Behavioral Pediatrics, 14,* 81–87.

Schuengel, C., Bakermans-Kranenburg, M. J., & van IJzendoorn, M. (1999). Frightening maternal behavior linking unresolved loss and disorganized infant attachment. *Journal of Consulting and Clinical Psychology, 67,* 54–63.

Selye, H. (1952). *The story of the adaptation syndrome.* Montreal: Acta.

Spangler, G., Fremmer-Bombik, E., & Grossmann, K. (1996). Social and individual determinants of attachment security and disorganization during the first year. *Infant Mental Health Journal, 17,* 127–139.

Spangler, G., & Grossmann, K. E. (1993). Biobehavioral organization in securely and insecurely attached infants. *Child Development, 64,* 1439–1450.

Spangler, G., & Grossmann, K. (1999). Individual and physiological correlates of attachment disorganization in infancy. In J. Solomon & C. George (Eds.), *Attachment disorganization* (pp. 95–124). New York: Guilford Press.

Spangler, G., Johann, M., Ronai, Z., & Zimmermann, P. (2009). Genetic and environmental influence on attachment disorganization. *Journal of Child Psychology and Psychiatry, 50,* 952–961.

Spangler, G., & Schieche, M. (1998). Emotional and adrenocortical responses of infants to the Strange Situation: The differential function of emotional expression. *International Journal of Behavioral Development, 22,* 681–706.

Sroufe, L. A. (1979). The coherence of individual development: Early care, attachment, and subsequent developmental issues. *American Psychologist, 34,* 834–841.

Starr, R. H. (1988). Pre- and perinatal risk and physical abuse. *Journal of Reproductive and Infant Psychology, 6,* 125–138.

Ursin, H., Baade, E., & Levine, S. (1978). *Psychobiology of stress: A study of coping men.* New York: Academic Press.

van IJzendoorn, M. H., & Bakermans-Kranenburg, M. J. (2006). DRD4 7–repeat polymorphism moderates the association between maternal unresolved loss or trauma and infant disorganization. *Attachment and Human Development, 8,* 291–307.

van IJzendoorn, M. H., Schuengel, C., & Bakermans-Kranenburg, M. J. (1999). Disorganized attachment in early childhood: Metaanalysis of precursors, concomitants, and sequelae. *Development and Psychopathology, 11,* 225–249.

Vaughn, B. E., Bost, K. K., & van IJzendoorn, M. E. (2008). Attachment and temperament: Additive and interactive influences on behavior, affect, and cognition during infancy and childhood. In J. Cassidy & P. R. Shaver (Eds.), *Handbook of attachment: Theory, research, and clinical applications* (2nd ed., pp. 192–216). New York: Guilford Press.

von Holst, D. (1986). Vegetative and somatic components of tree shrews' behavior. *Journal of the Autonomic Nervous System,* Suppl., 657–670.

Zimmermann, P., Mohr, C., & Spangler, G. (2009). Gene–attachment interaction in adolescents' regulation of autonomy with their mothers. *Journal of Child Psychology and Child Psychiatry, 50,* 1339–1347.

PART II
NEW DIRECTIONS

Chapter 6

Caregiving Helplessness

The Development of a Screening Measure for Disorganized Maternal Caregiving

CAROL GEORGE and JUDITH SOLOMON

One of the main goals of our work over the past 20 years has been to define the caregiving system, in accordance with Bowlby's (1982) view that the behavior of the child's attachment figure is guided by a caregiving behavioral system reciprocal to and separate from attachment (George & Solomon, 1989, 1996, 2008; Solomon & George, 1996, 2000). This chapter presents in writing for the first time information about the development, validation, and use of the Caregiving Helplessness Questionnaire (CHQ), a screening tool that is intended to assist researchers and clinicians who are interested in studying parent–child relationships from an attachment perspective. By way of important background to the development of this tool, we begin this chapter with a summary of our work and that of others on the construct and measurement of caregiving helplessness and its relation to disorganized child attachment.

THE CAREGIVING SYSTEM

The caregiving system is a biologically based motivational system that guides a parent's protective responses to his or her child and influences parental sensitivity and responsiveness to the child's attachment signals (Bowlby,

1982; Solomon & George, 1996). We have emphasized that the organization of the caregiving system requires the caregiver to make a fundamental shift away from being the one who *seeks* protection and care in order to become the person who *provides* protection and care for a child. Caregiving is a complex balancing act. The parent must be vigilant in detecting real and potential sources of danger and threat so as to respond to the child's needs and situational demands. This must be balanced against competing demands of other adult motivational systems, including peer relationships and friendships (affiliative system), sexual relationships (sexual system), work (exploratory system), and, importantly, the parent's own needs for comfort and care (attachment system). The complexities of caregiving are compounded by ecological, cultural, individual, and developmental constraints, including a parent's and a child's place on the lifespan continuum (i.e., infant, child, adolescent, adult).

The attachment system is generally understood to be guided by a cognitive control system, termed the "internal working model" (Bowlby, 1982; Bretherton & Munholland, 2008; Hinde, 1982). We have stressed the importance of an analogous but distinct internal working model for the caregiving system, conceived in terms of representational processes that evaluate, appraise, and organize parental behavior, expectations, and affects (George & Solomon, 1989, 2008). This *internal working model of caregiving* reflects the intersection of several sets of influential relationship experiences, including current and past experiences with a child and a parent's own experiences with childhood attachment figures (Slade & Cohen, 1996; Solomon & George, Chapter 2, this volume).

Interest in the link between parenting representation and child attachment has burgeoned since its emergence in the 1980s. Today, attachment researchers and clinicians use a range of approaches to examine a broad set of parenting dimensions. These include assessing the parent's affective responses to the child (Slade, Belsky, Aber, & Phelps, 1999; Slade, Grienenberger, Bernbach, Levy, & Locker, 2005); the parent's perception or "working model" of the child's personality (Zeanah & Anders, 1987; Zeanah, Benoit, Hirschberg, & Barton, 1993, 1994) or developmental status (Marvin & Pianta, 1999; Barnett & Ganiban, 1999; Barnett et al., Chapter 9, this volume); and the parents's capacity for insightful self-reflection (Slade et al., 2005). These studies, as well as our own, have demonstrated links between maternal representations and sensitivity to the child and indicate that representational sensitivity may be an important mechanism in the transmission of attachment patterns across generations (Atkinson et al., 2005; Solomon & George, 1996)

Our work is unique in that we incorporate Bowlby's ethologically based attachment systems perspective in our approach to the development and organization of caregiving. In addition, we conceive of representations of the caregiving system as resulting from the action of a set of defensive processes that filter experiences and regulate emotions related to caregiving strategies (Bowlby, 1980; George & Solomon, 1989, 2008; Solomon & George, 1996, 2000). These defensive processes have systematic parallels in attachment behavior and representation, resulting in the coadaptation of parent and child, or in Bowlby's terms, the "goal-corrected" partnership.

DISORGANIZED CAREGIVING

In order to define disorganized caregiving, we must return to our fundamental view of the development of the caregiving system as the transformation from the need to seek protection of the self (i.e., the goal of attachment) to that of providing care and protection for one's child. This transformation appears to be disrupted for mothers of disorganized children. These mothers "seem to have abdicated *psychologically* the caregiving role or [are] struggling without success to maintain control and provide protection" (George & Solomon, 2008, p. 192). Caregiving is therefore incoherent and inverted—literally, disorganized—and undermines the mother's ability to carry out the protective function of the attachment–caregiving relationship (Solomon & George, 1996; Chapter 2, this volume). We have described the caregiving system of mothers of disorganized children as disabled and the associated overarching quality of care as *failed protection* (Solomon & George, 1996).

With respect to the defensive processes underlying caregiving representation, we understand disorganized caregiving in terms of the rigid exclusionary defenses Bowlby (1980) termed *segregated systems*. For Bowlby, segregated systems entail exclusionary processes that work to isolate painful attachment-related experience and emotion from consciousness along with "the specific patterns of behavior that go to make up attachment behavior together with the desires, thoughts, working models and personal memories integral to them" (p. 348). As such, segregated systems maintain a separate representational self that is rigidly barred from consciousness and thereby blocks the thoughtful integration processes that are required to maintain organized, integrated attachment behavior and self-representation. Bowlby (1980) emphasized that this unintegrated self is not protected from experiential or affective triggers that may unleash behavioral or representational disintegration and disorganization. Contemporary cognitive and neurological models have provided new support for Bowlby's midcentury concept, derived from information-processing theory (Buchheim et al., 2006, 2008; Hesse & Main, 2006), albeit with somewhat different views of mechanisms (Liotti, 2004; Chapter 14, this volume; Lyons-Ruth, Yellin, Melnick, & Atwood, 2005; Spiegel, 1990).

The foundation of caregiving disorganization is segregated attach-ment-related fear (George & West, 2001, in press; George, West, & Pettem, 1999; Solomon, George, & De Jong, 1995). One of the central questions in understanding disorganization, then, is to understand the source of fear. This has been approached predominantly from an intergenerational per-spective, by examining how frightening experiences from a mother's child-hood influence how she views and responds to her child. There are sev-eral overlapping approaches, all of which are consistent with the model of failed integration processes that Bowlby suggested were the hallmark of segregated systems.

Main and Hesse view the foundation of disorganization as related to a mother's unresolved mourning of loss or abuse (Hesse & Main, 2006; Main & Hesse, 1990), following Bowlby's (1980) association between mourning and psychiatric "dissociative" symptoms (e.g., fugue states, memory lapses). This approach stresses that the primary mechanism that disorganizes a child's attachment is the absorbed and dissociated representations associ-ated with "unresolved" states of mind. Research supporting this mechanism is mixed, and studies suggest that psychological absorption and dissociation is associated with attachment disorganization for some, but not necessarily all, children (e.g., Madigan, Moran, & Pederson, 2006; McMahon, Barnett, Kowalenko, & Tennant, 2006; Solomon & George, 2006; for overview, see Lyons-Ruth & Jacobvitz, 2008; Solomon & George, Chapter 2, this volume).

Lyons-Ruth and colleagues view the foundation of disorganization as related to unintegrated representations of maltreatment and characterized by hostile or helpless states of mind regarding past experience. A mother who is hostile or helpless with respect to attachment figures is unable to integrate positive and "malevolent" representation of attachment figures and, sometimes also, identifies with the aggressive attachment figures; these representational states markedly disrupt parent–child interaction (Lyons-Ruth & Jacobvitz, 2008; Madigan et al., 2006).

Solomon and George (Solomon & George, 2006; Chapter 2, this vol-ume) have extended the class of attachment experiences leading to disor-ganized caregiving behavior and representation to include a wide variety of events from which it is difficult for a child to find adequate protection. These would include, for example, strong or unpredictable parental rage or out-of-control behavior such as that observed when parents are alcoholics with some psychiatric diagnoses. They have found that a mother who *has not been protected from* these experiences appears to carry forward seg-regated fears that contribute to a literal disorganization of her caregiving behavior and failure to protect her own child.

Disorganized caregiving likely develops in the context of a complex synthesis of past and current experience. For example, we have described elsewhere the contribution of current disorganizing or frightening experiences, which we conceive as "assaults to the caregiving system" (Solomon & George, 2000). These potentially include experiences such as miscarriage and death of a baby, premature birth, a child's accidental injury, child disability, parent divorce, and experiences of violence (Almqvist & Broberg, 2003). In sum, theory and research addressing past and present experience support the view that fear is at the center of disorganized caregiving. Defensively segregated fear threatens to dysregulate caregiving. Once triggered, a mother is at risk of becoming helpless and frightened and may lash out, retreat, or seek comfort and protection from her child (i.e., role-reversed).

Representations of Caregiving

Mothers' mental representations of caregiving as assessed using our Caregiving Interview are characterized by two different manifestations of segregated systems processing: dysregulation and constriction (George & Solomon, 1996, 2008). Both of these forms reflect a failure to integrate attachment with caregiving at the representational level and both forms are associated with evaluations of self-as-caregiver that we view as parental abdication of care. Dysregulation is identified during the interview when a mother's descriptions of caregiving show that she has become flooded by anger or fear and overwhelmed by feelings of vulnerability, inadequacy, and feeling out of control. We have found too that a "dysregulated" mother often portrays her child as an adversary—a "devil" child whose wild, evil, or malicious behavior is uncontrollable. Care for this child can be so difficult that the mother figuratively and often literally throws up her hands in helpless abdication or becomes confrontational herself. Similar portraits are presented by other researchers studying parental representations associated with disorganization. In two studies, mothers of disorganized children were evaluated as being highly emotional and they described their children as critical and hostile (Green, Stanley, & Peters, 2007; Jacobsen, Hibbs, & Ziegenhain, 2000).

Constriction is evidenced by the mother abruptly stopping an interview response or not engaging in the topic presented by the interviewer. A mother appears or reports herself suddenly to "go blank." We interpret constriction as a mechanism associated with segregated systems processing. Instead of becoming dysregulated, constriction serves as an effective defensive blockade against memories and affects that would otherwise be too painful or threatening to describe. These may sometimes be dissociative moments, similar to those observed by Hesse and Main (2006), but are not necessarily so. We have found that a "constricted" mother often portrays her child as an "angel," a precocious and perfect child that is so developmentally capable that the child is viewed as not really needing the mother's care. A constricted mother may also sometimes portray the child as a physical or psychological extension of the self (e.g., as part of the mother's body). In these dyads, representations of caregiving present mother and child as merged in perfect union. The angel child's capacity to be sensitive to and care for self and others is evaluated by the mother as a glorious quality in this child, which also releases this mother from parenting responsibilities. The mother can abdicate the "stronger and wiser" role because her child is safe and protected; she is released from the responsibility of situations and feelings that would otherwise render her helpless and severely inadequate as a parent.[1]

To summarize, helplessness can appear in dysregulated or constricted forms and, in either form, the reciprocal goals of the caregiving and attachment systems are out of balance and in a state of suspended breakdown. Mother and child are trapped in a cycle of mutual abandonment, isolation, and aloneness that, from a behavioral systems view, constitutes the most frightening human experience (Bowlby, 1973; Solomon et al., 1995).

Mother–Child Interaction

Attachment disorganization is primarily identified based on reunion behavior in the Strange Situation. In attachment theory, reunion represents a critical moment for emotional reintegration following separation. In disorganized dyads, reintegration is blocked by the infant's conflict between seeking and avoiding the parent (Main & Solomon, 1990). Organized attachment strategies of contact seeking and contact maintaining collapse, evidenced during reunion by approach–avoidance movements and behavior, fear and apprehension, and disoriented and trance-like confusion (Main & Solomon, 1990). Beginning in the preschool years, disorganization is identified with three forms of reunion behavior. For most children, the classic disorganized infant behavior is transformed into one of two controlling strategies—punitive and caregiving—that longitudinal research suggests are consolidated by age 5 (Cassidy, Marvin, & the MacArthur Attachment Working Group, 1992; Main & Cassidy, 1988; Moss, Cyr, Bureau, Tarabulsy, & Dubois-Combois, 2005). For a third subgroup, attachment behavior appears to be similar to the incoherent behavior patterns observed in infancy; children in this subgroup are called insecure–other or unclassifiable. This latter subgroup is not well understood; however, there is some suggestion that children in this subgroup are at especially high risk (Moss, Cyr, & Dubois-Comtois, 2004).

The quest to understand the caregiving contributions to attachment disorganization is ongoing. Main and Hesse (1990) suggest that attachment behavior collapse is the result of the infant's experience of a parent as frightened, frightening, or dissociated. Maternal dissociation and disorientation was found in two studies to be especially related to high-risk attachment, including indiscriminate attachment in infants and the insecure–other subgroup in the preschool years (Britner, Marvin, & Pianta, 2005; Lyons-Ruth, Bureau, Riley, & Atlas-Corbett, 2009).

Lyons-Ruth and colleagues view disorganization as a disruption of the balance of parent–infant communication. Their studies showed that infant disorganization is associated with maternal failure to reestablish emotional synchrony following hostile and disruptive exchanges that disrupt communication and interaction (Lyons-Ruth, Bronfman, & Parsons, 1999; Lyons-Ruth & Jacobvitz, 2008; Lyons-Ruth et al., 2005). Disrupted interaction patterns have also been found to characterize controlling mother–child dyads in the preschool and middle childhood years. Mothers of controlling children were observed to be more disruptive, conflict-laden, disengaged, and hostile than mothers of children with organized attachments (Easterbrooks, Biesecker, & Lyons-Ruth, 2000; Humber & Moss, 2005; Moss, Cyr, & DuBois-Comtois, 2004; Moss, Rousseau, Parent, St-Laurent, & Saintonge, 1998). Mothers of punitive and caregiving children, but not mothers of insecure–other children, were notably role-reversed (Britner et al., 2005; Humber & Moss, 2005; Macfie, Fitzpatrick, Rivas, & Cox, 2008; Moss, Cyr, & DuBois-Comtois, 2004; Moss et al., 1998). Mothers in punitive dyads had the most problems with interactive cooperation and joint engagement (Moss, Cyr, & DuBois-Comtois, 2004; Moss & St-Laurent, 2001).

We find the concept of maternal helplessness to be helpful in thinking about the underlying representational and behavioral processes that disorganizes caregiving. Bowlby (1982) emphasized that the protective function of attachment requires the attachment figure to assume a position of being older, wiser, and more powerful than the child. Helplessness and abdicated care undermine a mother's ability to maintain this position in the relationship. The controlling strategies observed in children past infancy seem to us to be desperate attempts by the child to reestablish the protective caregiving–attachment relationship, especially when the attachment system is activated and the child is feeling frightened, vulnerable, and as if on the brink of abandonment (George & Solomon, 2008). The signature of the punitive strategy is "baiting" a helpless combative mother to engage in a duel for power. A mother who engages in this power struggle signals to the child that she is involved (i.e., not abandoning the child), even if their battle is not in the mother's or the child's best interest in the long run. The signature of the caregiving strategy is the child nurturing the mother in order to reinstate her to the protective role. The signature of the insecure–other or unclassifiable child is infantile behavioral collapse. This response suggests that children in this subgroup may experience maternal helplessness somewhat differently than children who develop controlling strategies. The family histories of children judged unclassifiable in our middle childhood studies suggested these mothers may be experiencing tremendous recent or ongoing caregiving distress, such as a recent miscarriage or the child's hospitalization due to a life-threatening accident. This observation is consistent with Moss and colleagues' report that ongoing distress was more characteristic of mothers of insecure–other children than mothers of children in any of the other attachment groups (Moss, Cyr, & DuBois-Comtois, 2004). The mothers of children in the insecure–other group in this study reported the highest levels of marital discord and concurrent threatening life events (e.g., parent hospitalization). Thus, current assaults to the caregiving and attachment systems may render mother and child in these relationships mutually helpless. How these factors undermine a child's ability to engage in controlling strategies is as yet unknown.

Developmental Correlates

Two decades of research have firmly established that children with disorganized attachments in infancy and childhood are at higher developmental risk than those with organized attachments. This risk has been demonstrated in infancy through adolescence across the developmental spectrum, including reports of problems with affect regulation, peer interaction, cognitive development, language, school achievement, internalizing and externalizing behavior, and elevated psychiatric symptoms (e.g., dissociation, suicidal risk; Aikins, Howes, & Hamilton, 2009; Fearon, Bakermans-Kranenburg, van IJzendoorn, Lapsley, & Roisman, 2010; Lyons-Ruth & Jacobvitz, 1999, 2008; West, Adam, Spreng, & Rose, 2001; West, Spreng, Rose, & Adam, 1999; Willemsen-Swinkels & Buitelaar, 2000).

Relatively little research addresses the risk status and adjustment of mothers of disorganized children. The two main maternal adjustment problems in the attachment literature are maternal depression and stress. The findings for depression are mixed. Some studies reported attachment disorganization to be related to depression and other studies failed to find a definitive link (Atkinson et al., 2005; Martins & Graffan, 2000; McMahon et al., 2006; Moss, Cyr, & DuBois-Comtois, 2004; van IJzendoorn, Schuengel, & Bakermans-Kranenburg, 1999). Study outcomes were related in part to the risk status of the sample, the child's age, and the duration of the mother's depression (Campbell et al., 2004; Easterbrooks et al., 2000; Espinosa, Beckwith, Howard, Tyler, & Swanson, 2001; Hughes, Turton, McGauley, & Fonagy, 2006; Lyons-Ruth, Connell, & Grunebaum, 1990).

Notably in relation to the study described in this chapter, Campbell and colleagues (2004) reported that chronic symptoms of maternal depression were not clearly associated with disorganization until children were 3 years old.

Research on "stress" suggests that elevated maternal stress is increasingly associated with attachment disorganization during the preschool and middle childhood years. Bergman and colleagues reported no attachment group differences in maternal stress when babies were a year old (Bergman, Sarkar, Glover, & O'Connor, 2008). Moss and colleagues reported greater levels of perceived maternal stress during middle childhood for mothers of disorganized/controlling children than mothers of secure children (Moss, Cyr, & DuBois-Comtois, 2004; Moss, Bureau, St-Laurent, & Tarabulsy, Chapter 3, this volume). These researchers also found stress-related differences among the disorganized subgroups. Mothers of punitive and insecure–other children reported equally high stress levels. Longitudinal follow-up assessment showed, however, that only mother of the punitive children reported stress increases between the preschool and middle childhood (ages 5–7) assessment. These researchers interpreted the increased stress as related to mothers' reports that these children were becoming increasingly moody and difficult in middle childhood, a phenomenon consistent with the devil-child representation that we described earlier. Perceived maternal stress was stable between the preschool and middle childhood assessments for mothers of insecure–other children. Mothers of caregiving–controlling children reported being stressed; however, their stress levels decreased between the preschool and middle childhood assessments and these mothers did not perceive the child stressful. Mothers in this study described caregiving children as become increasingly adaptable, qualities that are consistent with the angel-child representation that we described earlier.

THE DEVELOPMENT OF THE CHQ

The remainder of this chapter describes the development and validation of the CHQ. One goal in creating this questionnaire was to develop a screening tool for caregiving disorganization for researchers and clinicians. All of the caregiving assessments currently used in the field are labor-intensive and costly (see George & Solomon, 2008). The other goal was to use the questionnaire to explore a dimensional, as opposed to a categorical, approach to understanding maternal helplessness and its correlates. Convergent validity for the questionnaire was assessed with respect to Caregiving Interview helplessness ratings (i.e., representational helplessness); disciminant and predictive validity were assessed using maternal reports of depression and life and caregiving stress, as well as children's behavior.

Method

Questionnaire and Scale Development

In our original work in defining the caregiving system, we developed the helplessness rating scale for the Caregiving Interview to reflect caregiving disorganization and abdication of care and the underlying representational process of segregated systems. This rating scale integrated four domains of helplessness: view of self, child or caregiving circumstances as out of control (including representations of overcontrol associated with worry of becoming out of control); mother or child as frightened; role-reversed caregiving; and psychological merging with and/or glorification of the child. Interview helplessness ratings scored above the midpoint successfully differentiated between mothers of disorganized/controlling and organized children in our two middle childhood samples (George & Solomon, 1996; Solomon & George, Chapter 2, this volume.).

The CHQ was developed using a construct approach (Loevinger, 1957). We began by constructing a pilot or "development" questionnaire that was comprised of an overinclusive set of items derived from mothers' verbatim responses to the Caregiving Interview. The present psychometric validation study was designed following promising preliminary research (Béliveau & Moss, 2005; Coulson, 1995; Magaña, 1997). The selection of the final question pool was based on evaluation of items for theoretical relevance and empirical strength, including face validity to the helplessness construct, internal reliability, and discriminant and predictive validity.

Participants and Recruitment

The development sample was a culturally diverse group of 208 mothers of children ages 3–11 (mean age = 6 years) living in northern California. Cultural representation included Caucasian (43%), Asian (15%), Hispanic (11%), and African American (3%) mothers; 28% of the sample reported their cultural backgrounds as mixed. Mothers ranged in age from 20 to 52 years (mean age = 38 years), with 103 mothers of girls (48%) and 105 mothers of boys (52%). Mothers were predominantly middle class (69%), married (82%), college educated (62%), and worked outside the home (72%). The participation rate of the mothers who expressed interest in the study was 83%.

Mothers were recruited between 1996 and 2000 through advertisement in parenting publications and notices posted in the community (e.g., school or community bulletin boards). The study was advertised as research investigating mother's experiences as a parent. Mothers who were interested in participating in the study were asked to contact the researchers for more information.

Construct, discriminant, and predictive validity were examined using a randomly selected subsample comprised of one-third of the mothers in the development sample ($n = 59$). The participation rate for the validity sample was 60%. The most frequent reason for declining to be in the validity sample was the extra time commitment required for the validity portion of the study. All mothers who declined to participate in this group participated in the questionnaire development sample.

The demographic characteristics of mothers and children who did and did not agree to participate in the validity group were examined using t-tests. There were no differences between the groups. Mothers in the validity group ranged in age from 21 to 51 years (mean age = 38 years), with 25 mothers of girls (42%) and 32 mothers of boys (58%). Their children ranged in age from 3 to 11 years (mean age = 7 years).

Procedures

All mothers were asked to complete consent forms, the Development CHQ and a family background questionnaire. Study materials for mothers in the development sample were delivered and returned in person or by mail, according to their preference. Mothers in the validity sample scheduled appointments with research assistants for the Caregiving Interview. Study materials were mailed to these mothers in advance and collected by the interviewer at the beginning of the interview session.

The Caregiving Interview was administered in a private, quiet location in the mother's home or the Mills College Developmental Research Laboratory. Interviews took approximately 75 minutes and were audiorecorded for later transcription. Mothers were reimbursed for babysitting costs as needed.

Measures

FAMILY BACKGROUND QUESTIONNAIRE

This questionnaire was developed for this study to obtain basic demographic information about mothers and their children. Questions addressed mothers' age, marital status, education, family income, cultural background, and information about the target child and the presence of any other children in their family.

DEVELOPMENT CHQ

The development questionnaire comprised 45 items, including six filler questions.[2] The items were generic statements that reflected mothers' descriptions and responses to Caregiving Interview questions. The questionnaire, like the Caregiving Interview, is designed to be relationship-specific. Mothers are instructed to think about what it is like when she and a particular child are together as she responds to the questions. Items are self-report on a 5-point scale ranging from *not at all characteristic* to *very characteristic*.

CAREGIVING INTERVIEW

The Caregiving Interview (George & Solomon, 1989) is an intensive clinical-style interview designed to tap the experiences and feelings associated with being a parent, and was adapted with permission from the Parent Development Interview (Aber, Slade, Berger, Bresgi, & Kaplan, 1985). Parents are asked to describe themselves as parents and to describe the affective aspects of their experiences being the parent of a particular child (e.g., joy, guilt, anger), five adjectives that describe their relationship with their child, and their experiences coping with attachment-relevant situations (e.g., separation, beginning school). Interviews are audiorecorded for verbatim transcription.

The Caregiving Interview is typically evaluated using four 7-point rating scales that we developed to identify the patterns of defensive processes that differentiate mothers of secure, avoidant, ambivalent, and disorganized/controlling children. These scales are secure base, rejection/deactivation, uncertain/cognitive disconnection, and helplessness/segregated systems. The scales have demonstrated concurrent construct and predictive validity (Fisher, 2000; George & Solomon, 1989, 1996, 2008; Solomon & George, 1999).

The interviews in the current study were rated only for helplessness/segregated systems. Reliability ratings were completed by two blind judges on 25% of the sample (*n* = 15 cases); the raters were the first author and a second rater who was trained to reliability by the first author on a separate sample. Interrater agreement was calculated using Pearson's *r*. The correlation was .86. Rater agreement within 1 rating point was 93%.

PARENTAL STRESS INDEX

The Parental Stress Index (PSI; Abidin, 1995) is a 102-item questionnaire developed to measure parents' perceived level of stress in three domains: parent characteristics, child characteristics, and situational/demographic life stress. Items are self-report using a 5-point scale indicating presence and severity of response. Items in the parent stress domain tap depression, feelings of parental competence, attachment (i.e., investment in maternal role), couple relationships, social isolation, role restriction, and health. Items in the child stress domain tap parents' subjective view of the child as adaptable, demanding, moody, hyperactive, acceptable (conforms to parents' expectations), and reinforcing. Items in the situational/demographic life stress domain ask parents to indicate using a predetermined list all stressful life events that have occurred in the past 12 months. This list includes events such as changes in the family system (e.g., marriage, divorce), financial or work-related experiences, and health. The PSI has established validity and reliability (e.g., Abidin, 1995; Moss, Bureau, Cyr, Mongeau, & St-Laurent, 2004).

BECK DEPRESSION INVENTORY

The Beck Depression Inventory (BDI; Beck, Ward, Mendelson, Mock, & Erbaugh, 1961) is a 21-item questionnaire that taps perceived symptoms of cognitive, affective, and physiological stress. Items are self-report using a 4-point scale and the total score represents prevalence and severity of depression symptoms. The BDI has established validity and reliability (Beck, Epstein, Brown, & Steer, 1988).

CHILD BEHAVIOR CHECKLIST

The Child Behavior Checklist (CBCL; Achenbach & Edelbrock, 1990) is a standardized measure that assesses children's emotional and behavioral problems. Items are self-report evaluations of the child using a 3-point scale indicating presence and severity of the problem. The CBCL provides an index of the child's internalizing (e.g., anxious, depressed) and externalizing (e.g., aggressive, noncompliant) behavior problems and has established validity and reliability (e.g., Achenbach & Edelbrock, 1990; Moss, Bureau, et al., 2004). The present study used the mother report form.

Statistical Analysis

The first objective of this study was to develop the scales for the CHQ through factor analysis and evaluating scale empirical strength. The remaining objectives were to evaluate the validity of the CHQ scales based on the validity sample assessments. These objectives were:

1. To investigate the discriminant validity of CHQ scales. We hypothesized that CHQ scores would not be related to mothers PSI reports of stress originating in affiliative relationships (i.e., friends, peers), sexual relationships (i.e., husband, partner), or health issues. These sources of stress are conceived as having an indirect, rather than direct, effect on the parent–child relationship (e.g., Cowan, Cowan, & Mehta, 2009; Crowell, Treboux, & Brockmeyer, 2009; George & Solomon, 2008). The isolation scale com-

prises six items that address feelings of social isolation from friends and peers (e.g., does not have friends, is not able to enjoy herself at a party, peers do not enjoy mother's company, has not been able to make new friends). The spousal relationship scale comprises seven items that address problems related to the mother's romantic partner (e.g., partner not helpful, problems with partner, don't spend as much time together, less interest in sex). The health scale comprises five items that address the mother's general health (e.g., aches and pains, changes in sleep or sickness patterns).

2. To investigate the convergent concurrent validity of the CHQ scales with respect to ratings of maternal helplessness derived from the Caregiving Interview.

3. To investigate the predictive validity of the CHQ as related to variables that have been empirically associated with disorganization. Predictive validity in the maternal domain was evaluated for depression, reported subjective experiences of parental stress, and frequency of attachment life stress events in the past year. Attachment life events included only life events related to building and breaking relationships (e.g., divorce, loss, pregnancy). Also included, following our most recent work (Solomon & George, 2006; Chapter 2, this volume), were alcohol and drug problems. Events on the PSI stress list that were related to work, finances, school, or legal problems were excluded. Predictive validity in the child domain was evaluated for mother's perception of the child as a source of stress and reports of child behavior problems on the CBCL.

Results

Factor Structure of the CHQ

The final CHQ is presented in Appendix 6.1. Factor analysis using a principle component analysis with varimax rotation yielded a five-factor solution that accounted for 42% of the variance. The seven items in the first factor pertained to caregiving helplessness and constitute the Mother Helpless scale. The items in the other four factors pertained to the constructs of fear and child caregiving. We combined the items in these remaining scales to produce two new scales: Mother–Child Frightened (six items) and Child Caregiving (6 items), conceived as the scales that corresponded to children's punitive and caregiving controlling strategies, respectively. The CHQ scales and factor loadings are shown in Table 6.1. The scales are internally consistent, with alpha coefficients of .85 for Mother Helpless, .66 for Mother–Child Frightened, and .64 for Child Caregiving. The empirical structure of the CHQ scales is shown in Table 6.2. Analysis of variance showed no significant differences for child gender or mother and child age. The empirical structure of the CHQ for child gender is shown in Table 6.3.

TABLE 6.1. Factor Weightings of CHQ Scales

Item No.	1 Mother Helpless	2 Mother– Child Frightened	3 Child Caregiving
1. Mother is out of control.	.68		
5. Mother cannot discipline my child.	.76		
7. Child is out of control.	.75		
10. Mother feels she is a failure.	.62		
18. Mother is helpless to make changes in her life.	.67		
20. Mother feels life is chaotic.	.59		
22. Child is rude.	.60		
3. Mother is frightened of her child.		.71	
4. Child hits, kicks, bites mother.		.72	
12. Mother punishes too harshly.		.60	
13. Mother cannot soothe child.		.51	
14. Child loses it when separated from mother.		.57	
15. Child is afraid of mother.		.65	
2. Child is caregiving.			.76
6. Child puts others at ease.			.67
8. Child is a great actor.			.56
9. Child is sensitive to others.			.77
11. Child is a clown.			.83
17. Child makes others laugh.			.84

Note. Only items with loadings greater than .5 and Eigenvalues greater than 1.5 were selected.

TABLE 6.2. Empirical Structure of the CHQ Scales

	CHQ scales		
	Mother Helpless	Mother–Child Frightened	Child Caregiving
Number of items	7	6	6
Alpha[a]	.85	.66	.64
Mean	9.67	8.71	18.62
SD	4.19	3.02	4.35
95% confidence interval	9.14–10.24	8.30–9.12	18.03–19.21
Interscale correlations[b]			
With CHQ M Helpless	—	.58**	.07
With CHQ M/C Frightened	—	—	.15*
With CHQ C Caregiving	—	—	—

Note. n = 208.
[a]Chronbach's alpha coefficient of internal reliability.
[b]Pearson's correlations. *p < .05; **p < .01; ***p < .001.

TABLE 6.3. The Empirical Structure of the CHQ Scales for Mothers of Boys and Girls

	CHQ scales		
	Mother Helpless	Mother–Child Frightened	Child Caregiving
Girls (n = 102)			
Mean	9.57	8.98	18.86
SD	3.98	2.96	3.89
95% confidence interval	8.79–10.35	8.40–9.56	18.10–19.63
Boys (n = 106)			
Mean	9.80	8.55	18.31
SD	4.42	3.11	4.71
95% confidence interval	8.95–10.65	7.95–9.15	17.40–19.22
	F(1,207) = 0.16	F(1,207) = 1.06	F(1,207) = .86
	p = .69	p = .30	p = .35

Convergent Validity

Convergent validity of the CHQ was evaluated by examining the Pearson product–moment correlations between CHQ scales scores and Caregiving Interview helplessness ratings. The helplessness ratings in this sample ranged from *limited helpless* (2 rating) to *very helpless* (7 rating) (mean score = 4). As shown in Table 6.4, significant positive correlations were found between the helplessness rating and two CHQ scales—Mother Helpless ($r = .45$) and Mother–Child Frightened ($r = .30$). The correlation between the helplessness rating and the Child Caregiving scale was not significant.

Discriminant Validity

Three subscales of the PSI that were unrelated to the mother–child relationship were used to evaluate CHQ discriminant validity: maternal isolation, spousal relationship, and health. As shown in Table 6.5, there were no significant correlations between the CHQ scales and these noncaregiving dimensions of parental stress.

Predictive Validity

We predicted a significant positive correlation between CHQ scale scores and both mother and child domain scores. We did not include Isolation, Spouse, and Health scores in the sum for the mother domain, as these items were used in the discriminant validity analysis. We expected a significant positive correlation between the CHQ scales and mothers' reports of depression symptoms (BDI), stress, and the number of stressful attachment life events experienced within the past year. In the child domain, we expected a significant positive correlation between the CHQ scales and mother's subjective experiences of her child as stressful (PSI-child domain and CBCL externalizing and internalizing problems).

We first examined the intercorrelations among these variables and demographic variables. There were significant positive correlations between both child and maternal age and maternal stress (i.e., PSI-parent domain), and between maternal age and depression (BDI). Maternal and child age were used as covariates in the analyses of maternal stress and depression.

The results of these analyses of interest are shown in Table 6.6. As predicted, there were significant positive correlations between two of the CHQ scales, Mother Helplessness and Mother–Child Frightened, with maternal depression (BDI) and the PSI mother and child domains. The Child Caregiving scale showed positive correlations with the three maternal scales—maternal depression, PSI mother stress, and number of attachment

TABLE 6.4. Convergent Validity: Correlations between the CHQ Scales and the Caregiving Interview Helplessness Ratings

| | | CHQ scales | | |
	Mean (SD)	Mother Helpless	Mother–Child Frightened	Child Caregiving
Caregiving Interview	4.0	.45**	.30*	.12
Helplessness Rating	(1.49)			

Note. n = 54. Five interviews could not be rated due to inaudible recording. Pearson's r (two-tailed). *p < .05; **p < .01.

TABLE 6.5. Discriminant Validity: Correlations between the CHQ Scales and Mother's Personal Stress

| | | CHQ scales | | |
PSI personal stress scales	Mean (SD)	Mother helpless	Mother–child frightened	Child caregiving
Isolation	14.40 (3.40)	–.21	–.17	–.12
Spouse	18.26 (6.03)	–.13	–.23	–.11
Health	13.59 (2.55)	.11	.17	.02

Note. n = 58. Not all mothers in the validity sample completed the PSI. Pearson's r (two-tailed).

TABLE 6.6. Predictive Validity: Correlations between the CHQ Scales and Maternal Life Stress, Depression, and Attachment Life Events

| | | CHQ scales | | |
	Mean (SD)	Mother Helpless	Mother–Child Frightened	Child Caregiving
Mother domain				
BDI[a]	7.8 (8.04)	.58***	.56***	.28*
PSI—Mother Stress[b]	112.28 (19.39)	.64***	.63**	.24+
No of attachment life events[b]	.63 (.96)	.43**	.32*	.24+
Child domain				
PSI—Child Stress[b]	96.79 (18.96)	.73***	.69***	.09
Internalizing Problems, CBCL[c]	6.94 (6.96)	.02	.16	.07
Externalizing Problems, CBSL[c]	6.01 (5.24)	.41*	.36*	–.22

Note. n's differ for the mother and child domain measures because not all mothers in the validity sample completed all measures.
Pearson's r (two-tailed). +p < .10; *p <.05; **p <.01; ***p < .000.
[a]n = 56; [b]n = 58; [c]n = 37.

life events—but only the correlation with maternal depression was signifi-cant. Child Caregiving was not related to either of the variables in the child domain.

Exploratory Analyses

These results led to two exploratory analyses. The first examined the three CHQ scales in relation to the PSI mother and child domain subscales. Moss and colleagues (2004) reported meaningful subscale differences among mothers of the three disorganized groups (i.e., punitive, caregiving, inse-cure–other). In particular, the controlling–caregiving pattern, in contrast to the other patterns, was associated with *lower* maternal and child-related stress past the preschool years. We wondered if subscale scores would show a similar pattern of correlations with the CHQ scales. The results of these analyses were partially consistent with those of Moss and colleagues, and are shown in Table 6.7. There were no clear distinctions in the pattern of correlations for the Mother Helpless and Mother–Child Frightened scales. There were significant positive correlations between Child Caregiving and the PSI mother scales for depression, attachment, and role restriction; com-petence was the only variable in the mother stress domain that was not significantly related to Child Caregiving. Child Caregiving was unrelated, however, to any of the child stress subscales.

Thus, these results suggested that Child Caregiving was positively related to maternal stress but the mother did not identify her child as the source of that stress. Nevertheless, if high scores in Child Caregiving are indicative of a role-reversed "angel child," we would have expected to see both low maternal stress and high child adjustment scores associated with this group. This raised the possibility that the dimensional approach was missing important variability.

We explored this possibility by creating four groups based on scores from two of the scales, Mother–Child Frightened and Child Caregiving. High and low groups on each dimension were defined by using the upper quartile as a cutoff for high scores (scores of 9 and 22, respectively). The resulting groups were named Frightened and Caregiving (scores above the cutoff on both Mother–Child Frightened and Child Caregiving), Frightened (scores above the cutoff for Mother–Child Frightened only), Caregiving (scores above the cutoff for Child Caregiving only), and Neither Frightened nor Caregiving (no scores above the cutoff). To see if the distinctions among these groups were meaningful, we examined the Kruskal–Wallace rankings of the groups with respect to the convergent and predictive validity vari-ables.

The results of this analysis are shown in Table 6.8. The n's for these analyses are small and the results must be interpreted with caution. Nev-

TABLE 6.7. CHQ Scale Correlations with PSI Mother and Child Stress Domains Subscales

| | | CHQ scales | | |
	Mean (SD)	Mother Helpless	Mother–Child Frightened	Child Caregiving
Mother domain[a]				
Depression	18.69 (6.09)	.64***	.61***	.28*
Attachment	14.12 (3.31)	.49***	.71***	.32*
Role restriction	18.60 (6.02)	.63***	.54***	.38**
Competence	33.60 (4.89)	.39**	.51***	.14
Child domain				
Adaptability	22.84 (5.60)	.51***	.42**	.01
Acceptability	11.79 (3.28)	.42**	.37**	−.03
Demandingness	17.53 (5.55)	.58***	.68***	.21
Mood	9.34 (3.10)	.55***	.53***	−.01
Distractibility/ hyperactivity	22.83 (5.21)	.60***	.50***	.18
Reinforces parent	12.45 (2.68)	.41**	.53***	−.09

Note. Pearson's r (two-tailed). **$p < .01$; ***$p < .000$.
[a] $n = 58$.

ertheless, the results were intriguing. The Frightened and Caregiving group ranked highest for all adjustment problems: helplessness, depression, mother and child stress, and child behavior problems. The Frightened and the Child Caregiving groups ranked second and third, respectively, in all mother dimensions except attachment life events. With respect to the child domain, the Caregiving group ranked even lower than the Neither Frightened nor Caregiving group on child behavior problems. This latter finding in particular is consistent with the proposition that high Caregiving (in the absence of elevations on the remaining scores) may overlap closely with the controlling–caregiving child attachment group, identified on the basis of reunion behavior (Main & Cassidy, 1988). We speculate that the Frightened

TABLE 6.8. Comparison of Mothers' Subjective Experiences as Frightened and Child Caregiving

	CHQ combined scales				
	Frightened and Caregiving Rank n Mean (SD)	Frightened Rank n Mean (SD)	Caregiving Rank n Mean (SD)	Neither Frightened nor Caregiving Rank n Mean (SD)	Kruskal–Wallace df Significance
Mother domain					
CHQ Mother Helpless[a]	#1*** 9 18.56 (8.87)	#2 14 13.5 (3.41)	#3 10 10.80 (4.37)	#4 26 8.52 (1.85)	23.16 3 .000
BDI[b]	#1 9 14.11 (15.82)	#2 14 7.43 (3.76)	#3 9 8.00 (7.97)	#4 24 5.30 (3.94)	4.04 3 .26
PSI—Parental Stress[c]	#1** 9 130.56 (26.1)	#2 14 115.29 (13.16)	#3 10 114.40 (14.76)	#4 25 103.00 (16.78)	11.32 3 .01
No of attachment life events[c]	#1 9 1.33 (1.32)	#4 14 .36 (.63)	#2 10 .60 (.70)	#3 25 .67 (.99)	5.32 3 .18
Child domain					
PSI—Child Stress[c]	#1*** 9 119.22 (17.8)	#2 14 109.07 (15.79)	#3 10 91.10 (8.33)	#4 25 84.75 (11.18)	29. 50 3 .000
Internalizing Problems, CBCL[d]	#1 5 55.00 (9.75)	#2 9 51.11 (8.96)	#4 6 44.33 (9.63)	#3 17 49.41 (11.06)	.03 3 .26
Externalizing Problems, CBCL[d]	#1* 5 53.60 (5.94)	#2 9 53.78 (9.63)	#4 6 39.83 (7.41)	#3 17 47.47 (8.49)	9.40 3 .02

Note. n's differ for the mother and child domain measures because not all mothers in the validity sample completed all measures.

Kruskal–Wallace (two-tailed). *$p < .05$; **$p < .01$; ***$p < .000$.
[a]$n = 59$; [b]$n = 56$; [c]$n = 58$; [d]$n = 37$.

and Caregiving group comprises dyads in which the child has been unable to consolidate a coherent role-reversal strategy and is perhaps comparable to the Unclassifiable child attachment group.

Discussion

The main goal of this study was to develop and validate the CHQ as a screening tool for caregiving disorganization for mothers of children ages 3 to 11. The construction of the scale was based on our approach to understanding disorganized caregiving as the product of a breakdown in defensive processes, termed by Bowlby "segregated systems," leading to mothers' subjective appraisal of themselves as helpless with respect to their child (George & Solomon, 1989, 2008; Solomon & George, 1996, 1999, 2000; Chapter 2, this volume). Factor analysis of the items on the development questionnaire produced three CHQ scales that correspond conceptually to the major dimensions of relationship disorganization past infancy: Mother Helpless, Mother–Child Frightened (mother dysregulated, child punitive relationships), and Child Caregiving (mother constricted, child caregiving relationships). CHQ scale intercorrelations showed that the Mother Helpless scale overlapped significantly with the Mother–Child Frightened scale, but not with the Child Caregiving Scale. There was some overlap between the Mother–Child Frightened and the Child Caregiving scales, but the low positive correlation suggested that these two scales tapped different dimensions of maternal representation.

All three scales showed the expected discriminant validity. The CHQ scales were examined in relation to measures of maternal stress that a behavioral systems approach would suggest are only indirectly related to the caregiving system. There were no significant correlations between the CHQ scales and maternal stress associated with the affiliative, sexual, and health domains.

The second objective was to examine the convergent or concurrent validity of the CHQ by examining the scale correlations with the helplessness ratings from the Caregiving Interview (George & Solomon, 1989; Solomon & George, Chapter 2, this volume). The correlations between the two measures were all in the positive direction, but only the results for two scales were statistically significant. The highest correlation was with the Mother Helpless scale, confirming our expectation that the Mother Helpless scale is the predominant indicator of disorganized caregiving on the CHQ. The Mother–Child Frightened and the Child Caregiving scales were conceived as tapping dysregulated and constricted caregiving representations, which we have previously reported to be the caregiving representational patterns associated respectively with children's punitive and children's caregiving controlling attachment strategies. The Mother–Child Frightened scale items reflect mothers' dysregulated representations of caregiving: combative, frightened, frightening, enraged, hostile, and out of control (George & Solomon, 2008; Solomon et al., 1995). It is likely that these are the representational elements that contribute to the prominent themes of hostility, conflict, and failed engagement that have been found to be characteristic of disorganized and controlling mothers and their children, especially those in punitive dyads (Britner et al., 2005; Easterbrooks et al., 2000; Humber & Moss, 2005; Moss, Cyr, & Dubois-Comtois, 2004; Moss et al., 1998; Moss & St-Laurent, 2001).

The correlation between the third CHQ scale, Child Caregiving, and the Caregiving Interview helplessness rating was not statistically significant. This suggests that this CHQ scale did not fully tap the constricted dimension of disorganized caregiving. The CHQ scale items describe cheering the mother, representations consistent with but not fully capturing the representation of the caregiving angel child (George & Solomon, 2008). These items do not capture a mother's inability to talk about caregiving, psychological merging with the child, or constricted interactive behavior (e.g., sudden and complete withdrawal under stress), all of which are associated in the Caregiving Interview with constricted representation. Future research using the CHQ should examine whether introducing items that capture these other features of constriction improves the convergent validity of this scale. Below we discuss exploratory analyses that suggest, that as currently constructed, this scale is most useful when used in categorical analyses based on patterns of scores on both the Child Caregiving and the Mother–Child Frightened scales.

Predictive validity of the CHQ scales was investigated by examining the correlations between the CHQ scales and mother and child adjustment risk. In the domain of maternal risk, there were significant positive correlations between the Mother Helpless and the Mother–Child Frightened scales and every dimension of risk, including maternal depression, and maternal caregiving stress, especially that related to problems in attaching to the child (e.g., emotional bonding, reading their child's cues), role restriction, and parenting incompetence. We interpret these findings as indicating patterns of risk that are associated with maternal helplessness, especially the dysregulated punitive relationship.

The correlation patterns between the mother adjustment variables and the Child Caregiving scale were less robust. Mothers who endorsed items on the Child Caregiving scale also described themselves as having problems with depression, attachment to the child, and role restriction. They apparently did not blame the child for these problems, however. Rather their PSI scores indicated that they experienced themselves to be competent as parents. This finding supports the view that child caregiving behavior indeed may be an effective attachment strategy that functions to reinstate the mother to the role of providing protection and care. The positive associations between stressful attachment life events (e.g., loss, divorce, pregnancy) and all three caregiving scales is consistent with the results of other studies (Moss, Cyr, & Dubois-Comtois, 2004; Solomon & George, 2006; Chapter 2, this volume); although again this relation was less robust for the Child Caregiving scale, where it only reached a trend level.

Investigators have persistently searched for a link between attachment disorganization and maternal depression, but findings have been inconsistent, including both positive associations (Campbell et al., 2004; Espinosa et al., 2001; Lyons-Ruth et al., 1990; Teti, Gelfand, Messinger, & Isabella, 1995) and inconclusive or negative ones (Atkinson et al., 2005; Easterbrooks et al., 2000; Hughes et al., 2006; Humber & Moss, 2005; Martins & Graffan, 2000; McMahon et al., 2006; Moss, Cyr, & Dubois-Comtois, 2004; Moss et al., 1998; van IJzendoorn, Schuengel, & Bakermans-Kranenburg, 1999). We found positive correlations between all three CHQ scales and maternal depression. One explanatory factor may be the older average age of the child in this study, which would be consistent with Campbell et al.'s (2004) finding that maternal depression assessed in the child's first 15 months was not related to depressive symptoms when the child was 3 years old. Another explanatory factor may be related to measurement factors. The CHQ scales may be more likely to reveal differences on the disorganized caregiving dimensions than analyses based on discrete classification groups. In line with this idea, Moss et al. (1998) found depression most prominent for mothers of ambivalent–resistant children, yet these same children in their longitudinal follow-up study were described by their mothers with qualities that were found in subsequent research to be associated with disorganized attachment (Moss, Cyr, & Dubois-Comtois, 2004). Another explanatory factor may be related to the caregiving type of controlling relationship that may function to soothe mothers' depressive feelings.

In the child domain, only mothers with high scores on the Mother Helpless and the Mother–Child Frightened scale reported child adjustment problems. Mothers who endorsed these scales described their children as not adaptable, not acceptable, demanding, moody, distractible, overactive, not providing positive reinforcement, and as having externalizing problems. The correlation patterns for the Child Caregiving scale suggested that these mothers viewed their children neither as stressful nor as having adjustment problems.

These results have implications for our understanding of caregiving disorganization. In this study elevated scores on the Mother–Child Frightened scale are associated with overall elevated risk for children, as is consistent with research findings for the punitive–controlling attachment (Moss, Cyr, & Dubois-Comtois, 2004; Moss et al., 1998). Indeed, mothers of children in the controlling group are likely to view their children as becoming increasingly difficult and out of control between the preschool and school-age years (Moss, Cyr, et al., 2004). Also consistent with work by Moss and colleagues, elevated scores on the Child Caregiving scale were associated with an absence of child adjustment problems. This finding was punctuated by the results of the exploratory analyses showing that mothers who endorsed only the highest scores for Child Caregiving, and who had low scores on the other two CHQ scales, viewed themselves and their children as having the lowest adjustment problems. A child who cheers mother up may indeed be unlikely to "act up," but these findings do not reveal the developmental costs that might be expected to be associated with role-reversal. Developmental assessments for childhood, most of which were developed before attachment theory and research became prominent, may not be refined enough to detect the problems of caregiving role-reversal (see Hazen, Jacobvitz, Higgins, Allen, & Jin, Chapter 7, this volume). It is also possible that the sequelae of the child caregiving strategy may not surface until these children are older, for example, during the self-transformations that are associated with adolescence or the transition to parenthood (Allen, 2008; George & Solomon, 2008).

The exploratory analyses showed that relationships characterized by the combination of elevated frightened and caregiving elements were at the highest risk. Mothers who reported high scores for both the Mother–Child Frightened and the Child Caregiving scales also reported the highest Mother Helpless scores in the sample. Our sample was low risk; and the depression scores, stress, and child behavior problem scores in this sample were rarely elevated to clinical cutoffs (the mean BDI score was 7.59; range 0–50, SD = 7.93). However, even in this sample, children's caregiving strategies apparently were not effective and the maternal caregiving system seemed to be the most highly compromised in these dyads. We suggest that this group represents the insecure–other or unclassifiable children in the preschool and middle childhood years. These mothers ranked highest for number of attachment life events in the past year, and their children ranked highest for externalizing behavior, consistent with other reports of insecure–other children (Moss, Cyr, & Dubois-Comtois, 2004; Moss, Bureau, St-Laurent, Tarabulsy, Chapter 3, this volume). Although there is yet little additional research with the CHQ, we find it encouraging that the patterns of findings in this study conform well to the literature that is based on reunion behavior classifications (e.g., Bureau, Easterbrooks, & Lyons-Ruth, 2009) and mother–infant interaction (Ellitsdotir, Bertha, Bureau, & Lyons-Ruth, 2009). We are hopeful that use of this instrument by other researchers and clinicians will lead to additional verification and facilitate the study of caregiving and attachment in circumstances that are not conducive to the use of the more extensive Caregiving Interview and classification system (George & Solomon, 1993/1996/2002/2008).

NOTES

1. We note here the unfortunate overlap in terms between our work and that of Lyons-Ruth that may lead to some confusion. We have termed both dysregulated mothers and constricted ones as "helpless," while Lyons-Ruth describes mothers of disorganized infants as "hostile vs. helpless." The different usages reflect in large part the slightly different research protocols. In our case, "helpless" captures the way these mothers evaluate themselves in interaction with the child, regardless of whether they lash out or withdraw. Lyons-Ruth's use of terms seems to reflect both mothers' attitudes toward their own caregivers and what can be observed in their interaction with their children. Interestingly, this confusion in terms mirrors the confusion in sense of self-as-caregiver that we refer to elsewhere (Solomon & George, Chapter 2, this volume).

2. Two variations of this final questionnaire were developed for student research projects. The results of these two studies established basic predictive validity for this approach (Coulson, 1995; Magaña, 1997).

REFERENCES

Aber, J. L., Slade, A., Berger, B., Bresgi, I., & Kaplan, M. (1985). *The Parent Development Interview*. Unpublished manuscript, Barnard College, Columbia University, NY.

Abidin, R. A. (1995). *Parental Stress Index* (3rd ed.). Odessa, FL: Psychological Assessment Resources.

Achenbach, T. M., & Edelbrock, C. (1990). *Manual for the Child Behavior Checklist and Revised Child Behavior Profile*. Burlington, VT: University of Vermont Department of Psychiatry.

Aikins, J. W., Howes, C., & Hamilton, C. E. (2009). Attachment stability and the emergence of unresolved representations during adolescence. *Attachment and Human Development, 11*, 491–512.

Allen, J. P. (2008). The attachment system in adolescence. In J. Cassidy & P. R. Shaver (Eds.), *Handbook of attachment: Theory, research, and clinical applications* (2nd ed., pp. 419–435). New York: Guilford Press.

Almqvist, K., & Broberg, A. G. (2003). Young children traumatized by organized violence together with their mothers: The critical effects of damaged internal representations. *Attachment and Human Development, 5*, 367–380.

Atkinson, L., Goldberg, S., Raval, V., Pederson, D. R., Benoit, D., Moran, G., et al. (2005). On the relation between maternal state of mind and sensitivity in the prediction of infant attachment security. *Developmental Psychology, 41*, 42–53.

Barnett, D., & Ganiban, J. (1999). V. Maltreatment, negative expressivity, and the development of type D attachment from 12–24. *Monographs of the Society for Research in Child Development, 64*, 97–118.

Beck, A. T., Epstein, N., Brown, G., & Steer, R. A. (1988). An inventory for measuring clinical anxiety: Psychometric properties. *Journal of Consulting and Clinical Psychology, 56*, 893–897.

Beck, A. T., Ward, C. H., Mendelson, M., Mock, J., & Erbaugh, J. (1961). An inventory for measuring depression. *Archives of General Psychiatry, 38,* 381–390.

Béliveau, M.-J., & Moss, E. (2005). Contribution aux validités convergente et divergente du projectif de l'attachement adulte [Contribution of convergent and divergent validity to the Adult Attachment Projective]. *La Revue Internationale de l'Education Familiale, 9,* 29–50.

Bergman, K., Sarkar, P., Glover, V., & O'Connor, T. G. (2008). Quality of child–parent attachment moderates the impact of antenatal stress on child fearfulness. *Journal of Child Psychiatry and Psychiatry, 49,* 1089–1098.

Bowlby, J. (1973). *Attachment and loss: Vol. 2. Separation: Anxiety and anger.* New York: Basic Books.

Bowlby, J. (1980). *Attachment and loss: Vol. 3. Loss: Sadness and depression.* New York: Basic Books.

Bowlby, J. (1982). *Attachment and loss: Vol. 1. Attachment.* New York: Basic Books. (Original work published 1969)

Bretherton, I., & Munholland, K. A. (2008). Internal working models in attachment relationships. In J. Cassidy & P. R. Shaver (Eds.), *Handbook of attachment: Theory, research, and clinical applications* (2nd ed., pp. 102–127). New York: Guilford Press.

Britner, P. A., Marvin, R. S., & Pianta, R. C. (2005). Development and preliminary validation of the caregiving behavior system: Association with child attachment classification in the preschool Strange Situation. *Attachment and Human Development, 7,* 83–102.

Buchheim, A., Erk, S., George, C., Kächele, H., Kircher, T., Martius, P., et al. (2008). Neural correlates of attachment dysregulation in borderline personality disorder using functional magnetic resonance imaging. *Psychiatry Research: Neuroimaging, 163,* 223–235.

Buchheim, A., Erk, S., George, C., Kächele, H., Ruchsow, M., Spitzer, M., et al. (2006). Measuring attachment representation in an fMRI environment: A pilot study. *Psychopathology, 39,* 144–152.

Bureau, J.-F., Easterbrooks, A., & Lyons-Ruth, K. (April, 2009). *The association between middle childhood controlling and disorganized attachment and family correlates in young adulthood.* Paper presented at the biennial meeting of the Society for Research in Child Development, Denver, CO.

Campbell, S. B., Brownell, C. A., Hungerford, A., Spieker, S. J., Mohan, R., & Blessing, J. S. (2004). The course of maternal depressive symptoms and maternal sensitivity as predictors of attachment security at 36 months. *Development and Psychopathology, 16,* 231–252.

Cassidy, J., & Marvin, R. S., with the MacArthur Attachment Working Group. (1992). *Attachment organization in preschool children: Coding guidelines.* Unpublished manuscript, University of Virginia, Charlottesville.

Coulson, W. (1995). *Disruptive caregiving strategies in mothers with symptoms of posttraumatic stress.* Unpublished undergraduate thesis, Mills College, Oakland, CA.

Cowan, P. A., Cowan, C. P., & Mehta, N. (2009). Adult attachment, couple attachment, and children's adaptation to school: An integrated attachment template and family risk model. *Attachment and Human Development, 11,* 29–46.

Crowell, J. A., Treboux, D., & Brockmeyer, S. (2009). Parental divorce and adult children's attachment representations and marital status. *Attachment and Human Development, 11*, 87–101.

Easterbrooks, M. A., Biesecker, G., & Lyons-Ruth, K. (2000). Infancy predictors of emotional availability in middle childhood: The roles of attachment security and maternal depressive symptomatology. *Attachment and Human Development, 2*, 170–187.

Ellitsdotir, L., Bertha, E., Bureau, J.-F., & Lyons-Ruth, K. (2009). *Cross-validation of self-report and direct observational measures of parent–child role confusion in young adulthood.* Paper presented at the biennial meeting of the Society for Research in Child Development, Denver, CO.

Espinosa, M., Beckwith, L., Howard, J., Tyler, R., & Swanson, K. (2001). Maternal psychopathology and attachment in toddlers of heavy cocaine-using mothers. *Infant Mental Health Journal, 22*, 316–333.

Fearon, R. P., Bakermans-Kranenburg, M. J., van IJzendoorn, M. H., Lapsley, A.-M., & Roisman, G. I. (2010). The significance of insecure attachment and disorganization in the development of children's externalizing behavior: A meta-analytic study. *Child Development, 81*, 435–456.

Fisher, N. K. (2000). *Mental representations of attachment and caregiving in women sexually abused during childhood: Links to the intergenerational transmission of trauma?* Unpublished doctoral dissertation, City University of New York, New York.

George, C., & Solomon, J. (1993/1996/2002/2008). *Caregiving representation rating manual: Rating scales and Caregiving Interview protocol.* Unpublished manuscript, Mills College, Oakland, CA.

George, C., & Solomon, J. (1989). Internal working models of caregiving and security of attachment at age six. *Infant Mental Health Journal, 10*, 222–237.

George, C., & Solomon, J. (1996). Representational models of relationships: Links between caregiving and attachment. *Infant Mental Health Journal, 17*, 198–216.

George, C., & Solomon, J. (2008). The caregiving system: A behavioral systems approach to parenting. In J. Cassidy & P. R. Shaver (Eds.), *Handbook of attachment: Theory, research, and clinical applications* (2nd ed., pp. 833–856). New York: Guilford Press.

George, C., & West, M. (2001). The development and preliminary validation of a new measure of adult attachment: The Adult Attachment Projective. *Attachment and Human Development, 3*, 30–61.

George, C., & West, M. (in press). *The Adult Attachment Projective Picture System.* New York: Guilford Press.

George, C., West, M., & Pettem, O. (1999). The Adult Attachment Projective: Disorganization of adult attachment at the level of representation. In J. Solomon & C. George (Eds.), *Attachment disorganization* (pp. 462–507). New York: Guilford Press.

Green, J., Stanley, C., & Peters, S. (2007). Disorganized attachment representation and atypical parenting in young school age children with externalizing disorder. *Attachment and Human Development, 9*, 207–222.

Hesse, E., & Main, M. (2006). Frightened, threatening, and dissociative parental behavior in low-risk samples: Description, discussion, and interpretations. *Development and Psychopathology, 18,* 309–343.

Hinde, R. A. (1982). *Ethology.* New York: Oxford University Press.

Hughes, P., Turton, P., McGauley, G. A., & Fonagy, P. (2006). Factors that predict infant disorganization in mothers classified as U in pregnancy. *Attachment and Human Development, 8,* 113–122.

Humber, N., & Moss, E. (2005). The relationship of preschool and early school age attachment to mother–child interaction. *American Journal of Orthopsychiatry, 75,* 128–141.

Jacobsen, T., Hibbs, E., & Ziegenhain, U. (2000). Maternal expressed emotion related to attachment disorganization in early childhood: A preliminary report. *Journal of Child Psychology and Psychiatry, 41,* 899–906.

Liotti, G. (2004). Trauma, dissociation, and disorganized attachment: Three strands of a single braid. *Psychotherapy: Theory, Research, Practice, Training, 41,* 472–486.

Loevinger, J. (1957). Objective tests as instruments of psychological theory. *Psychology Reports, 3,* 635–694.

Lyons-Ruth, K., Bronfman, E., & Parsons, E. (1999). Maternal frightened, frightening, or atypical behavior and disorganized infant attachment. In J. I. Vondra & D. Barnette (Eds.), Atypical patterns of early attachment: Theory, research, and current directions *Monographs of the Society for Research in Child Development, 64*(3, Serial No. 67), 67–96.

Lyons-Ruth, K., Bureau, J.-F., Riley, C. D., & Atlas-Corbett, A. F. (2009). Socially indiscriminate attachment behavior in the Strange Situation: Convergent and discriminant validity in relation to caregiving risk, later behavior problems, and attachment insecurity. *Development and Psychopathology, 21,* 355–372.

Lyons-Ruth, K., Connell, D. B., & Grunebaum, H. U. (1990). Infants at social risk: Maternal depression and family support services as mediators of infant development and security of attachment. *Child Development, 61,* 85–98.

Lyons-Ruth, K., & Jacobvitz, D. (1999). Attachment disorganization: Unresolved loss, relational violence, and lapses in behavioral and attentional strategies. In J. Cassidy & P. R. Shaver (Eds.), *Handbook of attachment: Theory, research, and clinical applications* (pp. 520–554). New York: Guilford Press.

Lyons-Ruth, K., & Jacobvitz, D. (2008). Attachment disorganization: Unresolved loss, relational violence, and lapses in behavioral and attentional strategies. In J. Cassidy & P. R. Shaver (Eds.), *Handbook of attachment: Theory, research, and clinical applications* (2nd ed., pp. 666–697). New York: Guilford Press.

Lyons-Ruth, K., Yellin, C., Melnick, S., & Atwood, G. (2005). Expanding the concept of unresolved mental states: Hostile/helpless states of mind on the Adult Attachment Interview are associated with disrupted mother–infant communication and infant disorganization. *Development and Psychopathology, 17,* 1–23.

Macfie, J., Fitzpatrick, K. L., Rivas, E. M., & Cox, M. J. (2008). Independent influences upon mother–toddler role reversal: Infant–mother attachment disorganization and role reversal in mother's childhood. *Attachment and Human Development, 10,* 29–39.

Madigan, S., Moran, G., & Pederson, D. R. (2006). Unresolved states of mind, disorganized attachment relationships, and disrupted interactions of adolescent mothers and their infants. *Developmental Psychology, 42,* 293–304.

Magaña, L. (1997). *Unresolved trauma and environmental stress in relation to the caregiving behavioral system: Disorganization of caregiving strategies.* Unpublished undergraduate thesis, Mills College, Oakland, CA.

Main, M., & Cassidy, J. (1988). Categories of response to reunion with the parent at age 6: Predictable from infant attachment classifications and stable over a 1-month period. *Developmental Psychology, 24,* 1–12.

Main, M., & Hesse, E. (1990). Parents' unresolved traumatic experiences are related to infant disorganized attachment status: Is frightened and/or frightening parental behavior the linking mechanism? In M. T. Greenberg, D. Cicchetti, & E. M. Cummings (Eds.), *Attachment in the preschool years* (pp. 161–182). Chicago: University of Chicago Press.

Main, M., & Solomon, J. (1990). Procedures for identifying infants as disorganized/disoriented during the Ainsworth Strange Situation. In M. T. Greenberg, D. Cicchetti, & E. M. Cummings (Eds.), *Attachment in the preschool years* (pp. 121–160). Chicago: University of Chicago Press.

Martins, C., & Graffan, E. A. (2000). Effects of early maternal depression on infant–mother attachment: A meta-analytic investigation. *Journal of Child Psychiatry and Psychiatry, 41,* 737–746.

McMahon, C. A., Barnett, B., Kowalenko, N. M., & Tennant, C. C. (2006). Maternal attachment state of mind moderates the impact of postnatal depression on infant attachment. *Journal of Child Psychology and Psychiatry, 47,* 660–669.

Moss, E., Bureau, J., Cyr, C., Mongeau, C., & St-Laurent, D. (2004). Correlates of attachment at age 3: Construct validity of the Preschool Attachment Classification System. *Developmental Psychology, 40,* 323–334.

Moss, E., Cyr, C., Bureau, J., Tarabulsy, G. M., & Dubois-Combois, K. (2005). Stability of attachment during the preschool period. *Developmental Psychology, 41,* 773–783.

Moss, E., Cyr, C., & Dubois-Comtois, K. (2004). Attachment at early school age and developmental risk: Examining family contexts and behavior problems of controlling–caregiving, controlling–punitive, and behaviorally disorganized children. *Developmental Psychology, 40,* 519–532.

Moss, E., Rousseau, D., Parent, S., St-Laurent, D., & Saintonge, J. (1998). Correlates of attachment at school age: Maternal reported stress, mother–child interaction, and behavior problems. *Child Development, 69,* 1390–1405.

Moss, E., & St-Laurent, D. (2001). Attachment at school age and academic performance. *Developmental Psychology, 37,* 863–874.

Slade, A., Belsky, J., Aber, J. L., & Phelps, J. L. (1999). Mothers' representations of their relationships with their toddlers: Links to adult attachment and observed mothering. *Developmental Psychology, 35,* 611–619.

Slade, A., & Cohen, L. (1996). The process of parenting and remembrance of things past. *Infant Mental Health Journal, 17,* 217–238.

Slade, A., Grienenberger, J., Bernbach, E., Levy, D., & Locker, A. (2005). Maternal reflective functioning, attachment, and the transmission gap: A preliminary study. *Attachment and Human Development, 7,* 283–298.

Solomon, J., & George, C. (1996). Defining the caregiving system: Toward a theory of caregiving. *Infant Mental Health Journal, 17*, 183–197.

Solomon, J., & George, C. (1999). The caregiving system in mothers of infants: A comparison of divorcing and married mothers. *Attachment and Human Development, 1*, 171–190.

Solomon, J., & George, C. (2000). Toward an integrated theory of caregiving. In J. Osofsky & H. Fitzgerald (Eds.), *World Association of Infant Mental Health handbook of infant mental health* (pp. 323–368). New York: Wiley.

Solomon, J., & George, C. (2006). Intergenerational transmission of dysregulated maternal caregiving: Mothers describe their upbringing and childrearing. In O. Mayseless (Ed.), *Parenting representations: Theory, research, and clinical implications* (pp. 265–295). New York: Cambridge University Press.

Solomon, J., George, C., & De Jong, A. (1995). Children classified as controlling at age six: Evidence of disorganized representational strategies and aggression at home and at school. *Development and Psychopathology, 7*, 447–463.

Spiegel, D. (1990). Hypnosis, dissociation, and trauma: Hidden and overt observers. In J. L. Singer (Ed.), *Repression and dissociation: Implications for personality theory, psychopathology, and health* (pp. 121–142). Chicago: University of Chicago Press.

Teti, D. M., Gelfand, D. M., Messinger, D. S., & Isabella, R. (1995). Maternal depression and the quality of early attachment: An examination of infants, preschoolers, and their mothers. *Developmental Psychology, 31*, 364–376.

van IJzendoorn, M. H., Schuengel, C., & Bakermans-Kranenburg, M. J. (1999). Disorganized attachment in early childhood: Meta-analysis of precursors, concomitants, and sequelae. *Development and Psychopathology, 11*, 225–249.

West, M., Adam, K., Spreng, S., & Rose, S. (2001). Attachment disorganization and dissociative symptoms in clinically treated adolescents. *Canadian Journal of Psychiatry, 46*, 627–631.

West, M., Spreng, S., Rose, S. M., & Adam, K. S. (1999). Relationship between attachment-felt security and history of suicidal behaviours in clinical adolescents. *Canadian Journal of Psychiatry, 44*, 578–583.

Willemsen-Swinkels, S. H. N., & Buitelaar, J. K. (2000). Insecure and disorganized attachment in children with a pervasive developmental disorder: Relationship with social interaction and heart rate. *Journal of Child Psychology and Psychiatry, 41*, 759–767.

Zeanah, C. H., & Anders, T. F. (1987). Subjectivity in parent–infant relationships: A discussion of internal working models. *Infant Mental Health Journal, 8*, 237–250.

Zeanah, C. H., Benoit, D., Hirschberg, L., & Barton, M. L. (1993). *Working model of the Child Interview: Rating scales and classification.* Unpublished manuscript, Lousiana State University School of Medicine, New Orleans.

Zeanah, C. H., Benoit, D., Hirschberg, L., & Barton, M. L. (1994). Mothers' representations of their infants are concordant with infant attachment classification. *Developmental Issues in Psychiatry and Psychology, 1*, 1–14.

APPENDIX 6.1. Caregiving Helplessness Questionnaire

Directions: This section of questions will explore how it feels to be _____ [name of child]'s parent and, more specifically, how it feels when you and your child are together. The following statements describe how some parents feel about their relationships with their child. Read each statement carefully and circle the number that most clearly reflects your relationship with your child.

1	2	3	4	5
Not characteristic at all		Somewhat characteristic		Very characteristic

1. When I am with my child, I often feel out of control.　　1 2 3 4 5
2. My child is good at tending to and caring for others.　　1 2 3 4 5
3. I am frightened of my child.　　1 2 3 4 5
4. My child hits, kicks, or bites me.　　1 2 3 4 5
5. I often feel that there is nothing I can do to discipline my child.　　1 2 3 4 5
6. My child knows how to put other people at ease.　　1 2 3 4 5
7. When I am with my child, I often feel that my child is out of control.　　1 2 3 4 5
8. I feel that my child is a great actor/actress.　　1 2 3 4 5
9. My child is very sensitive to the feelings and needs of others.　　1 2 3 4 5
10. I feel that I am a failure as a mother.　　1 2 3 4 5
11. My child likes to be a clown or family comedian.　　1 2 3 4 5
12. I feel that I punish my child more harshly than I should.　　1 2 3 4 5
13. My child becomes so upset or distressed that he can't be soothed.　　1 2 3 4 5
14. My child loses it when he/she is separated from me.　　1 2 3 4 5
15. Sometimes my child acts as if he/she is afraid of me.　　1 2 3 4 5
16. I enjoy doing things with my child that make him or her happy.　　1 2 3 4 5
17. My child is always trying to make others laugh.　　1 2 3 4 5
18. I feel that my situation needs to be changed but am helpless to do anything about it.　　1 2 3 4 5

19. I would describe myself as a reliable person.   1   2   3   4   5

20. I feel that my life is chaotic and out of control.   1   2   3   4   5

21. I am rarely bored when I am with my child.   1   2   3   4   5

22. My child treats me in a rude or sarcastic way.   1   2   3   4   5

23. I am happy with myself just the way I am.   1   2   3   4   5

24. I rarely feel guilty about my actions.   1   2   3   4   5

25. I can easily express myself to others.   1   2   3   4   5

26. I frequently talk to others about my child.   1   2   3   4   5

Scoring instructions:

1. The following items are fillers and are not included in analyses: 16, 19, 21, 23, 24, 25, 26. Do not include these scores in the factor totals.
2. Helplessness scores = summary score for each factor.

Three conceptual groupings of five factors, acceptable Bartlett's and Kaiser–Meyer–Olkin, Varimax rotation, Eigenvalues ≥ 1.5, explained 42% variance, loadings ≥ .5, alpha coefficient, .59–.85

Factors:

Factor 1: Mother Helpless
1 M out of control
5 M can't discipline
7 C out of control
10 M feels she's a failure
18 M feels helpless to make changes
20 M feels life chaotic
22 C is rude

Factor 2: Mother and Child Frightened

3 M is frightened	(original factor = Mother frightened)
4 C hits M	(original factor = Mother frightened)
12 M punishes too harshly	(original factor = Child frightened)
13 M can't soothe C	(original factor = Child frightened)
14 C loses it when separated from M	(original factor = Mother frightened)
15 C acts afraid of M	(original factor = Child frightened)

Factor 3: Child Caregiving

2 C caregiving	(original factor = Child caregiving)
6 C puts others at ease	(original factor = Child caregiving)
8 C is a great actor	(original factor = Child cheers mother)
9 C sensitive to others	(original factor = Child caregiving)
11 C is a clown	(original factor = Child cheers mother)
17 C makes others laugh	(original factor = Child cheers mother)

Chapter 7

Pathways from Disorganized Attachment to Later Social–Emotional Problems

The Role of Gender and Parent–Child Interaction Patterns

NANCY L. HAZEN, DEBORAH JACOBVITZ,
KRISTINA N. HIGGINS, SYDNYE ALLEN, and MI YOUNG JIN

A growing number of studies suggest that children who had disorganized attachment relationships with their mothers in infancy are at risk for the development of social–emotional problems by middle childhood. However, results differ as to whether they find that infant–mother attachment disorganization predicts later externalizing problems, internalizing problems, or both. The primary purpose of this chapter is to present a case for considering the role of child gender in predicting whether and how disorganized children develop particular types of social–emotional problems by middle childhood. We argue that by middle childhood, boys and girls may develop different strategies for coping with caregivers who seem frightening due to helpless, dissociative, and/or hostile behavior. These strategies may stem from biologically based differences in the reactions of boys and girls to frightening maternal behavior early in development as well as from the differential socialization of boys and girls over the course of early and middle childhood.

We first present a theoretical rationale for this idea, beginning by reviewing the literature on the relation of attachment disorganization to the later development of internalizing and externalizing symptoms, and then arguing that disorganized boys and girls are likely to follow different pathways in the development of such problems and to experience different outcomes by middle childhood. Next, we use data from our recent longitudinal study to examine these ideas both quantitatively and qualitatively. In Study 1, we examine whether disorganized attachment interacts with gender to predict children's internalizing and externalizing problems in middle childhood, and whether maternal caregiving patterns in infancy differ for disorganized girls and boys. In Study 2, case studies of disorganized girls and boys who were rated by their teachers and/or parents as being in the clinical or borderline range for internalizing or externalizing problems are examined to look for early patterns of mother–child interaction that might be used to generate hypotheses for future research concerning why some children take a path toward having primarily externalizing problems while others develop internalizing problems.

THE SEQUELAE OF ATTACHMENT DISORGANIZATION

According to attachment theory, the adaptive function of the attachment relationship is to protect infants from harm; thus, infants monitor their caregiver's whereabouts and seek proximity or signal for help when faced with real or perceived danger (Bowlby, 1982). Infants who are securely attached have experienced caregivers who have generally responded sensitively to their cues; thus, they internalize a mental representation of the self as worthy of care and others as able to provide reassurance in times of distress. This is not true of insecure–avoidant infants, whose caregivers often ignore or reject their signals for comfort, and insecure–resistant infants, whose caregivers are typically inconsistently available. Nonetheless, these infants are theorized to develop consistent strategies for coping with caregivers who provide inadequate care: avoidant infants try to minimize attachment cues such as crying or seeking proximity when distressed, so as to please caregivers who are uncomfortable with displays of needy negative emotions, whereas resistant infants maximize attachment cues, showing high levels of fussing and clinging to keep their inconsistent caregivers nearby (see Cassidy & Shaver, 2008, for more lengthy discussion).

However, in the case of disorganized attachment, the infant is believed to fear the caregiver herself. According to Main and Hesse (1990), the caregiver appears to enter into trance-like dissociative states during which she may display frightening behavior such as grabbing the infant from behind, using a haunted tone of voice, or acting frightened of the infant. George and Solomon (2008) proposed that caregivers who have disorganized infants appear helpless. Finally, Lyons-Ruth and her colleagues (Lyons-Ruth, Bronfman, & Parsons, 1999) proposed that these caregivers' hostile and helpless representations of their own childhood attachment relationships contribute to intrusive, disruptive, and often hostile interactive communication with children. All of these patterns of care are likely to be frightening to infants who must rely on their caregivers for protection and comfort in the face of perceived threat. When the infant needs comfort, he or she is trapped in a paradoxical situation: the person who should be the infant's source of comfort in stressful or frightening situations is simultaneously a source of fear (Main & Hesse, 1990). Disorganized infants thus experience a collapse of behavioral strategies for dealing with that fear, resulting in the signs of fearfulness, disoriented behaviors (e.g., postural stilling and dazed affect), and mistimed movements associated with disorganized attachment (Main & Solomon, 1990).

Studies using laboratory reunion procedures designed to assess attachment security in early childhood have found that most children who were disorganized in infancy are classified as controlling by 6 years of age (Marvin & Britner, 2008; Solomon & George, 2008). The majority of these children have been found to shift their focus away from their unsuccessful attempts at seeking comfort for their own needs to develop role-reversed controlling strategies to cope with their inadequate caregivers, although some persist in showing disorganized behaviors, indicating that they still have not developed a coping strategy (Moss, Bureau, St-Laurent, & Tarabulsy, Chapter 3, this volume). Controlling children develop either controlling–punitive strategies, using hostile, power-assertive tactics to gain the caregiver's attention, or controlling–caregiving strategies, suppressing their own negative affect and acting cheerfully overbright and solicitous to the caregiver.

Because disorganized infants lack a strategy for obtaining the comfort they need and relieving their distress, they would be expected to be at high risk for emotional dysregulation, and ultimately, for developing behavior problems related to such dysregulation, including internalizing and externalizing disorders (Lyons-Ruth & Jacobvitz, 2008). Even though most disorganized children do eventually adopt role-reversed controlling strategies, these strategies are theorized to be relatively inadequate for getting the caregiver to attend to the child's emotional needs, provide comfort when needed, and thereby assist the child in developing self-regulation. Controlling strategies, whether punitive or caregiving, are based on maintaining engagement with the caregiver by focusing on *her* emotional needs, either exploiting her emotional vulnerabilities with humiliating, punitive attacks, or attempting to please or cheer her up when she appears unhappy or distant. Although these strategies may often succeed in engaging the caregiver, thus giving the child some sense of predictability and control, they fail to draw the caregiver's attention to meeting the child's *own* emotional needs (Lyons-Ruth, Easterbrooks, & Cibelli, 1997). In fact, controlling children may feel added pressure to appear supercompetent to their caregivers, while at the same time receiving no relief for their own distress (Moss, Cyr, & Dubois-Comtois, 2004; Moss, Bureau, St-Laurent,& Tarabulsy, Chapter 3, this volume). Thus, controlling and persistently disorganized children should be at risk for later development of emotional and behavior problems related to emotional dysregulation.

A growing body of literature suggests that this is the case. A meta-analysis of 12 studies published in 1999 (van IJzendoorn, Schuengel, & Bakermans-Kranenburg, 1999), as well as an updated meta-analysis of 34 studies (Fearon, Bakermans-Kranenburg, van IJzendoorn, Lapsley, & Roisman, 2010), indicated a robust association between both disorganized attachment assessed in infancy and controlling attachment assessed in childhood, and children's later development of externalizing symptoms. Disorganized or controlling attachment has also been linked to internalizing symptoms in early childhood (Shaw, Keenan, Vondra, Delliquadri, & Giovannelli, 1997; Moss, Bureau, Cyr, Mongeau, & St. Laurent, 2004) and middle childhood (Carlson, 1998; Moss, Rousseau, Parent, St. Laurent, & Saintonge, 1998; Moss, Cyr, & Dubois-Comtois, 2004; Moss et al., 2006), although there is less data linking early attachment disorganization to internalizing problems than to externalizing problems.

Although disorganized and controlling attachment clearly puts children at risk for developing social–emotional problems, it is less clear why some studies find links only with externalizing problems (e.g., Lyons-Ruth et al., 1997; Solomon, George, & DeJong, 1995), while others find links only with internalizing problems (e.g., Carlson, 1998), and still others find links with both (e.g., Moss et al., 2004, 2006; Shaw et al., 1997). The meta-analytic studies examining the relation between disorganized/controlling attachment and later externalizing problems found a wide range of effect sizes, suggesting that the relationship between these factors is complex (van IJzendoorn et al., 1999; Fearon et al., 2010). Thus, the growing literature on the sequelae of attachment disorganization indicates that there are diverse pathways from disorganized attachment to the development of externalizing or internalizing problems (Moss et al., Chapter 3, this volume).

Lyons-Ruth et al. (1997) speculated that the type of controlling strategy used by disorganized children—punitive or caregiving—may influence the extent to which these children develop later externalizing or internalizing problems. Although both types of strategies result in frustration of attachment needs and emotional dysregulation, controlling–punitive children may be at greater risk for exhibiting externalizing problems since the hostile control strategies they used with their mothers may carry over to interactions with peers. In one of the few studies that examined controlling–punitive and controlling–caregiver groups separately, controlling–punitive children ages 5–7 were rated concurrently by their teachers as higher in externalizing symptoms, and controlling–caregiving children were rated as higher on internalizing symptoms, compared to other children (Moss, Cyr, & Dubois-Comtois, et al., 2004). A study by George and Solomon (Chapter 6, this volume) suggested that mothers of punitive children report their children's externalizing behavior as a major source of parental stress, whereas mothers of caregiving children do not report that they are stressful or have problems.

But what factors might influence whether a child adopts a caregiving or a punitive stance? And why do some children respond to emotional stress by externalizing their negative emotions, showing hostility and overt aggression, while other children suppress their fearful, negative emotions and strive to please? Abundant evidence suggests that gender differences may be one important factor leading to divergent developmental outcomes.

DISORGANIZED GIRLS AND BOYS: DIFFERENT PATHWAYS AND DIFFERENT OUTCOMES?

Disorganized girls and boys may experience different developmental outcomes for two key reasons: (1) based on biological predispositions, they may respond differently to the stress brought on by maternal disorganized caregiving during their early development; and (2) socialization agents, particularly parents at first, and later teachers and peers, may respond differentially to children's expressions of emotion, particularly negative emotions such as fear and anger, in accordance with gender-role stereotypes. Concerning the first reason, David and Lyons-Ruth (2005) found that as maternal behavior becomes more frightening, infant girls are more likely to approach their mothers than are infant boys. Citing a hypothesis proposed by Taylor and her colleagues (2000), they proposed that whereas male infants are more likely to respond to stress with "flight or fight," female infants are more likely to "tend and befriend" the source of stress. Taylor and her colleagues argued that for female primates, fleeing or attacking is less adaptive than "tending and befriending," that is, attempting to appease or affiliate with the source of threat, since it would interfere with protecting offspring. They presented evidence indicating that hormones that facilitate mother–infant attachment, particularly oxytocin, are implicated in the female tendency to tend and befriend.

More recently, del Guidice (2009) presented an evolutionary biological model suggesting that links between attachment security and differential reproductive strategies could lead to different developmental trajectories for insecurely attached boys versus girls beginning in middle childhood. Based on data indicating that attachment measures obtained in middle childhood (but not earlier) indicate that boys are more likely to show avoidant patterns of attachment and girls to show ambivalent patterns (del Guidice, 2008), he suggested that early insecure attachment acts as a cue for environmental risk, which in turn acts as a biological trigger to predispose insecure children toward reproductive strategies emphasizing earlier reproduction and less parental investment. He further argued that an optimal strategy for males would be an avoidant-type strategy in romantic/sexual relationships, emphasizing short-term relationships with little emotional commitment. In contrast, it may be more adaptive for insecure females to adopt an ambivalent-type strategy by coupling impulsive mating with high requests for commitment. Finally, del Guidice suggested that adrenarche, a period of intense endocrine development beginning at about age 6, may be the hormonal mechanism underlying the shift toward these different developmental trajectories. His model did not address attachment disorganization per se, but given that attachment disorganization should also be a strong signal of environmental risk, the same mechanisms ought to apply. The biological models proposed by David and Lyons-Ruth and by del Guidice share similarities in that both models propose that males and females respond to stress differently—males with aggression and/or avoidance (fight or flight), and females by showing a stronger tendency to affiliate—and both models propose that these differential stress responses are hormonally mediated. At present, both models are quite speculative and need further empirical testing.

Concerning the second reason for differential gender outcomes, to the extent that there are hormonally based tendencies toward flight or fight versus tend and befriend that begin at birth and/or at the beginning of middle childhood, they are likely to become stronger as children develop gender identity and are increasingly socialized by parents, teachers, and peers in accordance with gender-role stereotypes. Decades of research on gender-role socialization indicates that parents provide differential experiences and reinforcement for sons and daughters that promote the development of self-assertive, competitive, and dominant behaviors in sons and compliant, relationship-enhancing behavior in daughters (e.g., Fagot & Leinbach, 1987; Leaper, 1992). For example, during the toddler and preschool years, parents are more likely to encourage dependent behavior in daughters and autonomy in sons (Lytton & Romney, 1991). Fathers in particular are more likely to engage sons in rough physical play (Lindsey, Mize, & Pettit, 1997), but may actively discourage such play in daughters (Fagot, 1978). Through the play materials they provide their children as well as in their play interactions, parents encourage gender-typed pretend play, centered around domestic and caregiving themes with girls and action and adventure themes that often involve enactment of conflict and aggression with boys (Lytton & Romney, 1991). Parents also socialize gender-typed differences in emotional expression. For example, as early as infancy, mothers are more likely to disapprove of the expression of anger by daughters (e.g., by frowning) and support it in sons (e.g., by expressing empathy) (Malatesa & Haviland, 1982).

As children enter peer groups, peer socialization is likely to reinforce these emerging gender differences. Beginning around age 3–4 and continuing throughout middle childhood, children's peer groups become increasingly gender-segregated and children's social behavior becomes increasingly gender-typed; girls' peer groups are characterized by more compliance and negotiation, whereas boys' peer groups are characterized by more competition, dominance, and conflict (Maccoby, 1990). Preschool children also show reliable gender differences in how they cope with anger during peer conflict, such that boys are more likely to react with aggressive retaliation and to vent their anger (Fabes & Eisenberg, 1992), whereas girls are more likely to try to mask their anger (Underwood, Coie, & Herbsman, 1992), to diffuse conflict, or to seek social support or adult help (Miller, Danaher, & Forbes, 1986; Wertlieb, Weigel, & Feldstein, 1987).

These normative gender differences in coping styles have clear parallels to the flight or fight versus tend and befriend strategies described by Taylor et al. (2002). Externalizing and internalizing symptoms can be viewed as extreme, maladaptive versions of these two gender-typed coping styles. Thus, in extremely dysregulated children (such as disorganized children), boys may tend to develop externalizing symptoms and girls to develop internalizing symptoms. Numerous studies of clinically referred adolescents support this idea: boys referred for externalizing disorders outnumber girls by a ratio of about 2 to1, whereas the reverse is true for internalizing disorders (Huselid & Cooper, 1994; Whitley & Gridley, 1993).

Because attachment theory did not propose a role for gender, and also because disorganized groups are typically too small to effectively examine interactions between attachment and gender, studies of the relation of early attachment to later developmental outcomes have rarely examined the possibility that girls and boys with disorganized attachment might experience different developmental outcomes. However, a few studies indicate that child gender and attachment security do interact in predicting preschool children's developmental adaptation with peers. For example, Cutler and Hazen (1995) found that when 4-year-olds were taught how to complete a difficult task and later paired with a same-age, same-sex peer who had never experienced the task, both boys and girls who had been securely attached in infancy showed more balanced interactions with the peer and were more likely to work cooperatively while completing the task than did children classified as insecure. In contrast, insecure boys tended to dominate and control the task, typically telling the peer that he was doing it incorrectly and taking over the task completely, while insecure girls tended to let the peer dominate, often standing by passively and giggling awkwardly while the peer repeatedly tried to do the task incorrectly. Similarly, Turner (1991) found that insecure 4-year-old boys were more disruptive, aggressive, and attention seeking in peer interaction than secure boys, whereas insecure 4-year-old girls were more compliant, dependant, and pleasing with peers compared to more assertive secure girls. Thus, insecure attachment may accentuate gender-role stereotypes of male dominance and aggression, and female submission and compliance, whereas secure attachment may predict more flexible, balanced patterns of peer interaction for both boys and girls.

Although infant disorganization was not examined in these studies, we hypothesized that similar gender-related patterns might be found among disorganized children; that is, infants with disorganized attachment strategies should be more likely than infants with organized strategies to develop externalizing or internalizing behavior problems by middle childhood. In addition, boys and girls should show exaggerated gender-role stereotypes in their maladaptive outcomes, such that boys should be more likely to develop externalizing problems and girls to develop internalizing problems.

To test the above hypothesis, we examined both quantitative data (Study 1) and qualitative case study data (Study 2) from our longitudinal study, the Partners and Parents Project, following infants who were disorganized with their mothers in the Strange Situation until they were 7 years old. In Study 1, we examined whether disorganized attachment assessed in infancy predicts later externalizing problems primarily for boys and internalizing problems primarily for girl. Given that studies have shown that maternal frightened–frightening (FR) caregiving behavior predicts infant attachment disorganization (Schuengel, van IJzendoorn, & Bakermans-Kranenburg, 1999; Abrams, Rifkin, & Hesse, 2006), we also examined whether mothers show different levels of frightening caregiving to boys versus girls, and whether such differences predict later internalizing and externalizing problems for boys versus girls. Moreover, we examined attachment disorganization and gender as possible predictors of teacher- and mother-rated social problems and thought problems. *Social problems* assesses peer rejection and other peer problems (e.g., doesn't get along with peers, not liked by peers, teased), and *thought problems* assesses odd behaviors including obsessions, compulsions, and nervous or strange behaviors, both of which have been linked with disorganized attachment in previous studies (e.g., Jacobvitz & Hazen, 1999; Carlson, 1998). In Study 2, we examined case studies of girls and boys who were disorganized in infancy and rated at age 7–8 by parents or teachers as within the clinical or borderline-clinical range for internalizing or externalizing problems, or both, to generate testable hypotheses concerning possible family-based explanations for why different disorganized children experience different outcomes by age 7–8, and whether child gender helps explain these differences.

STUDIES 1 AND 2: THE PARTNERS AND PARENTS PROJECT

Method

Participants

The primary purpose of this longitudinal study has been to investigate the relationship of parents' attachment representations to their subsequent marital, caregiving, parent–child attachment, and family interaction patterns, and to investigate the relation of all these factors to children's developmental outcomes. When the women were in their third trimester of pregnancy, 125 couples were recruited through birthing classes, public service radio announcements, and flyers distributed at maternity stores in the Austin area. Only couples expecting their first child and living together (94.4% were married) were included in the study. Couples were mostly middle class, with a median family income of $30,000–$45,000, and the mean age of participants was 30.5 years. The majority reported education beyond the high school level, with 60% earning a bachelor's or graduate degree and another 30% reporting some college or trade/business school coursework. Ethnic distribution was predominantly Caucasian (85%), but also included Hispanic (8%), African American (3%), and "other" (4%).

By the 8-month visit (Phase 2), 121 of the original 125 mothers remained in the study. By the time children were 7–8 years old (Phase 4), 85 families from the original sample remained in the study. Of the 40 subjects that left the study, 21 had moved away and could not be home-visited, 14 could not be located, and five dropped out for personal reasons. Lower income families were more likely to drop out of the study than middle-class families; however, the sample available at Phase 4 did not differ significantly from the sample at 8 or 12–15 months in gender ratio, maternal FR caregiving scores, or distribution of attachment classifications.

Procedures and Measures

Families participated in four phases of data collection. During Phase 1 (Prenatal, when the mother was in her third trimester of pregnancy), couples were videotaped in their homes during a marital interaction task and completed several self-report measures. Later, during a lab visit, the Adult Attachment Interview (George, Kaplan & Main, 1985/1996) was separately administered to both members of each couple.

During Phase 2 (Infancy), mothers and fathers were videotaped separately while interacting with their 8-month-old infants in their own homes for about 30 minutes to assess their caregiving quality. Parents were asked to feed and play with their infant and change his or her clothes as they normally would. Later, videotapes of 121 mother–infant interactions were rated on a 9-point scale using the FR coding system developed by Main and Hesse (1995). Half of the videotapes were rated by two different coders for reliability (intraclass correlation = .68.) Couples were also videotaped in another marital interaction task.

When infants were 12 and 15 months old, they were assessed in a lab setting for security of attachment with both mother and father using the Strange Situation procedure (Ainsworth, Blehar, Waters, & Wall, 1978). The order in which mothers and fathers were observed in the Strange Situation with their infant was counterbalanced. Classification of organized (secure, avoidant, and resistant, or A, B, C) attachment was based on Ainsworth et al.'s (1978) coding system, and classification of disorganized (D) attachment was based on Main and Solomon's (1990) system. Usable data was obtained from 111 mother–infant dyads and 66% of these were double-coded for interrater reliablity (kappa = .79, $p < .001$, for A-B-C attachment and kappa = .95, $p < .001$, for D vs. not-D).

During Phase 3 (Toddlerhood), the 108 remaining families participated in two visits. During the home visit, mothers, fathers, and their 24-month-old toddlers participated together in a triadic interaction task in which parents were required to change the child's clothes, prepare and eat a snack together, and jointly complete a task while keeping their child occupied. Parents were also observed again in a marital interaction task, and each parent was individually administered a caregiving interview (George & Solomon, 1993) to assess each parent's representation of his or her relationship with their child. During the lab visit, mothers and fathers were observed separately while interacting with their child in free play, cleanup, and structured teaching tasks. While one parent interacted with the child, the other parent was interviewed once again using the Adult Attachment Interview. Finally, to obtain assessments of the toddler's autonomy and emotion regulation independent of the parent, children were observed interacting with a research assistant in a challenging problem-solving task and in a frustrating situation (a Barrier Box task, in which attractive toys are displayed in a plexiglass box but are inaccessible without adult assistance).

Phase 4 (Childhood) focused on assessments of child outcomes when the children were 7 years old. Specifically, parents completed the Child Behavior Checklist (CBCL), and teachers who knew the child for at least 3 months completed the Teacher Report Form (TRF), to assess children's social–emotional problems (Achenbach, 1991). Father CBCLs were not included in the present study because fathers have been found to be less reliable reporters than teachers and mothers (Seiffge-Krenke & Kollmar, 1998), and also because many fathers failed to return their questionnaires. Usable CBCL data was obtained from 80 of the 85 families participating at this phase, and usable TRFs were obtained from 70 teachers. In addition, 74 children were interviewed in their homes using an abridged version of the Berkeley

Puppet Interview (BPI) to assess their perceptions of themselves and their relationships with parents and peers (Ablow & Measelle, 1993). The children were interviewed with two puppets, one making a positive statement and the other a negative statement, then asking the child which puppet he or she is most like (e.g., "My mommy likes to play with me,", "My mommy doesn't like to play with me", "How about you?"). After administering the interview, interviewers rated several aspects of the child's behavior during the interview procedure using 7-point Likert scales, including the extent to which each child seemed anxious about performing the task correctly and doing a good job. Only the rating of child anxiety in the interview will be examined in Study 1, since the primary goal of this study is to examine gender and attachment as predictors of social–emotional problems in middle childhood. However, in Study 2, children's views of self and others obtained from the puppet interview data will be examined at a qualitative level.

Study 1 Results

Descriptive Statistics

Table 7.1 shows the breakdown of attachment classifications for girls and boys at Phase 2, when Strange Situation data were administered, and at Phase 4, for the children for whom mother and teacher ratings were available. No gender differences in distribution of attachment classification, including disorganization, were found for either phase.

Significant correlations were found between teacher-rated and mother-rated internalizing problems, $r(22) = .50$, $p < .05$, thought problems, $r(22) =$

TABLE 7.1. Breakdown of Attachment Classifications by Child Gender

	Avoidant	Secure	Resistant	Disorganized	Total
Whole Strange Situation sample					
Girls	3	20	4	17	44
Boys	9	27	11	20	67
Sample with teacher ratings available					
Girls	1	13	3	9	26
Boys	6	13	8	13	40
Sample with mother ratings available					
Girls	3	16	3	10	32
Boys	6	15	9	15	45

.48, $p < .05$, and social problems, $r(22) = .61$, $p < .01$, but not externalizing problems, $r(22) = .07$, ns. Interestingly, however, mother ratings for social problems were highly correlated with teacher ratings for externalizing problems, $r(22) = .60$, $p < .01$, internalizing problems, $r(22) = .50$, $p < .05$, and thought problems, $r(22) = .61$, $p < .01$. No other mother and teacher ratings were significantly correlated.

Disorganized Attachment and Gender as Predictors of Social–Emotional Problems

To examine whether children who were classified at age 12–15 months as disorganized are more likely than children with organized attachment relationships to show social–emotional problems at ages 7–8, and whether these predictive relations interact with gender, we performed nine two-way ANOVAs (analysis of variance) in which attachment disorganization (disorganized vs. organized) and child gender were entered as independent variables and the dependant variables were teacher-rated T-scores from the TRF and mother-rated T-scores from the CBCL for *externalizing, internalizing, social,* and *thought problems,* as well as the interviewer ratings of children's performance anxiety in the puppet interview task (BPI). Table 7.2 shows the means and standard deviations for these dependant variables broken down by attachment classification (organized vs. disorganized) and gender, as well as the results of each analysis.

For the teacher ratings, disorganized children were rated by teachers as having significantly higher ratings for internalizing and social problems than children who had been classified as having organized attachment relationships (see Table 7.2). In addition, boys had significantly higher ratings for externalizing, social, and thought problems than did girls, but boys and girls did not differ in teacher-rated internalizing problems. However, as shown in Figure 7.1, these main effects were all qualified by interactions between attachment and gender, indicating that significant differences between organized and disorganized attachment were found only for boys, although the interaction was only marginally significant for internalizing problems.

Regarding the mother ratings, the results of the analysis for social problems was very similar to the results found for teacher ratings of social problems; in both cases, we found significant main effects for attachment and gender as well as a significant interaction between the two (see Table 7.2). As shown in Figure 7.2, disorganized boys were rated significantly higher in social problems than disorganized girls or children who had organized attachment classifications. No other relations between disorganized attachment and mother-rated social-emotional problems were found, although a significant effect for gender was also found for internalizing problems and

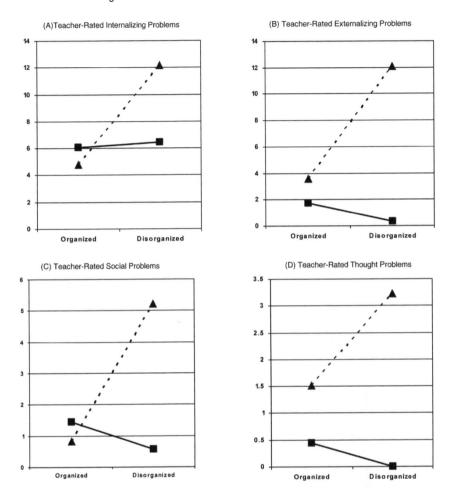

FIGURE 7.1. Interactions between disorganized attachment and gender for teacher ratings of social–emotional problems. - - -, boys; ———, girls.

a marginally significant effect for gender was found for thought problems, with boys being rated higher than girls in both cases.

Taken together, these data suggest that disorganized status was a significant risk factor for later social-emotional problems for boys, but not girls. In fact, mean levels of teacher-rated externalizing, social, and thought problems, as well as mother-rated social problems, are actually *lower* for girls who were classified in infancy as disorganized, compared to girls who had an organized attachment classification, although the differences in these ratings for organized versus disorganized girls were not statistically signifi-

TABLE 7.2. Means and Standard Deviations of Ratings of Children's Emotional/Behavior Problems at Age 7–8, by Attachment Classification (Organized vs. Disorganized) and Child Gender

Measures of emotional/ behavior problems		Organized		Disorganized		Significant results
		Boys	Girls	Boys	Girls	
Teacher ratings: ($n = 66$)						
Internalizing	Mean	51.78	52.35	62.15	53.11	Attach: $F(3,62) = 4.62$*
	SD	9.78	8.85	9.86	10.94	Gen × Att: $F(3,62) = 3.45$†
Externalizing	Mean	49.26	50.65	58.23	45.33	Gen: $F(3,62) = 7.37$**
	SD	7.56	6.80	11.26	4.69	Gen × Att: $F(3,62) = 11.37$**
Thought problems	Mean	55.70	53.24	62.92	50.00	Gen: $F(3,62) = 18.05$***
	SD	8.49	4.22	7.87	0.00	Gen × Att: $F(3,62) = 8.33$**
Social problems	Mean	52.59	54.59	63.69	52.11	Attach: $F(3,62) = 6.10$*
	SD	4.05	5.32	11.79	3.76	Gen: $F(3,62) = 7.54$**
						Gen × Att: $F(3,62) = 15.13$***

Measures of emotional/ behavior problems		Organized		Disorganized		Significant results
		Boys	Girls	Boys	Girls	
Mother ratings: ($n = 7$)						
Internalizing	Mean	53.77	49.09	54.64	46.40	Gen: $F(3,73) = 7.74^{**}$
	SD	8.63	9.78	8.55	11.24	
Externalizing	Mean	53.87	50.64	53.36	51.60	All n.s.
	SD	9.12	6.15	8.76	7.79	All n.s.
Thought problems	Mean	55.94	54.05	55.36	52.20	Gen: $F(3,73) = 3.64^{\dagger}$
	SD	6.18	5.25	4.57	2.44	
Social problems	Mean	52.06	53.36	57.71	52.80	Attach: $F(3,73) = 7.16^{**}$
	SD	3.33	4.03	5.20	1.99	Gen: $F(3,73) = 3.61^{\dagger}$ Gen × Att: $F(3,73) = 10.68^{**}$
Interviewer rating: ($n = 74$)						
Interview task performance anxiety	Mean	5.97	5.69	5.55	6.29	Gen × Att: $F(3,70) = 3.10^{\dagger}$
	SD	.18	.25	.32	.36	

Note. Attach, attachment classification; Gen, child gender,

$^{\dagger}p < .10$; $^{*}p < .05$; $^{**}p < .01$; $^{***}p < .001$.

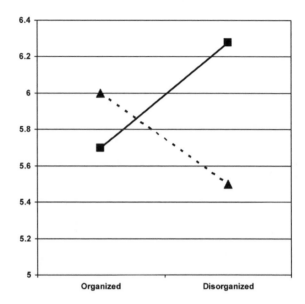

FIGURE 7.2. Interaction between disorganized attachment and gender for mother ratings of social-emotional problems. - - -, boys; ———, girls.

cant. However, results for interviewer-rated performance anxiety, shown in Figure 7.3, revealed a marginally significant interaction (see Table 7.2) between disorganized attachment and gender showing the *opposite* pattern for gender: girls classified as disorganized appeared to be the *most* anxious about performing well in the interview, and disorganized boys appeared to be the *least* anxious.

We next examined the relation of attachment disorganization and gender to *extreme* internalizing and externalizing problems (i.e., ratings within the clinical and borderline-clinical range). Of the 39 boys for whom teacher ratings were available, 6/13 (46%) of the boys with disorganized classifications but only 4/26 (15%) of the boys with organized classifications were rated as externalizing, $x^2(2, N = 39) = 10.87, p < .01$. Not one girl was rated by teachers in the clinical range for externalizing problems, and only two (one secure and one anxious–resistant) were rated as borderline. Mothers of disorganized children were *not* more likely to rate their children as extreme in externalizing scores than were other mothers, but mothers were more likely to rate boys as clinically externalizing then girls. No mother rated her daughter as clinically externalizing, and only one mother of a secure child rated her daughter as borderline. No significant relations between mother- or teacher-rated extreme internalizing scores and either attachment disorganization or gender were found.

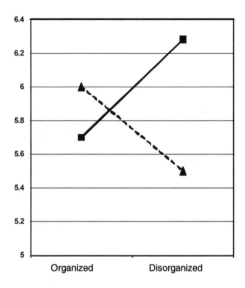

FIGURE 7.3. Interaction between disorganized attachment and gender for child anxiety during Berkeley Puppet Interview at age 7–8. - - -, boys; ——, girls.

Relation of Mother's FR Behavior to Gender, Attachment Disorganization, and Emotional/Behavior Problems

To see if FR behavior predicts disorganized attachment, and if mothers show more FR behavior to boys than girls at 8 months, a two-way ANOVA was conducted in which disorganized attachment status (organized vs. disorganized) and child gender were the independent variables and mothers' FR score was the dependent variable. Mothers were found to display significantly more FR behavior to boys ($M = 3.70$, $SD = .25$) than to girls ($M = 2.80$, $SD = .28$), $F(3,106) = 5.19$, $p < .05$. As expected, mothers' FR behavior was also associated with disorganized attachment (although the effect was marginal), $M = 3.59$ and $SD = 2.04$ for disorganized attachment versus $M = 3.01$ and $SD = 1.75$ for organized attachment, $F(3,106) = 3.30$, $p = .07$.

To examine the relation of maternal FR behavior to social–emotional problems, we correlated scores for FR behavior with mother and teacher ratings for internalizing and externalizing problems. Mother's FR behavior at 8 months was significantly correlated with teacher-rated internalizing problems, $r(69) = .33$, $p < .05$, and marginally correlated with mother-rated internalizing problems, $r(69), = .21$, p = .06. However, FR behavior was not found to predict externalizing problems.

Study 1 Discussion

As expected, we found that disorganized boys were more likely than disorganized girls, as well as children who were not disorganized in infancy, to show both higher externalizing scores and to be rated within the clinical range on externalizing problems, at least for the teacher ratings. Mother-rated externalizing problems were unrelated to attachment disorganization, but mothers also were more likely to rate boys than girls within the clinical range for externalizing problems. Mother and teacher ratings of externalizing problems were completely uncorrelated, but interestingly, mother-rated social problems were highly correlated with both teacher-rated social problems and teacher-rated externalizing problems. Also, mother-rated social problems showed the same pattern of results as teacher-rated social, thought, and externalizing problems in that disorganized boys were rated significantly higher on all these problem scales than other children. Thus, the children whom both mothers and teachers identified as being high on social problems (e.g., lonely, not liked by others, does not get along with others, teased) are the same children teachers viewed as being externalizing (e.g., aggressive and rule breaking), that is, disorganized boys. Perhaps mothers of these children recognize that their children are rejected by peers, but view this as more a result of unkind or bullying behavior by peers rather than as a result of their own child's externalizing problems. In this study, as in some other studies (Lyons-Ruth et al., 1997), mother ratings of social-emotional problems did not relate to attachment classifications, but teacher ratings did. Lyons-Ruth et al. (1997) reported that mothers of secure children tend to over-report child problems while mothers of insecure children tended to under-report them, and suggested that mothers of secure children may be more open to perceiving and acknowledging their children's emotional vulnerabilities than mothers of insecure (including disorganized) children.

We did not find internalizing problems to be higher in disorganized girls than disorganized boys; in fact, mothers rated *boys* higher on internalization. Also, although teacher ratings of internalizing problems did not differ between boys and girls, teachers tended to rate disorganized boys higher than other children on the internalizing scale. Taken together, the findings suggest that disorganized boys are at greater risk for developing all types of social-emotional problems, including internalizing problems, social problems and thought problems, as well as externalizing problems. However, we should not assume from this data that disorganized girls are not at risk. Even though mother and teacher ratings of internalizing behavior were correlated, teacher ratings but not mother ratings were related to disorganized attachment, suggesting again that mothers of disorganized children may be less open to perceiving social-emotional problems in their children. Other researchers have suggested that teachers, too, may underestimate children's internalizing problems since internalizing children are less disruptive and draw less attention in the classroom than those with externalizing problems (Kolko & Kazden, 1993).

We argue that internalizing problems may be underestimated in disorganized girls, particularly if girls are more likely than boys to eventually adopt controlling–caregiving strategies (see also George & Solomon, Chapter 6, this volume). Children using these strategies elicit caregivers' attention and approval by adopting a cheerful, supercompetent persona and thus are unlikely to give an outward appearance of being anxious or depressed. Perhaps disorganized attachment in girls might be more likely to forecast teacher ratings of children's high need for approval or perfectionism than ratings of internalizing problems. Our finding that trained, objective interviewers' ratings of children's anxiety about their performance on an interview task were higher for disorganized girls than for other children supports this idea. Of course, given that the finding is marginal and based on ratings from one relatively brief observation, it must be interpreted with caution and investigated further. The notion that girls who were disorganized as infants may eventually become overly pleasing and perfectionistic is also supported by our finding that disorganized girls were rated as extremely low on externalizing symptoms, and by results of the meta-analysis by Fearon et al. (2010) indicating that for one sample with only female participants, the relationship between attachment disorganization and externalizing behavior was actually significantly *negative*. Taken together, these data suggest that teachers viewed these girls as being near-perfect in the classroom, almost never showing any sort of disruptive behavior.

We also examined whether mothers of disorganized children are more likely to show FR behavior to boys than girls as a possible explanation of their different developmental outcomes. We did find that mothers of disorganized children show more FR behavior than other mothers, and they also are more likely to show FR behavior to boys than to girls. However, boys' higher scores in externalizing behavior did not directly result from their receiving higher levels of maternal FR caregiving in infancy, since FR behavior did not predict later externalizing problems. Rather, it predicted internalizing problems, which are likely outcomes for both disorganized boys and girls.

Perhaps maternal FR behavior, more so than disorganized attachment per se, is what leads to children's internalizing problems in particular. After all, fear of the caregiver, who is supposed to be the child's source of comfort, is assumed to be the driving force behind disorganized attachment patterns, and the source of the disorganized child's feeling that his or her emotional needs cannot be met. Thus, whereas frightening caregiving per se may predict internalizing problems for both boys and girls, mother–child interaction patterns characterized by hostility, which we expect is more characteristic of boys, may forecast externalizing problems.

In Study 2, we explore these possibilities by examining case studies of disorganized children who were rated as clinically internalizing and/or externalizing by teachers, mothers, or both by age 7, focusing in particular on the patterns of mother-child interaction that are emerging at 24 months. Unfortunately, we did not observe mother–child interactions between 24 months and 7 years. However, even in the first 2 years, mothers and children may show early signs of the sex-typed patterns we expect will become more pronounced later.

STUDY 2: CASE STUDIES OF DISORGANIZED BOYS AND GIRLS WITH EXTERNALIZING AND/OR INTERNALIZING PROBLEMS ABOVE BORDERLINE CLINICAL CUT-OFFS

Method

We first identified all cases of children who were classified as disorganized in infancy and later identified by their mothers, teachers, or both to have externalizing or internalizing problems above borderline clinical cutoffs. Ten boys and four girls met these criteria. These children were then grouped according to gender and shared social–emotional problems: Group 1 (n = 7) consists of boys rated as having both externalizing and internalizing problems (every boy rated as externalizing was also rated as internalizing); Group 2 (n = 3) consists of boys with internalizing problems who were not also externalizing; and Group 3 (n = 4) consisted of girls with internalizing problems (no disorganized girl was rated as externalizing). Three boys (two in Group 1 and one in Group 2) were dropped from the case study analysis because they lacked mother–child observational data from toddlerhood (24 months). Each case was examined in detail by two trained observers, the first author and either the third or fourth author. Data examined included parents' Adult Attachment Interviews, observations of mother–child and mother–father–child interactions at 8 and 24 months and during the Strange Situation at 12 or 15 months, mothers' caregiving interviews, and other child outcome measures (i.e., assessments of the child's performance in teaching tasks at 24 months, interviewer ratings of the child's performance anxiety in the BPI at age 7, and the child's views of self, family, and peers obtained from the BPI). Observers identified characteristic mother–child interaction patterns for each case and later met to discuss similarities and differences between the cases.

A summary of the data from each of the cases is shown in Table 7.3. The first column presents the type of social–emotional problem(s) reported for each child, whether the score was above the borderline or above the

TABLE 7.3. Summary Data: All Disorganized Children Rated within the Clinical Range for Externalizing or Internalizing Problems at Ages 7–8

	Problems in clinical range[a]	BPI anxiety[b]	BPI self/ other views	Mother AAI	Mother to infant	Infant to mother	Mother to toddler	Toddler to mother
Group 1: EXT/INT boys								
Jake	T: EXT, *Tht*, ADHD, *ODD*, *Anx*	Very low	Low self-esteem, peer rejection, marital conflict, low parent warmth	CC/E/D	Hostile–intrusive, angry punitive withdrawal	Avoidant or resistant (screams, struggles)	Hostile–intrusive, punitive withdrawal, power struggles	Avoidant or aggressive and defiant
Robert	T: EXT, INT, Tht, Soc, *Anx*, *ADHD* F: EXT, INT ODD, *Anx*	Very high	Peer rejection	U/E	Hostile, threatening, intrusive FR (scary faces), punitive withdrawal	Avoidant or resistant (hits mother)	Hostile-intrusive, punitive withdrawal, power struggles, child-like play	Avoidant or aggressive (hits mother)
Bryan	T: EXT, INT, *Tht*, Soc, *Aff*, Som, *ADHD*, ODD, *Con* F: EXT	Normative	Low self-esteem, peer rejection	D	Hostile–intrusive, punitive withdrawal	Avoidant or resistant (screams, struggles)	Hostile-intrusive, power struggles, child-like play	Avoidant or aggressive, often distressed
Clark	T: EXT, INT, Anx, *ADHD*, ODD F: *INT*, *Som*	High	Low self-esteem, peer rejection, socially withdrawn	No AAI	FR and intrusive (physically intrusive, loud, frightening faces)	Either engaged (screams back at mom) or avoidant	Intrusive, power struggles	Alternates between caregiving and punitive scolding

(*continued*)

TABLE 7.3. (continued)

	Problems in clinical range[a]	BPI anxiety[b]	BPI self/ other views	Mother AAI	Mother to infant	Infant to mother	Mother to toddler	Toddler to mother
Evan	M: *EXT*, INT, *Soc, Anx* F: *EXT, Soc*	No BPI	No BPI	U/F	FR (frightened), helpless, can't comfort or engage baby	Constantly fussy, stiff, disengaged	Very passive, asks child what she should do	Caregiving, very attentive to mom, but also bosses and scolds her
Group 2: INT boys								
Danny	T: *INT, Tht* F: INT, Tht, *Som* M: *Anx*	High	Peer rejection, marital conflict	U/CC/F	FR (extreme physical intrusions); otherwise sensitive	Inhibited, watchful, anxious	Child-like play, directs child in her play, acts helpless	Attentive to mom, compliant, controlling/ caregiving
Alex	T: *INT*	High	Marital conflict	F/U/E	FR (high physical intrusiveness); otherwise sensitive	Inhibited, watchful	Child-like play, directs child in her play, acts helpless	Attentive to mom, compliant, controlling/ caregiving
Group 2: INT girls								
Alice	T: INT, *Anx*	Very high	No negative views expressed	U/F	Very intrusive and misattuned, gets very upset and helpless when baby is distressed	Passive and watchful, or distressed by mom's intrusive behavior	Intrusive or punitively withdrawn	Attentive, compliant, caregiving, but passively resistant when she does not want to comply

188

Ella	T: *INT, Anx* M: INT, *Tht* F: *Tht*	Very high	No negative views expressed	U/CC	Intrusive, misattuned, FR (strange vocalizations, dissociating)	Passive and watchful, distressed by mom's FR and intrusive behavior	Intrusive or withdrawn	Very compliant and attentive to mom, but passively resistant when she does not want to comply
Mia	T: *INT, Aff, Som*	Very high	Socially withdrawn, marital conflict	E	Intrusive and misattuned, cannot comfort baby	Avoidant, crawls away from mom; puts head down and cries passively	Intrusive, tells child exactly what to do throughout play	Very compliant and attentive to mom, but often says "yes" to mom's orders and then does nothing
Karen	T: *INT*	Very high	No negative views expressed	No AAI	(From Strange Situation) Dissociating, misattuned, cannot comfort baby	(From Strange Situation) Inhibited, watchful	Child-like play, acts helpless, draws child into her play	Attentive to mom, very compliant

*a*Italics indicate scores in borderline clinical range; T = teacher-rated; M = mother-rated; F = father rated; EXT, externalizing problems; INT, internalizing problems; Soc, social problems; Tht, thought problems; Aff, DSM-IV affective problems, Anx, DSM-IV anxiety problems; Som, DSM-IV somatic problems; ADHD, DSM-IV attention-deficit/hyperactivity disorder; ODD, DSM-IV oppositional defiant disorder; Con, DSM-IV conduct problems.

*b*Very high = 6.5–7 on a 7-point scale; high = 5.5–6; normative = 4.5–5.5; low = 3–4; very low = below 3.

clinical level cutoff, and whether scores were reported by teacher, mother, or father. In addition to externalizing, internalizing, thought problems, and social problems, we also listed any DSM-IV scales that were rated above the cutoff. Next, child outcome measures are presented. Finally, brief descriptions are provided of mother and child behaviors during the 8-month mother–infant interactions and the 24-month mother–toddler interactions for each case.

We next chose one case with no missing data from each group to present in detail. These three cases were chosen because the three observers concurred that they seemed to present the most prototypic and complete example from each group. Following each case study, we drew general conclusions about the group from which that case was drawn, and compared that case with the group as a whole.

Study 2 Results

Group 1: Disorganized Boys with Externalizing and Internalizing Problems

THE CASE OF JAKE A

In many ways, Jake struck us as one of the most troubled children in our sample. At 24 months, he scored lower than any child in the autonomy and emotion regulation tasks. In both tasks, he would not even try to solve the problems. He simply collapsed on the floor and wailed, "No! No! No!" At age 7, Jake's teacher rated him within the clinical range on externalizing behaviors, attention problems, and the DSM-IV ADHD scale, and also within the borderline clinical range on thought problems, rule-breaking behavior, aggressive behavior, and on the DSM-IV anxiety problems and oppositional–defiant behavior scales. However, his mother, Mrs. A, rated Jake within the normal range on all scales. (His father did not complete the CBCL). His BPI at age 7 indicated that he has a low opinion of himself and of his relationships with his parent and peers. For example, when the puppets presented the choice, "Sometimes I think I'm stupid/I don't think I'm stupid," Jake firmly stated with a sad and serious expression, "Sometimes I think I'm an idiot." He also stated that his parents yelled at him, that his father was rough with him, and that his peers were mean to him and didn't want to sit next to him.

Jake's mother, Mrs. A, was classified on the AAI as "cannot classify," with an alternate classification of preoccupied. She discussed feeling responsible for protecting her mother from her father, who was alcoholic and sometimes abusive. She noted that she and her mother were "emotionally interdependent" and that she "worked hard to please [her mother]." Jake's father's prenatal AAI was inaudible and could not be scored, but his AAI at 24 months also revealed a history of abuse and inadequate care. Because he alternated between involving anger and sharp derogation when describing his childhood relationships with his parents, he was also rated as "cannot classify." Both Mr. and Mrs. A were children of divorce.

The A's marriage seemed troubled from the first prenatal marital interaction. By the 8-month triadic interaction, they openly bickered almost constantly. Their disagreements often focused on Jake, who was present:

> (8 months) When Jake approached his parents, fussing for attention, his father, Mr. A, pushed him back somewhat roughly, making him cry. Mrs. A said, "Don't treat him like that, you just make him cry every time you do that." Mr. A looked exasperated and stated that Jake "pisses everybody off sometimes." When Mr. A later criticized Mrs. A's parenting, she turned away and stared into space. Mr. A became angry and yelled, "I hate it when you do that, you zone out like you're on two thousand drugs or something!"

The amount of marital hostility displayed was the same at 24 months, and in the triadic mother–father–toddler interaction, the couple engaged in a very high degree of competitive coparenting, in which they often undermined each other's parenting in Jake's presence:

> (24 months) Jake turned on the television. Mr. A. said, "He shouldn't have that on now." Mrs. A responded, "It doesn't matter, let him if he wants to." Later, when Mr. A started to help dress Jake, Mrs. A remarked, "This never happens this way; I always do this myself." Mr. A later left to answer the phone, and Mrs. A said to Jake, "Now, this is real life. He's never here to help, right?"

The couple had divorced by the time we visited Jake for the puppet interview at age 7. In the interview, in response to the puppets' statement, "I think my parents' fights are about me," Jake stated with some relief, "They used to be, but not any more." Mrs. A probably had reason to be concerned about Mr. A's interactions with Jake, as his interactions with Jake at both 8 and 24 months were characterized by rough, hostile, and extremely frightening behavior; in fact, he was assigned a score of 9, the highest possible score, on the FR scale at 8 months.

Unlike Mr. A, Mrs. A was not rated high on the FR scale; however, she alternated between extreme emotional withdrawal, in which she did not interact or make eye contact with Jake for long periods, and hostile intrusiveness. Typically, Jake tried to avoid her or reacted with anger when she behaved in a hostile or controlling manner, and she often responded by withdrawing in a manner that seemed punitive. This pattern was observed in play interactions at 8 months, in the Strange Situation at 12 months, and again in play interactions at 24 months:

(8 months) After a long period of ignoring Jake, Mrs. A grabbed a dragon puppet, and made it "bite" his face while making growling sounds in his ear, then made a stuffed bunny "attack" him. Jake continually attempted to turn away and avoided eye contact. During the feeding session, when Mrs. A repeatedly tried to put the spoon in Jake's mouth, Jake covered his mouth, screamed, and tried to get out of his high chair. Mrs. A said, "I'll just let him sit there. Until you get hungry, and then you'll eat."

(12 months) When Mrs. A returned after the first separation, Jake started to approach her, then stopped, turned toward the wall, hung his head, then raced around the room while frantically pushing a push toy. Mrs. A did not greet or look at Jake, but walked straight to her chair. After a few minutes, Jake approached her and banged the push toy forcefully into her leg while yelling loudly and trying to grab the paper cup from which she was drinking. She said to Jake, "That's not for you." During the second reunion, Jake immediately ran to Mrs. A and grabbed her legs, but when she bent to pick him up, he backed away, staring up at her. Then, whimpering, he approached again with arms outstretched. She started to lift him by his arms, then stopped and said, "I'm not going to pick you up, then."

(24 months) Mrs. A smiled as she presented Jake with a doll to play with. Jake looked at the doll, said it was "yucky," and ran it over with a toy truck. Mrs. A laughed, and then said with a note of anger in her voice, "Don't run her [the doll] over!" Jake responded by hitting Mrs. A's leg with the truck.

Thus, by the time Jake was a toddler, he and his mother seem to have established a pattern in which Mrs. A responded to Jake with either hostile interference or emotional withdrawal, and Jake in turn responded with avoidance and ignoring, or with angry resistance or aggression.

In her caregiving interview, Mrs. A stated that she felt overwhelmed dealing with Jake much of the time, and was afraid to leave him because she feared he might accidentally die. She also expressed considerable frustration, for example, "I tried to make him this nice breakfast and he wouldn't have anything to do with it, and I had lots of things to do and, and didn't have enough time to pay the bills, and so he just, you know, screamed and threw a temper tantrum then I got mad at him and sent him to his room, you know that that's typical, that's the—, I'm stressed." As a child, Mrs. A experienced extreme role-reversal, caring for her mother and protecting her from her father; thus, she likely did not have her own needs met. Now, as a parent, she seems unable to meet the needs of her child, appearing helpless and ineffective. By criticizing her parenting rather than offering support, her husband probably adds to her feelings of helplessness and frustration.

GENERAL CHARACTERISTICS OF GROUP 1:
EXTERNALIZING AND INTERNALIZING BOYS

The case study of Jake suggests that disorganized boys whose mothers alternate between emotionally withdrawing from their children and becoming hostile and intrusive may be at risk for developing multiple problems, including *both* externalizing and internalizing problems. As shown in Table 7.3, four of the five boys in this group (all but Evan) experienced intrusive maternal care in infancy. These boys usually tried to avoid their mothers when they behaved intrusively, and when this was not possible, they typically responded by screaming or crying, struggling, and sometimes hitting their mothers (e.g., angry resistance). The mothers of these boys typically withdrew and did not respond to their infants when they behaved this way, whereupon the boys would display more anger.

During the 24-month mother–child interactions, the mothers of these four boys continued to show a pattern of intrusive care. They directed their children to play with the toys in particular ways and often set arbitrary limits. The boys usually ignored them and often behaved aggressively and even destructively toward the toys and other objects in the room. Three of the four boys (Jake, Bryan, and Robert) were already showing punitive, aggressive behaviors toward their mother, sometimes intentionally hitting or throwing toys at her. These three boys had experienced early care that was hostile as well as intrusive. However, the other two boys, Clarke and Evan, showed a mix of punitive and caregiving behaviors at 24 months, at times scolding their mothers in a parentified way when they did not follow orders (e.g., "No, Mommy! Bad Mommy!"), and at other times acting attentive to her needs. This may be because Clarke's mother was not hostile during their early interactions, and Evan's mother was neither hostile nor intrusive; in fact she acted frightened, passive, and helpless with him.

All the boys in Group 1 who had BPI data reported problems with peer relationships, particularly peer rejection. Interestingly, all of them said that they did not hit or tease kids at school, but all said that other kids hit or teased them. Also, all four boys with intrusive mothers were rated by their teachers over the borderline cutoff on the DSM-IV scale for ADHD.

Group 2: Disorganized Boys with Internalizing Problems (Not Externalizing)

THE CASE OF DANNY B

On the surface at least, Danny appeared much healthier in his social–emotional development than Jake. At 24 months, his language was very advanced, he spoke in full sentences, and he was one of the few children in our sample who was able to solve the autonomy task with virtually no assistance. In the barrier box task, he quickly assessed that the box was impossible to open without assistance, and immediately went to the research assistant and politely asked, "Please help me." Thus, Danny seemed exceptionally competent for his age in many ways.

However, at age 7, his teachers and parents all noted internalizing symptoms: his teacher gave him a borderline rating for internalizing and thought problems, his mother gave him a borderline rating on DSM-IV Anxiety Problems, and his father rated him in the clinical range for both internalizing and thought problems, as well as in the borderline range for anxious depression and somatic complaints. Also, in the puppet interview at age 7, Danny stated that his parents yell at him, they frequently fight, and he is "sad" and "worried" when they fight. He also indicated that "kids don't ask me to play with them" and "I don't have a lot of friends at school." Danny also expressed many worries and fears, including, "I worry about my mom or dad when I'm at school," "I worry my mom or dad will go away and never come back," "If my mom or dad isn't near my bed, I'm scared to go to sleep," and "I worry bad things are going to happen." The interviewer judged Danny to be very articulate and believable during the interview, but also high on anxiety. He seemed to be very concerned about the interview questions and eager to please.

Danny's mother, Mrs. B, was classified in the AAI as unresolved for both loss and trauma, reporting a history of physical and sexual abuse. His father, Mr. B, was classified as dismissing. Mr. B generally seemed to take control of the family interactions, taking on a paternal role with Mrs. B as well as with Danny. For example, before the triadic interaction tasks, he told Mrs. B, "You do that [the Q-sort task]," then he repeated the task instructions almost verbatim to her, as though she were a child who could not understand the research assistant. Although Mrs. B was usually sweet and sensitive in her interactions with Danny, she was rated as the most frightening mother in our sample. She received the highest possible score on the FR scale and displayed very frightening behaviors in both the 8-month play interactions and in the Strange Situation at 12 months:

> (8 months) While playing on the floor with Danny, Mrs. B said sweetly, "Do you love your teddy bear?" and then suddenly and inexplicably pressed a large stuffed bear over Danny's entire face, essentially smothering him for a moment, while shaking the bear and saying in a harsh, strange voice that sounded nothing like her normal gentle voice, "Love the bear!" Following this, Danny lay dazed and staring at her with wide eyes, breathing hard. Later, Mrs. B gently patted Danny with a spatula on his bottom. Suddenly her movements became more intense, and her voice again took on that same frightening tone, as she said, "Fry the baby!" Again, Danny looked alarmed and froze for a moment, but soon they were playing and laughing again.

(12 months) During the Strange Situation, when Mrs. B left for the first separation, Danny did not cry but hid behind Mrs. B's chair, then quietly walked up to her at the reunion and waited passively for her embrace. After she cuddled him and returned to her chair, he brought her a ball. She threw the ball and whispered "Go get it" in a low, haunted tone. He later climbed on her lap, still making no sound and staring up at her. She then said to him in the same haunted tone, "Get the doll, kiss the doll." When Mrs. B left for the second time, Danny was clearly extremely distressed. Breathing hard, he seemed to force himself to stop crying. He went to the chair and picked up her magazine, taking it to the door as though trying to use it to get her to come back. When she returned and sat back on her chair, he quietly approached and brought a tissue to her. She said, "Thank you, you're so helpful!" He then brought her a toy phone. As she filled out forms, he stared up at her and gently touched her hand.

Thus, by 12 months, Danny's pattern of dealing with stress and with his mother's unpredictable outbursts of frightening behavior was characterized by extreme watchfulness directed toward his mother, as well as inhibition of attachment behaviors and exploration. He seemed to adopt the "tend or befriend" strategy of approaching her with "gifts" of toys or tissues.

By age 2, Danny seemed well on the way to forming a controlling–caregiving interaction style with his mother. Mrs. B played with the toys in a dreamy, child-like way, while Danny let her set the agenda and responded quickly and eagerly to her suggestions. Often, Mrs. B distracted Danny from his interests, drawing attention to herself:

(24 months) Danny was riding on a toy car, wearing a fire hat and saying, "I'm a fireman! Mrs. B picked up a lei and called, "Look what I found in here! You want one?" Danny went quickly to Mrs. B, who said "Let me put it around your neck." He then politely said, "It's okay, you can wear it." She did, saying "Do I look pretty?" In the cleanup and teaching tasks, Danny watched Mrs. B carefully, followed her instructions, and seemed concerned with doing a good job.

Mrs. B viewed Danny as remarkably competent and special. In the caregiving interview, she noted, "He's real bright and he's very problem solving, he'll work on something and get it taken care of." She also said that he had been very helpful with his new baby sister but had also become more demanding, sometimes "whining" for attention. She said, "I hate when he does that, I just hate it." She also said that he is often sick, which makes her feel "helpless," and that she cannot handle it when he gets hurt. Recounting an incident when Danny fell and hurt his knee, she said, "It bled a little bit, and I was like (gasp), I didn't know what to do, I was like shaking because it just really scared me." Thus, Mrs. B is thrilled with Danny when he is compliant and helpful, but feels overwhelmed and helpless whenever he shows that he has needs of his own.

GENERAL CHARACTERISTICS OF GROUP 2: INTERNALIZING BOYS

There were only three children in this group, and since one lacks 24-month mother–child interaction data, only one boy, Alex, can be compared with Danny. Danny and Alex were quite different from the externalizing boys in Group 1 and remarkably similar to each other in terms of their interaction patterns with their mothers. First, the mothers of Danny and Alex were both scored as very frightening (scores of 7 or higher on the 9-point FR scale), but were generally warm and sensitive to their sons except for the brief periods when they seemed to dissociate and lapse into unprovoked, out-of-context bouts of frightening behavior. These caregiving patterns are concordant with both mothers' AAI classifications, since both were classified as unresolved but alternatively secure-autonomous. Mothers classified as unresolved in the AAI are more likely to show FR behaviors with their infants (Schuengel et al., 1999; Jacobvitz, Hazen, & Leon, 2006), and secure-autonomous mothers to be higher in sensitive caregiving (van IJzendoorn et al., 1999), compared to other mothers. Danny and Alex also both inhibited their attachment behaviors and watched their mothers almost constantly as if always on alert for a frightening outburst. By 24 months, both boys seemed well on the way to developing a caregiving–controlling coping style. Both of their mothers engaged in dreamy, self-absorbed child-like play, and both drew their sons' attention to their own play. Their sons, in turn, were very compliant and solicitous, trying hard to please.

Interestingly, one of the Group 1 boys, Evan, was more similar to Danny and Alex than to the other Group 1 boys in his interaction patterns with his mother. The mothers of all three boys were frightening but helpless rather than hostile. Also, although Evan was fussy and distressed rather than watchful and inhibited as an infant, by 24 months, he was very attentive and caregiving to his mother like Danny and Alex. It is unclear why he showed externalizing as well as internalizing problems by age 7. Possibly he has a more reactive temperament, or he and his mother formed a more punitive–hostile dynamic over time, or he may have had a mutually hostile relationship with his father, although that was not obvious in the 24-month family interactions.

Group 3: Disorganized Girls with Internalizing Problems

THE CASE OF ALICE C

Alice was rated by her teacher as being within the clinical range for internalizing problems, and as borderline for anxious depression and somatic complaints. Both her parents rated her as normal, and in fact, her mother gave her zeros on every scale, indicating she had no problems whatsoever. On the puppet interview at age 7, Alice seemed to share her parent's positive views of herself and of her relationships with parents and peers. The interviewer, however, rated her anxiety during the BPI at the highest possible level.

Alice's mother, Mrs. C, was classified on the AAI as unresolved for abuse, and her father, Mr. C, was classified as dismissing. In the AAI, Mrs. C reported that she hated her father, as he physically abused both her and her mother frequently and severely. She also reported that both of her parents were very controlling and that nothing she did was ever good enough for them. She said that she rebelled throughout childhood by acting out and was delinquent as a teen.

In all of the marital interactions assessed, Mrs. C alternated between dominating the interaction and becoming very quiet and withdrawn when things did not go her way. For example, when asked to discuss each other's strengths and weaknesses as parents, Mr. C cited only strengths for Mrs. C's parenting, but when it was her turn, although she first said that Mr. C is a "great dad," she then launched into a litany of criticisms of Mr. C's parenting. When Mr. C finally offered a mild criticism of Mrs. C, she became withdrawn, turning away from him and not answering. Mrs. C's control of the marital relationship was also apparent in the triadic interaction task at 24 months. Whenever Mr. and Mrs. C. disagreed on the placement of an item on the parenting Q-sort task, Mrs. C insisted on her choice until Mr. C accepted her decision.

Mrs. C displayed highly controlling, intrusive behavior toward Alice, and was also quite misattuned to Alice's signals, both in the 8-month home interaction and in the Strange Situation:

(8 months) When the researchers explained that the interaction tasks would include giving her child a snack, Mrs. C responded, "We just wait until she tells us she's hungry." Mrs. C then asked Alice if she wanted to eat. Alice did not respond, so Mrs. C did not try to feed her, but instead picked her up and sang into her face, even though Alice kept turning away. Several times, Mrs. C spoke for Alice (e.g., "We're not hungry yet"). Finally, Mrs. C put Alice in her high chair and very slowly gave her small amounts of finger food. Alice tried to grab the finger food and eat it quickly, but Mrs. C. would not let her feed herself, and continued to give her food very slowly. When Alice started crying, Mrs. C tried to calm her, saying loudly and repeatedly, "Oh, it's okay! We're so hungry!," but she did not give Alice more food. Alice's screaming increased until her face was red and she had difficulty catching her breath. Then Mrs. C suddenly left while Alice was crying, saying she was going to get more food. She was gone several minutes while Alice kept screaming.

(12 months) On the second reunion of the Strange Situation, Alice ran to Mrs. A with her head down, crashing into her legs. When Mrs. A picked her up, she stopped crying, but began again when Mrs. A quickly put her down. She raised her arms to be picked up again, but Mrs. A sat down again to fill out forms. Mrs. A still did not pick her up, but asked, "What's wrong? Are you hungry? Are you tired"?

In the 24-month dyadic interactions, Mrs. C continued to be misattuned to Alice's signals, particularly when Alice was distressed, and she placed high demands on Alice to play correctly and do well on tasks. Whenever Alice became frustrated or noncompliant, Mrs. C withdrew physically and emotionally:

(24 months) Mrs. C insisted that Alice use the cash register correctly and make a proper sandwich with the play food. When Alice wanted to put an object other than the plastic food into her pretend "sandwich," Mrs. C corrected her, "That's for toys, not for eating." Later, when Alice had difficulty with one of the teaching tasks and wanted to quit, Mrs. C sat silently, staring ahead.

By 24 months, Mrs. C. and Alice seemed to have established a pattern whereby Mrs. C. tried to control Alice's behavior (as well as Mr. C's behavior), and Alice was generally compliant. However, at times, Alice met Mrs. C's controlling, interfering behavior with passive noncompliance, and Mrs. C. generally responded with punitive emotional withdrawal, as illustrated in this example observed during the 24-month triadic interaction:

(24 months) Mr. C asked Alice if she wanted juice with her snack, and Mrs. C replied, "No, Daddy, just water please," even though Alice could speak clearly in full sentences. She then told Alice, "Let's eat first, then drink." Alice refused to eat and asked for juice. Mrs. C insisted, "You have to eat first." Alice still refused, closing her mouth tightly and turning away. Mrs. C begged, "Will you please eat some food?" As Alice continued to turn away with her mouth closed, Mrs. C withdrew, sitting with her arms crossed and looking down with a distressed expression. When it was time for the clothes changes, Mrs. C said tearfully, "She is not going to get up and get changed." She told Mr. C, "I need to take a break," and walked out, leaving him to change Alice's clothes.

Also at 24 months, Alice refused to separate from Mrs. C for the autonomy problem-solving task, so Mrs. C had to be present. When Alice still refused to try the task, Mrs. C (referring to the fact that the goal of the task was to push a small bag of Goldfish crackers through a plexiglass tube) said, "We don't use food as a bribe," so the task was terminated. When Alice became frustrated with the emotion regulation task (barrier box), Mrs. C again disparaged the task, saying, "She has never experienced something like this." Thus, Mrs. C seemed to feel that it was very important that Alice perform well, and made excuses for her when she did not.

The high standards that Mrs. C placed on Alice were also apparent in her caregiving interview. She stated that it was important to her that Alice "get into the best schools" and "make the best connections," and that she was already thinking about where Alice should go to school. She also said she felt it was important to keep track of exactly what Alice ate so she would know that Alice was getting a nutritionally balanced diet and would not develop weight problems. She indicated that she herself used to have an eating disorder and did not want that to happen to Alice. Interestingly, eating seemed to be one domain where Alice did exert her autonomy and passively refused to go along with Mrs. C's directives.

GENERAL CHARACTERISTICS OF GROUP 3: INTERNALIZING GIRLS

Like Alice, the other girls in Group 3 had mothers who were very controlling and emotionally misattuned both in infancy and toddlerhood. The mothers of Mia and Ella, like Mrs. C, were physically intrusive during their interactions with their infant daughters and seemed anxious to control their every move, and they too became very distressed when their daughters were distressed. Although they did not physically leave in such instances like Mrs. C did, they similarly abdicated their parental responsibilities by becoming very agitated and frantic, then emotionally withdrawing or spacing out. The fourth girl in this group, Karen, was not observed in mother–infant home interactions, but her mother was similarly misattuned to her daughter in the Strange Situation, although not intrusive.

At 24 months, like Mrs. C., the mothers of Ella and Mia were very directive and intrusive in the play interactions, telling their daughters exactly what to do and correcting them, often with physical intervention, when they did not perform correctly. Karen's mother was not intrusive but, like the mothers of Evan, Danny, and Alex, was more passive and child-like in the play situation. All four girls were very attentive and compliant with their mothers, showing early signs of developing caregiving–controlling strategies, and all but Karen were observed to use passive resistance when they did not want to follow a particular maternal directive. Interestingly, all of the girls in this group seemed to have a very high need for approval, not just from their mothers, but in general. They were all rated very high in performance anxiety in the BPI, and except for Mia, who expressed some worries about being shy and about her parents' fighting, gave "perfect" responses to the BPI, that is, for virtually every question, they gave the socially appropriate response.

GENERAL DISCUSSION AND CONCLUSIONS

Lyons-Ruth and her colleagues (1999) have argued that the interaction patterns of mother–child dyads with a history of attachment disorganization are characterized by a lack of balance and asymmetry of power, in which one partner's attachment-related needs and goals dominate those of the other partner. As such, one partner is in the position of being helpless and/or submissive, while the other is hostile and/or controlling. Supporting this view, our case studies suggest that this pattern can take multiple forms. When the parent is hostile and/or intrusive, as was the case with Jake and Alice, the child is helpless. We propose that boys, perhaps because they are more inclined to respond to threat with a flight-or-fight response, actively leaving and refusing to comply, or actively resisting and aggressing against the parent, are more likely than girls to try to gain control and put the parent in the helpless position, resulting in power struggles and the creation of a mutually hostile dynamic. To the extent these boys do manage to gain control, they may persist with a punitive–controlling pattern, displaying hostile, externalizing behaviors with teachers and peers by the time they are school-age.

Girls, on the other hand, seem more likely to respond to frightening, hostile, and/or intrusive parenting with tend-or-befriend responses, offering compliance, affiliation, and comfort. In this case, although the parent still dominates most of the time, the child may be rewarded with praise and attention for compliance and achievement. Also, when the parent is feeling overwhelmed, the controlling–caregiving child may gain control by taking over the parenting role. However, frightening and hostile parents are not likely to relinquish the position of control for long. Children continually forced into a helpless and vulnerable position may be particularly at risk for developing internalizing problems. Some, like Alice, may use passive resistance to regain a small degree of control. Also, to the extent that children in these relationships are able to gain some control with a frightening and hostile parent by taking on a caregiving role, they may be less likely to be perceived by parents and teachers as having internalizing problems.

In contrast, parents who seem emotionally withdrawn and lapse into trance-like states but are not hostile, or who are normally sensitive but lapse unpredictably into frightening behavior, seem to elicit watchful vigilance, worry, and concern for the parent among both boys and girls. Such children are likely to feel considerable fear and anxiety as well, sensing that they cannot count on their parent for protection. This may lead both boys and girls, like Danny and Karen, to gain some control by trying hard to please and help the parent, adopting an early caregiving–controlling strategy. Such children are thus forced into a position of control far before they are developmentally ready to assume such responsibility, putting them at risk for developing internalizing problems.

In sum, these quantitative and qualitative data suggest that particular externalizing or internalizing outcomes for children may depend not only on the gender of the child, but also on whether or not the parent's frightening caregiving also involves hostility, including punitive and/or intrusive patterns of care, or involves withdrawn behaviors that include a sense of helplessness, vulnerability or dissociating patterns of care that are often otherwise sensitive. Researchers should longitudinally explore possible links between infant disorganization, the development of different types of coping strategies (caregiving and punitive) in early childhood, and different types of problematic outcomes (internalizing and externalizing) in middle childhood and beyond.

Further examination of the role that a child's gender plays in the pathway from infant disorganization to later social–emotional problems is also essential. In many ways, the mothers of most of the clinically internalizing girls (Group 3) are similar to the mothers of most of the externalizing boys (Group 1). Most of the mothers in both groups are intrusive, controlling, and emotionally misattuned, and they tend to withdraw when their infants become distressed or when their toddlers are oppositional. The key difference seems to be that there is less hostility, anger, and punitive behavior in the mothers of the internalizing girls. It is unclear, though, whether that is because mothers are simply more likely to show more anger and hostility to boys, or because infant and toddler boys are more likely to react to maternal interference with angry avoidance or resistance whereas girls are more likely to react with passivity and watchfulness, and mothers respond in kind. Several studies examining the concurrent relation of disorganized/controlling attachment to aggressive or externalizing problems during preschool or early school age have not found gender differences in aggressive and externalizing outcomes (Solomon et al., 1995; Moss et al., 1998, 2006; Moss, Bureau, et al., 2004). Also, Moss, Cyr, & Dubois-Comtois (2004) did not find gender differences in children's use of punitive– versus caregiving–controlling strategies. Certainly some girls, for whatever reason, are more likely than others to respond to interfering mothers with angry resistance and aggression, and some boys are more likely to respond with compliance and caregiving. Such within-gender differences may be due to dispositional or temperamental differences in children, or differences in the extent to which children's parents or their social–cultural environments (including teachers and peers) impose gender-typed socialization pressures. For example, it is possible that children who grow up in Texas (e.g., our sample) experience more gender-typed socialization than children who grow up in northern California (e.g., Solomon et al.'s sample) or Montreal (e.g., Moss and her colleagues' samples).

Future studies should also investigate whether, for school-age children, it may be more difficult to diagnose internalizing problems in girls than boys. Although we found that boys were rated higher in internalizing problems than girls, girls may be more likely to inhibit expression of their fears and anxiety, or may be more effective than boys in doing so. Our findings that disorganized girls, unlike disorganized boys, rarely reported negative views of themselves or their relationships with parents and peers, but were more likely than boys to be rated by interviewers as anxious, support the idea that disorganized girls may try harder than boys to conceal their anxiety, bury their own emotional needs, and present a positive, supercompetent front.

Our case studies also indicate that future research examining disorganized attachment in the context of the whole family system, including father–child interactions patterns, the marital relationship, and whole family interactions, should help explain variations in pathways from infant disorganization to later social–emotional problems. A positive father–child relationship may serve as a protective buffer, leading to more positive outcomes for children in a disorganized mother–child relationship, whereas a negative father–child relationship is likely to be an additional risk factor. For example, Jake had disorganized and hostile relationships with both parents, and he also had perhaps the most negative outcomes of any child in our sample. A conflicted marital relationship also presents an additional risk for the disorganized child's development, as research has demonstrated strong links between marital conflict and the development of child externalizing problems (Cummings & Davies, 1994). Also, we found that family systems characterized by boundary disturbances and parent-child role-reversal present a risk for the later development of social–emotional problems (Jacobvitz, Hazen, Curran, & Hitchens, 2004). Boundary disturbances are more likely to occur when mothers are unresolved for loss or trauma (Hazen, Jacobvitz, & McFarland, 2005), indicating that disorganized children (whose mothers are often unresolved) may be more likely to grow up in family systems characterized by boundary disturbances.

Finally, researchers should investigate the developmental pathways of children who were classified as disorganized in infancy, but who are well adjusted later in childhood. In our sample, although 14/35 (40%) of the disorganized infants who remained in the study were viewed as having extreme social–emotional problems study by age 7–8, 60% were not. How do the children who were viewed as relatively well adapted differ from those who did develop problems? Did their relationships with their mothers improve, and if so, how did this happen? Did they develop secure relationships with alternative attachment figures, perhaps the father? Or are they simply more resilient due to intellectual or personality factors? Answers to these questions were beyond the scope of the present study, but would provide valuable information for clinicians and family therapists in designing family interventions for children with disorganized attachment.

REFERENCES

Ablow, J. C., & Measelle, J. R. (1993). *Berkeley Puppet Interview: Administration and scoring system manuals*. Berkeley: University of California.

Abrams, K. Y., Rifkin, A. T., & Hesse, E. (2006). Examining the role of parental frightened/frightening subtypes in predicting disorganized attachment within a brief observational procedure. *Development and Psychopathology, 18,* 344–362.

Achenbach, T. M. (1991). *Manual for the Child Behavior Checklist/4-18 and 1991 Profile*. Burlington: University of Vermont, Department of Psychiatry.

Ainsworth, M. D. S., Blehar, M. C., Waters, E., & Wall, S. (1978). *Patterns of attachment: A psychological study of the Strange Situation*. Hillsdale, NJ: Erlbaum.

Bowlby, J. (1982). *Attachment and loss: Vol. 1. Attachment*. New York: Basic Books. (original work published 1969)

Carlson, E. A. (1998). A prospective longitudinal study of attachment disorganization/disorientation. *Child Development, 69,* 1108–1128.

Cassidy, J., & Shaver, P. R. (Eds.). (2008). *Handbook of attachment: Theory, research, and clinical applications*. New York: Guilford Press.

Cummings, E. M., & Davies, P. T. (1994). *Children and marital conflict: The impact of family dispute and resolution*. New York: Guilford Press.

Cutler, K., & Hazen, N. L. (1995). *Linking parent–child and child–peer communication styles: The role of attachment and child gender*. Paper presented at the annual meeting of the Society for Research in Child Development, Indianapolis, IN.

David, D. H., & Lyons-Ruth, K. (2005). Differential attachment responses of male and female infants to frightening maternal behavior: Tend or befriend versus fight or flight? *Infant Mental Health Journal, 26,* 1–18.

del Guidice, M. (2008). Sex-biased ratio of avoidant/ambivalent attachment in middle childhood. *British Journal of Developmental Psychology, 26,* 369–379.

del Guidice, M. (2009). Sex, attachment, and the development of reproductive strategies. *Behavioral and Brain Science, 32,* 1–67.

Fabes, R. A., & Eisenberg, N. (1992). Young children's coping with interpersonal anger. *Child Development, 63,* 116–128.

Fagot, B. I. (1978). The influence of sex of child on parental reactions to toddler children. *Child Development, 49,* 459–465.

Fagot, B. I., & Leinbach, M. D. (1987). Socialization of sex roles within the family. In D. B. Carter (Ed.), *Current conceptions of sex roles and sex typing*. New York: Praeger.

Fearon, R. P., Bakermans-Kranenburg, M. J., Van IJzendoorn, M. H., Lapsley, A. M., & Roisman, G. I. (2010). The significance of insecure attachment and disorganization in the development of children's externalizing behavior: A meta-analytic study. *Child Development, 81,* 435–456.

George, C., Kaplan, N., & Main, M. (1985/1996). *Adult Attachment Interview.* Unpublished protocol (3rd ed.), University of California at Berkeley, Department of Psychology.

George, C., & Solomon, J. (1993). *Internal working models of caregiving.* Unpublished interview and coding manual, Mills College, Oakland, CA.

George, C., & Solomon, J. (2008). Attachment and caregiving: The caregiving behavioral system. In J. Cassidy & P. R. Shaver (Eds.), *Handbook of attachment: Theory, research, and clinical applications* (2nd ed., pp. 833–856). New York: Guilford Press.

Huselid, R. F., & Cooper, M. L. (1994). Gender roles as mediators of sex differences in expressions of pathology. *Journal of Abnormal Psychology, 103,* 595–603.

Jacobvitz, D., Hazen, N., Curran, M., & Hitchens, K. (2004). Observations of early triadic family interactions: Boundary disturbances in the family predict symptoms of depression, anxiety, and attention-deficit/hyperactivity disorder in middle childhood. *Development and Psychopathology, 16,* 577–592.

Jacobvitz, D., & Hazen, N. L. (1999). Developmental pathways from infant disorganization to childhood peer relationships. In J. Solomon & C. George (Eds.), *Disorganized attachment: The origins and consequences* (pp. 127–159). New York: Guilford Press.

Jacobvitz, D., Hazen, N., & Leon, K. (2006). Does expectant mothers' unresolved trauma predict frightening/frightened maternal behavior?: Risk and protective factors. *Development and Psychopathology, 18,* 363–379.

Kolko, D. J., & Kazdin, A. E. (1993). Emotional–behavioral problems in clinic and nonclinic children: Correspondence among child, parent and teacher reports. *Journal of Child Psychology and Psychiatry and Allied Disciplines, 34,* 991–1006.

Leaper, C. (1992). Parenting girls and boys. In M. H. Bornstein (Ed.), *Handbook of parenting* (2nd ed., Vol. 1, pp. 189–225). Mahwah, NJ: Erlbaum.

Lindsey, E. W., Mize, J., & Pettit, G. S. (1997). Differential play patterns of mothers and fathers of sons and daughters: Implications for children's gender role development. *Sex Roles, 37,* 643–661.

Lyons-Ruth, K. Bronfman, E., & Parsons, E. (1999). Maternal disrupted affective communication, maternal frightened or frightening behavior, and disorganized infant attachment strategies. In J. Vondra & D. Barnett (Eds.), Atypical patterns in infancy and early childhood among children at developmental risk. *Monographs of the Society for Research in Child Development, 64*(3, Serial No. 258), 172–192.

Lyons-Ruth, K., Easterbrooks, A., & Cibelli, C. (1997). Infant attachment strategies, infant mental lag, and maternal depressive symptoms: Predictors of internalizing and externalizing problems at age 7. *Developmental Psychology, 3,* 377–396.

Lyons-Ruth, K., & Jacobvitz, D. (2008). Attachment disorganization: Unresolved loss, relational violence, and lapses in behavioral and attentional strategies. In J. Cassidy & P. R. Shaver (Eds.), *Handbook of attachment: Theory, research, and clinical applications* (2nd ed., pp. 666–697). New York: Guilford Press.

Lytton, H., & Romney, D. M. (1991). Parents' differential socialization of boys and girls: A meta-analysis. *Psychological Bulletin, 51,* 267–296.

Macobby, E. E. (1990). Gender and relationships: A developmental account. *American Psychologist, 45,* 513–520.

Main, M., & Hesse, E. (1990). Parents' unresolved traumatic experiences are related to infant disorganized attachment status: Is frightened and/or frightening parental behavior the linking mechanism? In M. T. Greenberg, D. Cicchetti, & E. M. Cummings (Eds.), *Attachment in the preschool years: Theory, research, and intervention* (pp. 161–182). Chicago: University of Chicago Press.

Main, M., & Hesse, E. (1995). *Frightening, frightened, timid/deferential, dissociated, or disorganized behavior on the part of the parent: Coding system.* Unpublished manuscript, University of California at Berkeley.

Main, M., & Solomon, J. (1990). Procedures for identifying infants as disorganized/disoriented during the Ainsworth Strange Situation. In M. Greenberg, D. Cicchetti, & E.M. Cummings (Eds.), *Attachment during the preschool years: Theory, research, and intervention* (pp. 121–160). Chicago: University of Chicago Press.

Malatesa, C. Z., & Haviland, J. M. (1982). Learning display rules: The socialization of emotional expression in infancy. *Child Development, 53,* 991–1003.

Marvin, R. S., & Britner, P. (2008). Normative development: The ontogeny of attachment. In J. Cassidy & P. R. Shaver (Eds.), *Handbook of attachment: Theory, research, and clinical applications* (pp. 44–67). New York: Guilford Press.

Miller, P. M., Danaher, D. L., & Forbes, D. (1986). Sex-related strategies for coping with interpersonal conflict in children aged five and seven. *Developmental Psychology, 22,* 543–548.

Moss, E., Bureau, J.-F., Cyr, C., Mongeau, C., & St-Laurent, D. (2004). Correlates of attachment at age 3: Construct validity of the preschool attachment classification system. *Developmental Psychology, 40,* 323–334.

Moss, E., Cyr, C., & Dubois-Comtois, K. (2004). Attachment at early school-age and developmental risk: Examining family contexts and behavior problems of controlling–caregiving, controlling–punitive and behaviorally-disorganized children. *Developmental Psychology, 40,* 519–532.

Moss, E., Rousseau, D., Parent, S., St-Laurent, D., & Saintonge, J. (1998). Correlates of attachment at school age: Maternal reported stress, mother–child interaction, and behavior problems. *Child Development, 69,* 1390–1405.

Moss, E., Smolla, N., Cyr, C., Dubois-Comtois, K., Mazzarello, T., & Berthiaume, C. (2006). Attachment and behavior problems in middle childhood as reported by adult and child informants. *Development and Psychopathology, 18,* 425–444.

Schuengel, C., van IJzendoorn, M., & Bakermans-Kranenburg, M. (1999). Frightening maternal behavior linking unresolved loss and disorganized infant attachment. *Journal of Consulting and Clinical Psychology, 67,* 54–63.

Seiffge-Krenke, I., & Kollmar, F. (1998). Discrepancies between mothers' and fathers' perceptions of sons' and daughters' problem behaviour: A longitudinal analysis of parent–adolescent agreement on internalizing and externalising problem behaviour. *Journal of Child Psychology and Psychiatry, 39,* 687–697.

Shaw, D. S., Keenan, K., Vondra, J. I., Delliquadri, E., & Giovanelli, J. (1997). Antecedents of preschool children's internalizing problems: A longitudinal study of low-income families. *Journal of the American Academy of Child and Adolescent Psychiatry, 36,* 1760–1767.

Solomon, J., & George, C. (2008). The measurement of attachment in infancy and middle childhood. In J. Cassidy & P. R. Shaver (Eds.), *Handbook of attachment: Theory, research, and clinical applications* (2nd ed., pp. 383–416). New York: Guilford Press.

Solomon, J., George, C., & DeJong, A. (1995). Children classified as controlling at age six: Evidence of disorganized representational strategies and aggression at home and at school. *Development and Psychopathology, 33,* 447–463.

Taylor, S. E., Kein, L. C., Lewis, B. P., Gruenewald, T. L., Gurung, R. A. R., & Updegraff, J. A. (2000). Biobehavioral responses to stress in females: Tend-and-befriend, not fight-or flight. *Psychological Review, 107,* 411–429.

Turner, P. J. (1991). Relations between attachment, gender, and behavior with peers in preschool. *Child Development, 62,* 1475–1488.

Underwood, M. K., Coie, J. D., & Herbsman, C. R. (1992). Display rules for anger and aggression in school-age children. *Child Development, 63,* 366–380.

van IJzendoorn, M. H. (1995). Adult attachment representations, parental responsiveness, and infant attachment: A meta-analysis on the predictive validity of the Adult Attachment Interview. *Psychological Bulletin, 117,* 387–403.

van IJzendoorn, M. H., Schuengel, C., & Bakermans-Kranenburg, M. J. (1999). Disorganized attachment in early childhood: Meta-analysis of precursors, concomitants and sequelae. *Development and Psychopathology, 11,* 225–249.

Wertlieb, D., Weigel, C., & Feldstein, M. (1987). Stress, social support, and behavior symptoms in middle-childhood. *Journal of Child Clinical Psychology, 16,* 204–211.

Whitley, B. E., & Gridley, B. E. (1993). Sex role orientation, self-esteem, and depression: A latent variables analysis. *Personality and Social Psychology Bulletin, 19,* 363–369.

Chapter 8

Disorganized Attachment Behavior Observed in Adolescence

Validation in Relation to Adult Attachment Interview Classifications at Age 25

KATHERINE H. HENNIGHAUSEN, JEAN-FRANÇOIS BUREAU,
DARYN H. DAVID, BJARNE M. HOLMES,
and KARLEN LYONS-RUTH

I told you that my family conflict *is* all about me. I'm totally responsible. I told a friend on Saturday that I would just act worse and worse until I could get my mother to cry. Then when she did, I thought, "Good!" I *like* being in control of my family—it's much better than feeling helpless.... They control everything ... everything!"

Little research on disorganized or controlling parent–adolescent attachment relationships currently exists to help us understand this quote from a clinical session with a 16-year-old girl hospitalized for an eating disorder. The work presented in this chapter constitutes the first step in a program of studies to develop and validate a coding system for attachment patterns observed in adolescence, with a particular emphasis on the controlling and disorganized forms of attachment seen in high-risk and clinical samples. This new coding system builds on the research literature describing forms of attachment-related interactions at earlier ages, and creates a descriptive lexicon for the variations in functioning of a goal-corrected partnership that are seen among adolescents and their parents during stressful interactions, including disorganized and controlling forms of attachment.

Adolescence is a critical time of transition from a position of dependence on the family to a position of more autonomous functioning in the larger community (Allen & Hauser, 1996; Sroufe, Egeland, Carlson, & Collins, 2005). During this transition, adolescent activities expand into a variety of new domains, including increased intimacy and sexuality in relationships; increased involvement in paid work or career-related studies; and increased exploration of belief systems and lifestyle choices that may differ from those of their parents. There are also increased risks of making choices that place long-term constraints on further adult growth and development, choices such as early pregnancy, early school dropout, involvement in antisocial activity, or excessive use of drugs or alcohol (Dodge, 2000; Jimerson, Egeland, Sroufe, & Carlson, 2000; Miller & Moore 1990; Patterson & Bank, 1989; Shelder & Block, 1990; Sroufe et al., 2005; Steinberg & Morris, 2001). Psychiatric symptomatology also rises during the teen years, with increased depressive symptoms, suicidality, and eating disorders among girls and increased substance abuse and illegal activity among boys (Ge, Lorenz, Conger, Elder, & Simons, 1994; Patterson & Bank, 1989).

Attachment theory provides one framework for conceptualizing the psychological and relational resources that allow teens to negotiate the complexities of this phase of life. This theory posits that the adequacy of comfort and communication available in central relationships during infancy and childhood shapes the self-regulating resources of the individual over time, through the mediation of internal representational models of the caregiver's availability and responsiveness (Bowlby, 1982; Sroufe et al., 2005). During infancy, attachment security is mediated more heavily by physical proximity and contact with the caregiver, which calms the infant's distress and serves as a secure base for the resumption of exploration of the environment (Ainsworth, Blehar, Waters, & Wall, 1978; Bowlby, 1982; Sroufe et al., 2005). The appearance of language allows the child and parent to exchange ideas, as well as to correct possible erroneous perceptions of the child's or parent's intentions (Nelson, 1996). These new capacities facilitate communication about past and future interactive episodes, which may in turn foster the joint negotiation of plans between the child and the parent for the adjustment of proximity and the maintenance of the child's felt security when not in the immediate physical presence of the caregiver (Bowlby, 1988). This increased capacity for shared planning and negotiation between parent and child allows the emergence of what Bowlby (1982) referred to as "a goal-corrected partnership" during the preschool years, which forms the basis for secure attachment at later ages.

Kobak, Cole, Ferenz-Gillies, Fleming, and Gamble (1993) reasoned that if a goal-corrected partnership is established between parent and child during the early years, flexible strategies for negotiating between the needs of self and others will become established as internal working models available for guiding negotiations with others around increased autonomy during the transition through adolescence. Allen, Hauser, and Borman-Spurrell (1996) further hypothesized that a central attachment-related task in adolescence involves establishing autonomy of thought while maintaining relatedness in interactions with parents. They also point out that maintaining a balance between autonomy and relatedness in adolescence is functionally similar to the infant's task of balancing exploration of the environment with maintenance of a secure base in the parent–infant relationship (Bowlby, 1980). In light of this, disorganized attachment presents unique challenges to adolescent development because the internal working models of disorganized children for how to negotiate comfort and closeness with others are thought to be fear-imbued and contradictory, leaving little room for flexibility and collaborative dialogue in negotiating new developmental challenges.

In this chapter, we first examine current methodologies used to assess attachment in adolescence, particularly those used to assess disorganization. Then we review developmental pathways associated with disorganized or controlling attachment processes and consider how disorganization and/ or controlling behavior may present in adolescence and have an impact on development. Finally, we introduce a new classification system for observed adolescent–parent attachment that may be more sensitive to serious deviations in attachment relationships. We believe this system will be helpful for assessing how family relational factors do or do not interact with life events, peer influences, and biological predispositions to shape trajectories toward adult psychosocial adaptation or disorder.

CURRENT APPROACHES TO ASSESSMENT OF ATTACHMENT IN ADOLESCENCE

Most of the groundbreaking studies of adolescent attachment have used the Adult Attachment Interview (AAI; George, Kaplan, & Main, 1985), a semistructured interview designed to assess an individual's current state of mind about past parent–child experiences. In-depth qualitative analysis of the interview leads to an overall classification, which is usually one of four groups: Secure/Autonomous, Insecure/Dismissing, Insecure/Preoccupied, or Unresolved with Respect to Loss or Abuse (George et al., 1985). These categories parallel the infant attachment classifications of secure, insecure/avoidant, insecure/ambivalent, and insecure/disorganized, respectively (Ainsworth et al., 1978). Kobak and his colleagues (Kobak, 1993; Kobak et al., 1993; Kobak & Sceery, 1988), who coded the AAI using the Kobak Q-set method, found significant associations between attachment scores on the Q-set and adolescents' self-reports of distress, perceived competence, and social support in a normative sample. In a study assessing the associations between attachment and mother–teen problem solving, they found that teens with secure attachment strategies engaged in problem solving discussions characterized by less dysfunctional anger and less avoidance of problem-solving (Kobak et al., 1993). However, the Q-set has no items for discriminating the Unresolved states of mind that predict infant disorganized strategies in the next generation.

Using prospective longitudinal data, Allen and Hauser (1996) reported that overall coherence (an index of security on the AAI) in adults' states of mind regarding attachment at age 25 could be predicted from their mothers' behaviors promoting autonomy and relatedness during a family interaction task 11 years earlier. This prediction held after controlling for psychiatric history and global indices of functioning in both adolescence and adulthood. In contrast, passivity of thought processes (a marker of insecurity on the AAI) was predicted by the adolescent's enmeshing and lack of distancing behaviors during the family task. These findings support the position that learning to balance autonomy and relatedness may be an attachment-related developmental task of adolescence.

The very few attachment-oriented longitudinal studies extending from infancy to adolescence have also used the AAI to index attachment in late adolescence. Most of these longitudinal samples have involved low-risk cohorts with too few disorganized infants for separate analysis (Grossmann et al., 2002; Hamilton, 2000; Waters, Merrick, Treboux, Crowell, & Albersheim, 2000). Results have not been consistent across studies. Waters and colleagues (2000) interviewed 60 middle-class subjects using the AAI and found continuity in attachment patterns from infancy to young adulthood, as did Hamilton (2000). However, Grossmann and colleagues (2002) did not replicate those findings.

Main and colleagues (Main, Hesse, & Kaplan, 2005) are among the few to examine the continuity of disorganized attachment patterns from infancy to adulthood, but their sample of 42 middle-class families included only 15 infants who were classified as disorganized using the Strange Situation. They found a nonstatistically significant trend for disorganized infants to be classified as Unresolved or Cannot Classify (meaning the interview showed evidence of unresolved trauma or loss or of contradictory strategies) on the AAI at age 19, but more than half of the disorganized infants were later classified as Dismissing on the AAI.

Only the Minnesota Longitudinal Study of Parents and Children has involved a low-income sample with a higher incidence of disorganization in infancy (see Carlson, 1998). In their first report, little continuity was found from attachment classifications in infancy to AAI attachment classifications at age 19 (Weinfield, Sroufe, & Egeland, 2000), with 52% of all adolescents classified as Dismissing on the AAI. Therefore the majority of adolescents in the sample claimed little memory for childhood experiences, idealized their parents with limited support, and/or derogated attachment experiences. Weinfield, Whaley, and Egeland (2004) later found that disorganized infants were significantly more likely to be coded as either insecure or unresolved at age 19, rather than secure. Again, the majority of participants who were disorganized as infants were later coded as Insecure/Dismissing on the AAI rather than Unresolved.

Weinfield et al. (2004) speculated that the AAI may be somewhat less valid with disadvantaged adolescents, either because they assume particularly defensive stances or because they may not yet have developed the perspective-taking or reflective integration skills required by the task (see also Sroufe et al., 2005). In addition, current procedures for coding unresolved states of mind in adulthood require the reporting of loss or abuse experiences during the interview. However, many adolescents may not report abuse and/or may not have experienced significant loss or abuse, which might prevent the identification on the AAI of potentially long-standing patterns of disorganized cognition and behavior. Lyons-Ruth, Yellin, Melnick, and Atwood (2005) described this as a "transmission block" in the current conceptual and methodological models of intergenerational transmission of disorganized attachment.

An important conceptual and methodological problem arises, then, regarding how we should assess disorganized attachment patterns in adolescence or adulthood, especially when there has been no serious loss or abuse to inquire about on the AAI. In one approach to this dilemma, Hesse (2008) developed criteria for designating an AAI as Cannot Classify if it contains contradictory or incompatible content over the entire interview, regardless of the characteristics of discourse in relation to loss or abuse. Hesse also noted that Cannot Classify transcripts may include attempts to frighten the listener, such as unexpectedly describing a gruesome crime, or inexplicable refusals to respond to questions. Due to the rarity of these protocols, however, limited data exist to establish the coding reliability of this category or to demonstrate prediction from this adult classification to the transmission of disorganized attachment in offspring. Hesse (2008) did suggest that parents who have AAI transcripts deemed "globally incoherent and unorganized" (p. 572) may be more likely to have disorganized or unclassifiable children.

A second approach to coding interview-wide indices of disorganization on the AAI assesses the presence of a pervasively unintegrated Hostile-Helpless (HH) state of mind in regard to attachment relationships (Lyons-Ruth, Yellin, et al., 2005). In contrast to the Unresolved coding system, which indexes unresolved states of mind regarding loss or abuse, the Hostile-Helpless coding system indexes unintegrated and affectively polarized states of mind regarding attachment relationships as manifest over the entire interview, regardless of whether loss or abuse has occurred. HH states of mind have recently been validated in relation to infant disorganization, maternal disrupted affective communication, maternal experiences of abuse, maternal substance abuse, and borderline personality disorder (Finger, 2007; Lyons-Ruth, Yellin, et al., 2005; Lyons-Ruth, Yellin, Melnick, & Atwood, 2003; Lyons-Ruth, Melnick, Patrick, & Hobson, 2007; Melnick, Finger, Hans, Patrick, & Lyons-Ruth, 2008). In addition, HH states of mind regarding the attachment relationship show discriminative validity in that they do not overlap significantly with Unresolved or Cannot Classify states of mind, and they account for independent variance in infant disorganization (Lyons-Ruth, Yellin, et al., 2005; Melnick et al., 2008).

Other interview measures of attachment in adolescence and/or adulthood have been developed more recently. West, Rose, Spreng, and Adam (2000) designed the Adolescent Unresolved Attachment Questionnaire to assess the adolescent's perception of the care provided by the attachment figure; the fear generated by the adolescent's appraisal of failed attachment figure care; and the negative affective responses to the perceived lack of care from the attachment figure. These scales are all significantly associated with a composite group of Unresolved and Cannot Classify categories on the AAI in a clinical adolescent population. Using the Adult Attachment Projective (AAP), a projective task intended to reproduce the AAI categories, George and West (2001) reported good correspondence between the AAP and the AAI in a low-risk adult sample. In addition, Webster and Hackett (2005) reported a significant association between the Unresolved classification on adolescent AAPs and poorer adolescent social adaptation. However, a body of work using these alternative interview measures in adolescence has not yet emerged, nor have they been validated in relation to directly observed parent–infant interaction and attachment. Therefore, it remains unclear whether interview-wide coding systems can bridge the transmission block and adequately assess whether disorganized infants or controlling young children carry forward their controlling or disorganized behavior into adolescence and young adulthood, with the potential to transmit disorganization to the next generation.

A pressing need in the assessment of disorganized attachment is an observationally based measure of disorganized parent–child interactions present in adolescence and early adulthood. Direct observations during this period might provide a more powerful methodology for studies investigating how disorganized–controlling behaviors develop into adulthood. A viable attachment classification system for adolescents needs to integrate accumulated developmental work on presentations of secure, insecure, controlling, and disorganized behavior at earlier ages. In the next section, we review developmental pathways associated with disorganized or controlling attachment strategies and consider how these strategies may appear in adolescence.

ATTACHMENT DISORGANIZATION:
LONGITUDINAL TRAJECTORIES
FROM INFANCY TO ADOLESCENCE

Disorganization in Infancy

Secure attachment patterns, as well as insecure-avoidant and insecure-ambivalent patterns of attachment, are conceptualized as organized strategies for maintaining a modicum of felt security when under stress. Organization is inferred based on the similarity of these behavior patterns across infants and on the functional goals that activate or terminate these patterns of behavior (Ainsworth et al., 1978). In contrast, the term *disorganized* refers to the apparent lack of a consistent or coherent strategy for organizing attachment responses to the parent when under stress (Lyons-Ruth & Jacobvitz, 2008; Main & Solomon, 1990). The particular combinations of disorganized behaviors observed in human infants tend to be idiosyncratic from child to child but include apprehensive, helpless, or depressed behaviors; unexpected alternations of approach and avoidance toward the attachment figure; and other marked conflict behaviors, such as prolonged freezing or stilling, or slowed "underwater" movements (see Main & Solomon, 1990, for a full description).

These disorganized attachment behaviors in infancy have gained additional significance from studies relating attachment disorganization to elevated cortisol secretion after exposure to brief stressors (Hertsgaard, Gunnar, Erickson, & Nachmius, 1995; Spangler & Grossmann, 1993). In animal models, such elevated cortisol response is associated with the animal's inability to mobilize an effective strategy to cope with the stressor (Levine, Weiner, & Coe, 1993). These findings are consistent with Main and Solomon's (1986) view that disorganized infant behaviors reflect the lack of an effective attachment strategy for regaining some sense of comfort and security in the face of fearful arousal.

In this view, the attachment relationship functions as what might be called the "psychological immune system" in its role of buffering the effects of psychological stressors and maintaining psychophysiological arousal within acceptable limits (see also Spangler, Chapter 5, this volume). Using this metaphor, it is apparent that illness can result either from the virulence of the outside disease agent or from inadequate functioning of the immune response mounted to fight off the stressor. Vulnerability to stress-related psychological dysfunction, then, should be a joint function of at least three factors: (1) the characteristics of the threat or stressor, (2) the individual's genetic vulnerability to stress, and (3) the capacity of the attachment relationship to moderate a sense of threat and reduce arousal to acceptable levels. In such a model, the impact of traumatic attachment-related events, such as loss or abuse, is mediated in part by the degree of comfort and soothing available in close relationships (see also Solomon & George, Chapter 2, this volume).

Based on this model, we have developed a conception of the etiology of infant disorganization that does not depend on the caregiver's display of frightened or frightening behavior toward the infant (see Main & Hesse, 1990). We see infant fearful arousal as stemming from many sources in addition to the parent's own behavior, including the types of parental absences or separations demonstrated to enhance infant stress in the animal literature (e.g., Coplan, et al., 1996; Francis, Diorio, Liu, & Meaney, 1999; Kraemer & Clarke, 1996). In this view, disorganization of infant attachment strategies occurs in response to the parent's repeated inability to provide adequate comfort to the stressed infant (see also George & Solomon, 2008; Solomon & George, 1996). Such emotional unavailability can be communicated through a variety of aversive responses to the infant's attachment bids, including withdrawal, fearful disorientation, role-reversal, negative intrusive behavior, or contradictory responses (see also Beebe et al., 2010).

Why might the child's attachment signals evoke such uncomforting responses? There is an inherent, although not one-to-one, relation between the caregiver's experience of uncomforted fear and distress in her own history and the openness of the caregiving system to hear, to respond to, and to help modulate fear-related affects in the infant. If the caregiver has not experienced comfort and soothing in relation to her own past fear, the infant's fear and vulnerability will evoke her own unsoothed fearful affects. These affects, in turn, will be associated with the caregiver's helplessness to know how to find or give comfort, as well as her defensive adaptations developed over time to deal with the fear and helplessness (see also Fraiberg, Adelson, & Shapiro, 1975; George & Solomon, 2008). From this relational diathesis viewpoint, there should be a sizeable group of adults who have not experienced childhood loss or abuse, but whose experience of unintegrated fearful affects and disorganized attachment strategies are rooted in their childhood relationships with unresponsive caregivers (see also Solomon & George, Chapter 2, this volume).

This view of the ramifications of parental unsoothed fear on the process of the parent–child relationship leads to an important further postulate. If the parent must restrict her conscious attention to the infant's fear-related cues in order not to evoke her own uncomforted experiences of fear and distress, the parent's fluid responsiveness to the infant's attachment-related communications becomes restricted and distorted. The more pervasive these restrictions and distortions on the parent's attention and responsiveness, the more the parent's need to regulate her own negative arousal will take precedence over the flexible deployment of attention to the child's current states. When this occurs, the interaction between parent and child becomes more contradictory, less balanced, and less mutually regulated to meet the needs of the child. At the extreme, the parent abdicates a parental regulatory role entirely, as discussed by Solomon and George (1996).

Such unbalanced or contradictory relational processes provide a conceptually powerful construct that can explain many additional aspects of the findings regarding disorganized attachment patterns. Both Bowlby (1980) and his forebears in psychoanalytic scholarship emphasized that mental representations of relationships are inherently dyadic. What is represented is not only the individual's way of participating in the relationship, for example, as the distressed child, but also the entire dyadic relational pattern of distressed child–abandoning parent. The more skewed these relational roles become, that is, the more one partner's initiatives are ignored or overridden by the other, the more discontinuous and self-contradictory are the internalized models that accommodate both relational possibilities. In addition to contradictory internal models, highly unbalanced relational processes offer at least two contradictory and unintegrated behavioral possibilities that might become actualized in any given relational transaction. For example, if an early victim–victimizer model is never reevaluated, an abused child may become both a battered spouse and a battering parent by actualizing opposite poles of a single dyadic model in different relationships. Only if the underlying need or fear is acknowledged, and the old dyadic patterns found wanting, can new ways of being in relationship to others be constructed, and new and more responsive behavior toward the attachment-related needs of both the self and the other merge.

These unbalanced relational processes can be observed in a broad range of relational patterns. A dominant–submissive pattern in which the parent or child coercively opposes and counters the initiatives of the other is the most obvious example of an unbalanced relational pattern. However, overriding the initiatives of the child can occur in much more subtle forms that on the surface appear helpless rather than powerful. Profound withdrawal and unresponsiveness is an obvious example in which the unresponsive parent may look depressed and helpless rather than hostile and coercive, and yet the end result of the unresponsive stance is to defeat the attempts of the child to jointly regulate the attachment relationship (see also Liotti, Chapter 14, this volume).

The extreme end of unbalanced attachment-related interaction patterns due to withdrawal occurs in cases of prolonged infant separation from or loss of the parent. Kraemer and Clarke (1996) have described the extremely fearful behavior, alternating with discontrolled aggression, that characterizes the behavior of infant rhesus monkeys raised with peer companionship but no adult attachment figure. The disregulated fear appears to be a consequence of the absence of early maternal soothing responses to the infant's attachment behaviors. This evidence indicates that infant fearful and disorganized behavior can result from profound *lack of response*, as well as from specifically frightened or frightening behavior (see also Solomon & George, 1996, 1999). Lyons-Ruth, Bronfman, and Atwood (1999) pointed out that, in a related set of observations on film, entitled *John: Nine Days in a Residential Nursery*, Robertson and Robertson (1969) documented the progressive disorganization of the child's attachment behaviors over time in the context of a prolonged parental absence of 9 days, during which kindly but inadequately available nurses engaged in routine care. Thus, infant fear without resolution can come about through a variety of caregiving conditions that result in inadequately specific and balanced responses to the infant's attachment initiatives. Therefore, in this model, directly frightened or frightening parental behaviors are not privileged as solely causal of infant disorganization but are seen as only one subset of a broader class of caregiving responses that fail to provide adequate regulation of the infant's fearful arousal from whatever source.

Disorganized and Controlling Strategies in Childhood

As disorganized infants and toddlers make the transition into the preschool years, the signs of conflict, apprehension, or helplessness characteristic of disorganized attachment strategies in infancy often give way to various forms of controlling behavior toward the parent. These controlling behavioral strategies emphasize either caregiving behavior, including directing, organizing, and entertaining behavior, or punitive and coercive behavior. This developmental shift toward controlling behavior patterns with the parent has been documented in 6-year-old follow-up studies of two middle-income samples (Main & Cassidy, 1988; Wartner, Grossmann, Fremmer-Bombik, & Suess, 1994; see also Moss, Bureau, St-Laurent, & Tarabulsy, Chapter 3, this volume).

However, this apparent transformation from a disorganized to a controlling attachment pattern does not occur for all disorganized children. Studies show that 25–33% of disorganized babies do not adopt a controlling attachment pattern by age 6 (Main & Cassidy, 1988; Moss et al., Chapter 3, this volume; Wartner et al., 1994). Moreover, it has been shown that the proportion of disorganized infants who develop controlling strategies by the end of the preschool period is smaller in higher risk samples than in more advantaged samples (Cicchetti & Barnett, 1991). This suggests that developing a controlling strategy requires skills, such as perspective-taking and joint attention skills, that may not be developed enough among many preschool children living in very deprived environments; therefore, some children may develop forms of controlling behavior later than others. The developmental shift to controlling strategies is made more complex by the very different forms of controlling behavior emerging over the preschool period. Hence, there is considerable heterogeneity in the attachment behavior shown by preschool children that is associated with earlier disorganized behavior in infancy. This spectrum includes punitive–controlling behavior, caregiving–controlling behavior, and continued behaviorally disorganized forms of behavior in the presence of the parent (Main & Cassidy, 1988; Solomon, George, & De Jong, 1995; Wartner et al., 1994; see also Moss et al., Chapter 3, this volume).

Recent studies have also highlighted different developmental outcomes and trajectories for these three disorganized/controlling subgroups (controlling–punitive, controlling–caregiving, and behaviorally disorganized) over preschool and middle childhood (see Moss et al., Chapter 3, this volume, for a review). Interestingly, previous studies have not generally reported gender differences in the incidence of controlling attachment behavior during the preschool period (for an exception at age 3, see NICHD Early Child Care Research Network, 2001), nor have gender differences been reported in the *types* of controlling attachment behaviors displayed (i.e., caregiving vs. punitive), although small *N*'s limit the power of the latter analyses.

The controlling–caregiving pattern has been associated with more internalizing problems and with a history of maternal losses in the work of Moss and colleagues (Chapter 3, this volume). Recent work by Solomon and George (2006; Chapter 2, this volume) has also demonstrated an unusually high rate of complicated bereavement reported by mothers of controlling–caregiving children. This is consistent with the view that these children may be attempting to orient, contain, or cheer up their mothers, but that these caregivers are less available to their children to help them regulate their own emotions. The children who assume caregiving roles may also be more prone to anxiety, depression, and low-self worth (Teti, 1999), given the tendency to suppress their own needs in favor of meeting the needs of the parent.

In contrast to caregiving children, those demonstrating a controlling–punitive pattern of attachment are characterized by higher externalizing problems throughout childhood (see Moss et al., Chapter 3, this volume). This difference between controlling–caregiving and controlling–punitive children was also noted by Solomon et al. (1995), who found that the internal working models of caregiving children in a doll-play procedure were marked by inhibition and anxiety, while the models of punitive children were characterized by representations of chaos and violence.

For the controlling group as a whole, Solomon and George (George & Solomon, 1996, 2008; Chapter 6, this volume; Solomon & George, 1996) found that mothers of controlling children described themselves as lacking effective and appropriate resources to handle the child's behavior and to provide care. The majority of mothers of controlling children evaluated their child as being "out of control," but this evaluation took one of two forms. Some of these children were described by their mothers as being wild and acting out, while others were described as being precocious and caregiving (George & Solomon, 1996; Chapter 6, this volume). In either case, such ineffectiveness of the parental caregiving system leaves the child with the precocious need to care for and regulate him- or herself, as well as to regulate the relationship. One may speculate that among parents with histories of emotional or physical abuse, the child's increased willfulness emerging in toddlerhood may activate the mother's representations of prior unbalanced and/or abusive relational patterns and thereby increase parental tendencies toward hostile attributions regarding the child and toward coercive cycles of interaction. This hypothesis receives support from Solomon and George's (2006; Chapter 2, this volume) results showing that mothers' current reports of helplessness in their interactions with their children mediated the association between their own representations of abuse and the controlling behavior of their children.

Bureau, Easterbrooks, and Lyons-Ruth (2009) recently extended the assessment of disorganized/controlling attachment into middle childhood. Three scales were developed and validated evaluating the extent of controlling–punitive behavior, controlling–caregiving behavior, and behavioral disorganization among 8-year-olds during a reunion with their mothers following a 1-hour separation (Middle Childhood Disorganization and Control Scales; Bureau, Easterbrooks, Killam, Miranda, & Lyons-Ruth, 2006). Results indicated that children with higher ratings of *disorganized* behavior (e.g., fear, disorientation, sexualized behavior) were significantly more likely to come from families with a history of maltreatment and to produce disorganized representations on the Separation Anxiety Test (SAT; Main, Kaplan, & Cassidy, 1985). Higher scores on the *punitive* scale were associated with disorganized representations on the SAT, higher maternal disrupted communication scores in infancy on the AMBIANCE scales (Bronfman, Parsons, & Lyons-Ruth, 1992), and greater child unresponsiveness in a free-play session with mother. Children with higher ratings on the *caregiving* scale were more overresponsive to their mothers in the free-play session and had mothers who were more withdrawn in infancy on the AMBIANCE scales.

It is likely that such adaptations within the parent–child relationship at age 8 will continue to be evident in some form as the child makes the transition into adolescence. To the extent that an adolescent continues to experience punitive struggles with parents or continues to attend closely to the needs of a helpless or frightened parent, personal resources will be diverted from consolidating a coherent sense of self-identity, and a contradictory and unintegrated sense of self is likely to be reinforced. With the increased developmental complexity and capacities of the adolescent period, we might also expect heterogeneity in the manifestations of controlling or disorganized behavior to increase. To date, however, little is known about how these childhood controlling or disorganized behaviors may evolve from age 8 into adolescence and adulthood.

CONCEPTUALIZING AND ASSESSING SECURITY AND DISORGANIZATION IN ADOLESCENCE

Assessing Organized Attachment Strategies

The importance of the parent as a secure base and the attachment relationship as a goal-corrected partnership should continue during adolescence. However, developmental changes during adolescence pose two challenges for assessment (Allen, 2008; Kobak et al., 1993). First, the need for the availability of the attachment figure is less frequent and intense in adolescence than in earlier childhood (Bowlby, 1980; George & Solomon, 2008). This requires a shift from observing responses to separations to observing more subtle and ongoing secure base behaviors that occur in the process of interaction (Waters & Cummings, 2000). Second, during adolescence how caregivers and adolescents communicate about conflicts and about vulnerable topics that threaten self-esteem will constitute central aspects of the goal-corrected partnership. This suggests that assessment in adolescence needs to focus on the extent to which collaborative and balanced negotiation functions to maintain the adolescent's security and confidence in the caregiver's availability in the face of vulnerability, disagreement, and conflict (Bretherton & Munholland, 2008; Kobak & Duemmler, 1994).

Therefore, in developing the current instrument described in more detail below, we defined a goal-corrected partnership in adolescence as a sense of freedom to explore thoughts and feelings with the parent in a collaborative way. Secure base behavior comes into play as adolescents approach sensitive or conflicted topics and negotiate moments of vulnerability with the parent. In a secure dyad, while discussing an area of conflict, we would expect to see the parent communicate a strong sense of warmth and respect for hearing the adolescent's opinions, and both partners to show active attempts to understand the other's point of view, and to allow differences of opinion. Such collaborative interactions form the basis for the internalized representations of a facilitating attachment relationship that supports autonomous exploration of the larger environment.

In addition, there should be balanced turn taking and reciprocity in the parent–adolescent dialogue. We derive this emphasis from the work of Baldwin, Cole, and Baldwin (1982) in the large-scale Rochester study of children of psychiatrically hospitalized parents. They found that warmth and balance in the observed parent–child dialogue were the best predictors of child adaptation among children of mentally ill parents and were more important than any aspect of parental diagnosis or level of functioning. Balance did not imply equality of roles between parent and child, however, but instead an age-appropriate spontaneity of give-and-take in the parent–child relationship. Sroufe (1991) also identifies the importance of balance within a relationship system, including (1) balance between the individuals, or the ability to feel safe with each other and to retain a position despite disagreement; (2) balance between the relationship and the development of the individuals, such as when a parent is able to support the adolescent's bids for autonomy instead of making self-referential demands; and (3) balance between the relationship and the outside world, including the ability to address a need of the other without becoming bogged down by other concerns.

Finally, based on our observations of the importance of maternal withdrawal and role confusion in infancy (Lyons-Ruth, Bronfman, & Parsons, 1999), as well as on the emerging role confusion evident among controlling dyads by school age (Moss et al., Chapter 3, this volume), we view a secure base in adolescence as continuing to require the parent's maintenance of a parental role, which involves taking responsibility for flexibly monitoring and guiding the interaction, regulating vulnerable moments to protect the adolescent's self-esteem, and keeping track of task goals in the interaction. This concept is similar to the authoritative parenting identified by Baumrind (1971) that is associated with positive developmental outcomes.

Below is an example of how secure dialogue might present between a mother and her college-age son. They are discussing an area of conflict within their relationship as part of a revealed differences research task. The topic is whether or not the son is spending too much time working in a restaurant:

MOTHER: It's not so much the work, as I hope you realize, it's the consequence of having that time away from your schoolwork and the social environment of school. You don't have any free time for yourself or any time to have fun, and you stress out about your schoolwork. So I guess my basic thing is that, even though you like your job, you need to prioritize the things you can fit in your life and try to alleviate stress. That's the crux of it, don't you think?

ADOLESCENT: Yeah, but it's really nice having money and I really like working there and they are really cool. Sometimes it's just kind of like fun and mindless and easy.

MOTHER: So it's kind of a de-stressor as well?

ADOLESCENT: Yeah ... unless I have to do more than a 5-hour shift and then I get really wiped. See the thing is, since I've been working weekends, it's been much more exhausting since they don't have 5-hour shifts, they only have 6- or 7-hour shifts.

As their conversation progresses, the mother asks open-ended questions to help her son think about an ideal schedule (e.g., "If money was not a factor, how much would you like to work?") and the son decides to work only one weekend day instead of two. They both seem confident and candid about expressing their feelings about a genuine concern, and they seem to be actively listening to one another.

Organized but insecure attachment strategies should also be evident in adolescence, based on the replicated findings of continuity in organized attachment patterns from observed interaction patterns in infancy to interview responses on the AAI in young adulthood (Waters et al., 2000; Hamilton, 2000). Consistent with previous literature (Main & Cassidy, 1988; Main & Goldwyn, 1984; Moss, Cyr, & Dubois-Comtois, 2004; Moss et al., Chapter 3, this volume), deflecting/minimizing (avoidant) adolescents and their parents were expected to express opinions during conflicts, but with an overall tone of neutrality and distance. The interactive goal was conceived as one of limiting affective engagement by minimizing disagreement or avoiding too much exploration of potentially charged topics. Consistent with the organized nature of this strategy, however, we expected that both parents and adolescents would be active in monitoring more neutral aspects of the task goals and in structuring the interaction, and that parents in deflecting dyads would not reach the extreme of abdicating a parental role (Solomon & George, Chapter 6, 1996; George & Solomon, this volume), as might be seen among more traumatized or depressed parents. The following deflecting/minimizing exchange between a mother and her adolescent daughter highlights the effort to avoid potential disagreement or stress:

MOTHER: You should stop fighting with your brother.

DAUGHTER: Okay, I'll stop fighting

(*Both laugh.*)

MOM: I have no idea what else to say. We don't disagree.

DAUGHTER: Are we done?

With regard to ambivalent attachment patterns, and consistent with the large body of previous literature (e.g., Cassidy & Berlin, 1994; Main & Cassidy, 1988; Main & Goldwyn, 1984; Moss et al., 2004; Moss et al., Chapter 3, this volume), we expected adolescents and parents in organized entangled/oscillatory (ambivalent) interactions to be characterized by heightened but relatively low-level negative affect and tangential dialogue structure. What we observed among adolescents and parents classified as ambivalent was a pattern of bickering that seemed fruitless (e.g., haggling about irrelevant details; rehashing points from previous arguments) but that was regulated well enough not to escalate into actively hostile or derogatory interactions. The underlying goal was thought to be that of keeping the other involved emotionally through continued, mildly heated discussion at a superficial level. While parental leadership was less effective in this category, the parent avoided escalating anger or increasing the adolescent's potential moments of upset by moving the conversation in another direction or by not humiliating or attacking the adolescent. Therefore, although awkwardness or arguing often marked these interactions, the parent was actively involved and did not escalate the tension or leave the adolescent in charge, so that some sense of protection remained present.

The following entangled/oscillatory exchange between a mother and her adolescent son demonstrates the tendency to return to old topics and to focus on less pertinent points:

SON: Ah! The age-old argument of why Maria always gets to sit in the front seat of the car and I have to sit in the front seat with her. When I was her age I had to sit in the back and Mark got the front seat all the time. There's a good one! What do you have to say about that one?

MOTHER: Just what I've always told you—when you were small and Mark was the same age difference, I didn't have a three-seater, so there were only two seats in the front so somebody had to sit in the back. But this car, she could sit in between us for a long time.

SON: Yeah, I know, but you know it's uncomfortable for her to be there with me. You know how big I am. She's not a short kid and she's sitting in front there. That's not meant for somebody to sit there the whole time.

MOTHER: Why is there three seat belts there?

SON: It's like for when you have to bring a lot of people or something. The point is I always had to sit in the back and there is no reason why she shouldn't be made to sit in the back.

MOTHER: I remember what it was. She was in a booster seat and it was the front and she got used to sitting there ...

As can be seen, within all of the organized attachment strategies, even if insecure, the parent clearly remains in a parental role and the adolescent remains in an adolescent role. Recognizing this dynamic is important for recognizing the relational imbalances seen in the disorganized processes described below.

Disorganized/Controlling Attachment Strategies

Our conceptualization of the interaction patterns that constitute the disorganized/controlling spectrum in adolescence draws heavily on our prior work characterizing hostile–helpless relational processes. This conception was first developed in relation to patterns of interaction observed between mothers and infants (Lyons-Ruth, Bronfman, & Atwood, 1999) and was later further elaborated in describing hostile–helpless states of mind in adulthood shown in the AAI (Lyons-Ruth, Yellin, et al., 2005).

In this view, a core problem in disorganized attachment relationships lies in the hostile–helpless working model of interpersonal closeness that is transmitted intergenerationally from parent to infant. We have proposed that hostile–helpless dyadic models are actualized in unbalanced parent–infant relationships in which the parent's initiatives are elaborated at the expense of the infant's, either through dissociative, withdrawing responses or through hostile, overriding behavior. These nonreciprocal interaction patterns lead to a lack of development and/or a distortion in development of the child's initiatives in close relationships. The dyadic representational model that results is a highly polarized and contradictory model of how to be in relationships, one that combines representations of self-subjugation with representations of dominating and failing to respond to the other. Such polarized patterns of parent–child communication also increase the likelihood that the child will not be able to organize a consistent strategy for finding comfort and soothing from the parent when under stress. These unbalanced hostile–helpless relationships are also those relationships least likely to offer adequate protection and soothing to facilitate the mental integration and resolution of the traumatic affects associated with experiences of loss or abuse. Finally, particularly nonreciprocal and unbalanced relationships are those most likely to contribute to the development of contradictory behavioral and mental processes, as these unbalanced relationship processes are internalized as contradictory internal working models of relationship. In this model, then, we place patterns of parent–child interaction, rather than experiences of loss or trauma, as most central to the etiology of disorganized attachment behavior.

These nonreciprocal interactive processes become much more visible over the preschool years when clear role-reversal often occurs between parent and child, and the child is attending disproportionately to the parent's affective states (Moss et al., Chapter 3, this volume). So, in contrast to the more symmetrical roles of parent and adolescent in the earlier descriptions of secure and insecure-organized attachment patterns, in the disorganized/controlling spectrum we expected to see a markedly unbalanced, hostile–helpless role structure. In such unbalanced interactions, there is a pronounced disruption in both the goal-corrected partnership and the secure base functions of the parent–adolescent relationship.

In addition, in disorganized dyads over the adolescent years, the teen becomes increasingly capable of taking over guidance of the interaction in more subtle and apparently effective ways, by leading the discussion, using humor and self-revelation, monitoring the task goals, and smoothing over moments of tension. We therefore expected to continue to observe forms of caregiving and punitive control on the part of the adolescent, as well as forms of disorganized or disoriented behavior that failed to reveal an over-all strategy. However, in observing attachment in adolescence it becomes particularly important to track who takes responsibility for handling the crucial attachment tasks in the interaction, including who fosters give-and-take in the conversation and who defuses tensions when they arise. As shown below, a new controlling–containing attachment presentation emerged during adolescence in which the adolescent attempts to manage and parry humiliating, hostile, or dominating behaviors on the part of the parent by joking, entertaining, changing the subject, and attempting to steer the conversation back to the topic, while generally refraining from being overtly hostile in return. The overall sense was that the adolescent was working very hard to smooth over and maintain the interaction in the face of his or her increasing awareness of the vulnerability behind the parent's inappropriate behavior.

This was seen as a form of role-confused controlling behavior, but was not as actively directive and solicitous as in controlling–caregiving patterns and was not as overtly hostile and demeaning as controlling–punitive behavior. By late adolescence (18–23 years), this was the most prevalent behavior pattern observed in the disorganized spectrum in a separate longitudinal study of low-income young adults, and was particularly associated with borderline features and suicidality, underscoring the seriousness of the observed deviation in a goal-corrected partnership (Lyons-Ruth, Bureau, Hennighausen, Holmes, & Easterbrooks, 2009).

A second form of disrupted interaction that was present during adolescence but has not been prominent in earlier literature was a pattern of domineering control on the part of the parent accompanied by stifled, capitulating behavior on the part of the adolescent. This pattern was particularly prevalent in earlier adolescence (14–16 years) in the more socioeconomically advantaged sample reported on in this chapter.

DEVELOPMENT OF THE GOAL-CORRECTED PARTNERSHIP IN ADOLESCENCE CODING SYSTEM

The Goal-Corrected Partnership in Adolescence Coding System (GPACS; Lyons-Ruth, Hennighausen., & Holmes, 2005) was developed to fill the critical gap in the assessment of directly observed forms of disorganization in adolescence. The coding system is designed to be applied to a videotaped procedure between a parent and an adolescent that consists of a 5-minute unstructured reunion (following a 1- to 2-hour separation during which individual interviews take place) and a 10-minute revealed differences task based on an agreed-upon topic of disagreement between the adolescent and parent. A variety of other coding systems for adolescent–parent interaction were reviewed but these tended to focus more on coding specific affects or behaviors (Bullock & Dishion, 2007; Chen & Berdan, 2006; Wakschlag, Chase-Lansdale, & Brooks-Gunn, 1996) and did not fully capture the types of distortions in interaction documented in the disorganized attachment literature at earlier ages. More attachment-focused coding systems did not include overall classification systems (Allen, Hauser, Borman-Spurrell, & Worrell, 1990; Sroufe, 1991).

In creating the GPACS, our priority was to develop a coding instrument that was both clinically informative (i.e., descriptive categories) and research-useful (i.e., variable-level scales). Therefore, overall profiles or classifications of attachment strategy were developed, as well as scales for rating more specific aspects of parent and adolescent behavior. This chapter focuses on the overall classifications. The overall classifications were developed first, based on prior theory and research in the attachment area and by viewing videotapes and reading verbatim transcripts of adolescent–parent conflict discussions collected from previous adolescent studies in two other labs. These profiles are summarized as follows:

Secure Profile: Facilitating/Collaborative/Valuing Dyadic Strategy

As described above, both the parent and the adolescent are warm, respectful, and balanced about expressing opinions or feelings. The parent takes an appropriate parental stance in guiding the discussion (e.g., monitors task goals) and is sensitive to the adolescent's signals of vulnerability. The adolescent seems confident about advancing opinions and is able to raise vulnerable topics or emotions.

Insecure but Organized Profiles

Deflecting/Minimizing Dyadic Strategy

Both the parent and the adolescent express opinions, but seem neutral and distanced. They have rushed or limited discussions with little facilitation of the other's point of view. They seem to try to limit affective engagement around potentially charged issues by shifting or ignoring topics, putting on a positive spin, or coming to an abrupt agreement.

Entangled/Oscillatory Dyadic Strategy

Both the parent and the adolescent express opinions freely, but their discussions often have an argumentative, tense, and/or fruitless and tangential quality due to their self-focused stances and difficulty understanding and coordinating perspectives.

Disorganized/Unbalanced Profiles

Submissive Adolescent Stances

This stance is comprised of two subgroups.

1. *Hostile/Capitulating Pattern.* A dominant parent attempts to control the discussion by engaging in hostile or humiliating remarks while a capitulating adolescent responds with defensive, helpless, or odd/out-of-context comments or behaviors.

2. *Leading/Stifled Pattern.* The parent assumes an indirectly undermining stance by asking a string of leading questions to try to persuade the adolescent to validate the parent's opinion. The adolescent vacillates, appears extremely uncomfortable, and may withdraw from the situation by not participating or by engaging in other odd or out-or-context behaviors.

Controlling–Punitive Adolescent Stances

This stance is comprised of two subgroups.

1. *Punitive Strategy.* The adolescent engages in hostile/humiliating remarks while the parent capitulates with pacifying, helpless, or odd/out-of-context comments.

2. *Reciprocally Punitive Strategy.* Both parties attempt to control the discussion and override one another's contributions.

Caregiving–Containing Adolescent Stances

This stance is comprised of three subgroups.

1. *Caregiving Strategy.* The adolescent engages in caregiving, task managing, and/or entertaining behaviors. The parent may seem immature or petulant, nervous and deferential, helpless, and/or inappropriately intimate or seductive.

2. *Containing Strategy.* The parent ineffectively attempts to control the discussion, often with elements of hostility, while the adolescent manages the attempted control with impassiveness, diversionary tactics, entertaining, and/or odd, out-of-context behavior, possibly aimed at containing the level of negative affect in the interaction.

3. *Mixed Caregiving/Punitive Strategy.* The adolescent shows the above caregiving features combined with sporadic pointed references to parental inadequacies that seemed designed to embarrass or humiliate the parent.

Disoriented Adolescent Stance

The parent and/or the adolescent displays predominantly odd, out-of-context, disoriented behavior or confusing behavioral sequences that do not fit any of the above descriptors.

Emotionally Unavailable Parental Stance

The parent rarely participates in the discussion and may appear withdrawn, inwardly absorbed, and/or possibly depressed. The adolescent may attempt to engage the parent, but seems to give up. Both may lapse into prolonged periods of silence.

LONGITUDINAL VALIDITY STUDY OF THE GPACS AT AGE 14 IN RELATION TO THE AAI AT AGE 25

Forty adolescents and their families participated in the current study. Participants were randomly selected from Paths Over Time, a larger longitudinal study overseen by Drs. Stuart Hauser, Joseph Allen, Judith Crowell, and J. Heidi Gralinski-Bakker. The Paths Over Time sample consisted of two groups recruited in adolescence (M age = 14.43, SD = .87), one from a private psychiatric hospital (n = 70) and one from a public high school (n = 76).

The hospitalized adolescents carried primary DSM-III diagnoses (American Psychiatric Association, 1980; the psychiatric diagnostic system current at the time), including conduct or oppositional defiant disorder (50%), depressive disorders (22.9%), anxiety disorders (5.7%), or other disorders (20.6%), but none were identified as psychotic or organically impaired. The two groups did not differ significantly in terms of age, gender, birth order, or family structure and differed only moderately in socioeconomic standing (with higher socioeconomic status in the high school sample). Participants were predominantly white and from upper-middle-class families (M Hollingshead, 1975, socioeconomic status = 2.07, SD = 1.26).

At age 14, adolescents and their parents in the Paths Over Time study completed an audiotaped conflict resolution task in which they discussed possible solutions to moral dilemmas for 10–20 minutes. All audiotaped adolescent–parent discussions were transcribed. Transcripts were classified blind to all other data from the study using the GPACS classifications.

Two coders coded 19 transcripts and the interrater reliability kappa was .83 (Secure, Insecure, and Disorganized).

At age 25, participants in Paths Over Time completed AAIs (George et al., 1985), a semistructured interview about early experiences with caregivers designed to classify the individual's state of mind toward attachment relationships. Expert coders Eric Hesse and Judith Crowell classified the AAIs blind to all other data. The 40 adolescents in the present study were randomly selected from the larger study by personnel of the Paths Over Time study, sampling more heavily from the higher risk psychiatric group ($n = 24$) than the control group ($n = 16$) and from those assigned unresolved or other rare classifications on the AAI in order to include good representation of atypical classifications.

Results

Control analyses first established that there was no association between psychiatric status and GPACS classifications (Secure, Insecure, Disorganized), $tau_c = .10$, n.s. GPACS classifications by nonpsychiatric and psychiatric status, respectively, were as follows: Secure 19% versus 13%; Insecure 31% versus 29%; and Disorganized 50% versus 58%. There was also no significant relation between psychiatric status and AAI categorizations at age 25 in this study sample: Secure 38% versus 13%; Insecure 25% versus 33%; Disorganized (Unresolved or Cannot Classify) 38% versus 54%; $tau_c = .25$, n.s.

When the correspondence was examined between the four GPACS categories (Facilitating/Valuing, Deflecting/Minimizing, Entangled/Oscillatory, and Unresolved or Cannot Classify) and the four AAI categories (Secure/Autonomous, Insecure/Dismissing, Insecure/Preoccupied, and Unresolved/Cannot Classify) assessed 10 years later, a strong and significant association was found, kappa = .51, $p < .000$. The overall distribution is presented in Table 8.1.

We have previously proposed that the rare AAI categories Dismissing/Derogating (Ds2) and Fearfully Preoccupied (E3), as well as Cannot Classify (CC), represent parental states of mind likely to be associated with infant disorganization (Lyons-Ruth & Jacobvitz, 2008; Lyons-Ruth, Yellin, et al., 2005). Therefore, a second analysis grouped participants with Dismissing/Derogating and Fearfully Preoccupied states of mind at age 25 among those with Unresolved and Cannot Classify states of mind. That distribution is displayed in Table 8.2. All had been classified as disorganized in interaction with the caregiver at age 14, and the overall correspondence between the two classifications increased to kappa = .60.

As can be seen in Tables 8.1 and 8.2, there was significant agreement between the GPACS in midadolescence and the AAI at age 25 both overall

TABLE 8.1. Four-Way Agreement between GPACS Adolescent Classifications and AAI Classifications at Age 25

AAI classifications at age 25	GPACS adolescent classifications at age 14			
	Facilitating	Deflecting	Entangled	Disorganized
Autonomous AAI	5	2	1	1
Dismissing AAI	0	3	1	2
Preoccupied AAI	0	0	3	3
Disorganized AAI (U, CC)	1	0	2	16

Note. n = 40. Kappa = .51, *p* < .001.
*a*Unresolved or Cannot Classify.

and for each classification individually. From Table 8.2, it can be seen that 83% of the adolescents judged to be Facilitating/Valuing based on the GPACS coding were later classified as Secure/Autonomous on the AAI, z = 3.87, p < .05. Sixty percent of the adolescents judged to be Deflecting/ Minimizing on the GPACS were later classified as Insecure/Dismissing on the AAI, z = 3.98, p < .05. Forty-three percent of adolescents judged to be Entangled/Oscillatory on the GPACS were later classified as Insecure/ Preoccupied on the AAI, z = 2.67, p < .05. Eighty-six percent of the adolescents coded as disorganized on the GPACS at age 14 were later classified on the AAI as Unresolved due to Loss or Trauma (U) (six out of an n of eight Unresolved adults); Cannot Classify (10 out of an n of 11 CC adults); Dismissing/Derogating (two out of an n of two Ds2 adults); or Fearfully Preoccupied (one out of an n of one E3 adult), z = 4.41, p < .05.

The most important implication of these data is that lapses in coherence when discussing difficult experiences in adulthood, such as loss or abuse, are

TABLE 8.2. Four-Way Agreement between GPACS Adolescent Classifications and AAI Classifications at Age 25 Using Augmented Disorganized Grouping for AAIs

AAI classifications at age 25	GPACS adolescent classifications at age 14			
	Facilitating	Deflecting	Entangled	Disorganized
Autonomous AAI	5	2	1	1
Dismissing AAI	0	3	1	0
Preoccupied AAI	0	0	3	2
Disorganized AAI (U, CC, Ds2, E3)*a*	1	0	2	19

Note. n = 40.
Kappa = .60, *p* < .001.
*a*Unresolved, Cannot Classify, Dismissing/derogating, Fearfully Preoccupied

predicted by clearly disrupted patterns of interaction between parent and child in adolescence. This is one of the first demonstrations that patterns of observed parent–child interaction significantly predict later Unresolved status on the AAI. This finding grounds lapses of coherence in the interview within broader patterns of disruption in the observed dialogue between parent and adolescent. For example, looking backward from the AAI, 75% of adults classified as Unresolved Due to Loss or Trauma were classified as having had disorganized/controlling interactions with their parents in mid-adolescence. Our interpretation of this relation is that disrupted patterns of communication with caregivers around emotionally arousing topics in childhood and adolescence lead to similar disruptions in communication with the interviewer around emotionally arousing topics during the AAI. The particular forms of those observed disruptions are also revealing. Of the eight participants with Unresolved classifications in adulthood, Unresolved abuse was particularly associated with submissive, leading-stifled patterns of parent–adolescent interaction (3/5 Unresolved abuse). In contrast, unresolved loss was associated with controlling and disoriented patterns of interaction (1 disoriented, 1 reciprocally punitive, 1 punitive–controlling).

Another important aspect of this initial validity data is the link that emerges between disorganized/controlling patterns of interaction in adolescence and rare states of mind regarding attachment that have not been well understood in the past (Cannot Classify; Dismissing/Derogating; Fearfully Preoccupied). Empirical evidence indicates that these rare AAI classifications tend to be found more frequently in clinical samples. For example, the state of mind coded Cannot Classify has been associated with psychiatrically hospitalized criminal offenders (Levinson & Fonagy, 2004; van IJzendoorn, Feldbrugge, Derks, & de Ruiter, 1997), as well as with men who behave violently toward their wives (Holtzworth-Munroe, Stuart, & Hutchinson, 1997). The states of mind coded Fearfully Preoccupied and Cannot Classify have been associated with patients with borderline personality disorder and sexually abused psychiatric patients (Patrick, Hobson, Castle, Howard, & Maughan, 1994; Stalker & Davies, 1995). Allen and colleagues (1996) found a strong association between the Dismissing/Derogating classification and hard drug use.

As noted, we have speculated previously that these adult states of mind will be associated with the intergenerational transmission of disorganized attachments rather than with the organized–avoidant or organized–ambivalent strategies with which they are now grouped. These findings indicate that adults in these rare AAI subgroups are likely to have participated in very nonreciprocal, dyadically unbalanced forms of parent–child interaction during adolescence. Of the 11 adults in the AAI Cannot Classify group, four were classified disoriented in adolescence, three were hostile (mother)–capitulating (adolescent), two were punitive, and one was leading (mother)–

stifled (adolescent) on the GPACS. The remaining adolescent in the Cannot Classify group in the AAI was classified as Entangled on the GPACS in adolescence.

Two participants had been classified as Dismissing/Derogating on the AAI at age 25. At age 14, both had parents who dominated the problem-solving discussion and were classified leading (mother)–stifled (adolescent). In the first transcript, the parent is clearly domineering in insisting upon her opinions and overriding or belittling the adolescent's contributions; in the second case, the parent more indirectly insists on her point of view by reiterating it, failing to acknowledge input from the adolescent, and repeatedly attempting to lead the adolescent to agree with the parent.

The one young adult classified Fearfully Preoccupied on the AAI was classified as caregiving at age 14. This converges with findings from a previous study of patients with borderline personality disorder and depressed controls in which Fearfully Preoccupied states of mind in adulthood on the AAI were significantly related to reports of controlling–caregiving behavior toward the parent in childhood on the AAI (phi = .46), as coded by the Hostile–Helpless coding system (Lyons-Ruth et al., 2007).

EXAMPLES OF ADOLESCENT–PARENT DIALOGUE FROM DISORGANIZED GPACS CLASSIFICATIONS

In the final section of this chapter, we illustrate in more detail the caregiving, punitive, and submissive adolescent stances observed across several studies on the GPACS, as well as providing examples of disoriented or odd/out-of-context behavior.

Caregiving Stances

The GPACS caregiving profiles describe the caregiving stances observed among adolescents toward their parents. These stances include behaviors such as giving advice or making reassuring comments, taking responsibility for keeping track of the task goals, and engaging the parent through excessive or forced humor, clowning, coyness, or flirtatiousness. Our interpretation of the function of these behaviors is that these adolescents are taking undue responsibility for reading and regulating their parents' signs of vulnerability, discomfort, distress, or anger in order to manage the parents' hostility or helplessness. Adolescents in role-reversed dyads will often seem highly attuned to the states of their parents. They may seem exceptionally skilled at leading the conversation and/or giving directives to their parents, but may do so by surrendering their own opinions and feelings to advance the opinions of or conciliate their parents. There is also a strong sense that these adolescents are holding back from spontaneous expression, are exceptionally focused on their parents' offerings, feel their parents may be unable to cope with or manage the situation, and are subtly and indirectly helping to guide their parents. The parents may appear to expect or may directly ask their adolescents to provide reassurance, directives, insight, affection, and/or caregiving. They may treat the adolescents more like peers, romantic partners, or parental figures.

The following is an example of caregiving dialogue between a 14-year-old female adolescent and her father in which they are trying to decide upon a topic to discuss:

DAUGHTER: Time for going to bed. Now that's one for you and me both. (*Wags finger at father.*) I should go to bed earlier because I have to get up and you should go to bed earlier so you don't go to sleep on the couch. (*Laughs.*)

FATHER: Yeah. (*Laughs nervously.*) But I still get sleep though, right?

DAUGHTER: But there's times when I have to wake you up and neither of us is easy to get up. Mom would have a fit if she found you out of bed on the couch.

(*They try to identify another topic to discuss.*)

FATHER: I said talking back to your mother.

DAUGHTER: I didn't put that *(looks surprised)*.

FATHER: I did.

DAUGHTER: Elaborate on that. How much does it bother you? What bothers you?

FATHER: (*Lapses into silence for several seconds.*)

DAUGHTER: (*Lights a cigarette and begins to smoke.*) What I say to her or just talking back to her?

FATHER: (*nervously*) More what you say.

DAUGHTER: Half the stuff I don't mean, but there's sometimes I mean it because she says some pretty loaded stuff to me. Our stuff is pretty heated, but I usually apologize to her afterwards. I don't usually mean it, it just comes out of anger. Anything else? (*Smiles brightly.*)

The example illustrates how the adolescent takes responsibility for initiating and maintaining the discussion, keeping it on topic, and drawing her father out, as well as closing off topics. Her comments and laughter about sleeping habits have mildly seductive overtones. The father seems anxious or deferential to her. He does not attempt to structure their conversation or follow up on the issue he raised.

Punitive Stances

Adolescents may also assume more controlling punitive stances by attempting to override the opinions and feelings of their parents. The adolescents who assume control often seem hostile or derisive, and may escalate the conflict in hurtful and nonconstructive ways. This often involves making humiliating remarks to their parents, such as "You cannot stand up for yourself" or "You're useless." Another tactic observed among punitive adolescents was to attack, punish, or shame their parents about personal problems or weaknesses, such as criticizing a father for a recent suicide attempt. The punitive adolescent may laugh at painful situations instead of showing empathy or remorse. Other work using the Hostile–Helpless AAI coding system has found that parental laughter at pain during the AAI is a powerful marker of infant disorganization (Lyons-Ruth, Yellin, et al., 2005).

Capitulating parents may respond with brief or vague comments, or may simply echo their adolescents' points throughout the discussion. These parents often seem nervous, defensive, and uncomfortable, and may laugh at inappropriate times to try to diffuse tension. Signs of capitulation to their adolescents' aggression include pacifying, helpless, or odd/out-of-context comments. The main strategy of capitulating parents seems to be to placate or avoid provoking their adolescents.

In one such controlling–punitive exchange between a 17-year-old adolescent and his mother, they discuss how the son handles problems with peers:

SON: I like to argue with Rob because it always turns out to fighting, but not real fighting, just joking around, like slap boxing, and it's fun. And he never gets serious—that's why I like messing with him. It doesn't matter how much you hurt him, he won't get serious. Sometimes his nose bleeds. (*Laughs.*) We smack each other up bad.

MOTHER: (*Mutters.*) You guys are crazy, beating each other up.

SON: (*Laughs.*) It's fun, though. That's how you got to do it to get tough. Unless you want to get bullied your whole life.

MOTHER: To get tough?

SON: You want to get bullied? You want to get bullied your whole life?

MOTHER: (*softly*) No.

SON: (*leaning in and becoming increasingly menacing*) You want to get bullied?

The son uses a hostile tone of voice and threatening body language to intimidate his mother. He is amused while describing another person's physical pain. The mother seems afraid of the adolescent and unable to assume a parental stance to address what he is saying about his aggressive behavior toward others or his aggressive behavior toward her.

Submissive Stances

In contrast, some adolescents assume more submissive stances. For example, adolescents in leading–stifled dyads often vacillate in their opinions and seem extremely uncomfortable, anxious, or sad during discussions with parents. The adolescents' efforts to articulate feelings and opinions seems muffled, uncertain, and possibly incoherent. They may advance and retract a number of stances, give in to parents prematurely, or respond to inappropriate personal questions. These adolescents may appear to tune out or withdraw for prolonged periods (e.g., staring off, closing eyes). They seem resigned that they cannot be part of conversations with parents in any meaningful way. For some dyads there is the sense of an "elephant in the room," in that sensitive and significant topics for the adolescent (e.g., a parent's alcoholism, custody arrangements) may be indirectly mentioned, but are quickly dropped.

Parents in leading–stifled dyads assume control of the conversation, but do not support the voice of their adolescents. They prioritize their own agendas, which may never be stated directly, and try to advance their agendas by asking a string of leading and/or indirect questions. These parents seem to be indirectly pressuring the adolescents to validate their own opinions. The parent may not attack the adolescent directly, but clearly undermines the stance of the adolescent ("So you don't have any feeling, in other words, one way or another very much"). The parent may also engage in mind-reading ("Isn't that what you were really thinking?"). They may raise sensitive topics (e.g., bed wetting, conflicts with an estranged parent) and seem unaware of how emotionally vulnerable their adolescents feel about these topics. They may also use strong guilt induction. These parents may try to appear confident and capable while seeming anxious or uncomfortable.

In the following dialogue between a mother and her 15-year-old son, the son would like to discuss problems he is having with his younger siblings:

SON: They keep jumping on my bed and I can't sleep.

MOTHER: You got to remove yourself from the situation.

SON: How?

MOTHER: I can't just take and beat you all for everything you do wrong, can I? If I beat you all for every little thing you do, then I will be a child abuser. Then you will be removed from my house and then what?

SON: (*Shrugs.*)

MOTHER: I would have to work extra hard to prove I'm a good parent to get my kids back. So what do you think I should do? I can't give you all my undivided attention. I try to spread my love through all three of you all. What else can I do?

SON: (*Begins to cry silently.*)

MOTHER: Don't you think I'm hurting, too, huh? (*Starts to tear up.*)

SON: Yeah

MOTHER: I'm tired. I'm tired now. I'm tired every day. I just need you to give me a break.

The mother is so overwhelmed that she uses guilt to try to induce compliance and seems unaware of her adolescent's emotional vulnerability. The adolescent's efforts to articulate his feelings are stifled, and he becomes increasingly withdrawn and sad. The parent's need to seek validation for her own position from the adolescent is so strong that the needs and feelings of the adolescent are completely overlooked.

Disoriented Stances

Odd or out-of-context behaviors or remarks may be seen in any of the disorganized profiles, but are most prominent in the submissive or disoriented profiles. These behaviors or remarks may seem incoherent, disjointed, startling, and possibly inexplicable or difficult for an observer to understand. Examples in adolescence are similar to odd, out-of-context behaviors seen among disorganized children at younger ages and may include speaking in an odd, hushed, forced, high-pitched, or childish tone of voice; exaggerated, false, forced, or stilted affect; mistimed, stiff, or stilted gestures; unusual shifts away from the topic; and wandering aimlessly around the room (see Main & Solomon, 1990). Odd/out-of-context behavior or remarks may indicate poor self-regulation or disinhibition; a momentary shift in or lapse of strategy; and/or dissociative processes. They seem especially significant when they occur during stressful or vulnerable moments.

The following example of disoriented, odd, out-of-context behavior is from a dialogue between a 13-year-old girl and her mother. The mother is asking repeatedly why her daughter does not have more friends:

MOTHER: (*Looms forward, rests her elbows on the table, and props her chin in her hands; speaks in a sing-song voice.*) I think Miss Julie Rosalie Banks needs to have more friends.

DAUGHTER: No.

MOTHER: Yes. Yes, you do, Miss Julie Rosalie Banks.

DAUGHTER: No. There's Ann. There's Rory. There's Deedee. There's Jamie. There's Casey. There's Theresa. There's a bunch of other people.

MOTHER: You are too young not to have—why aren't you able to make friends?

DAUGHTER: I can make friends easy.

(The mother appears increasingly frustrated as she presses the issue about having friends for several minutes while her daughter becomes more restless.)

MOTHER: *(in a low, hushed tone)* You need ... to have ... more friends. You don't want to be a hermit crab like me. That is not a good way to live.

DAUGHTER: Anyway, if I play with my friends, I will go outside. You will get fresh air. You will get that clear stuff with oxygen and carbon dioxide *(pretending to gather air in her two hands and bringing her hands together)* combined to release AIR! *(Abruptly pushes her arms out and opens her hands in her mother's face.)*

In this example, the mother's looming body language is potentially threatening and her voice tone is unusual. She does not seem to listen to her daughter's point of view or seem attuned to her vulnerability. Her daughter initially tries to manage the interaction and deflect her by being flip or impassive, but she becomes increasingly flustered and disregulated herself, as revealed by the lapse into odd, out-of-context behavior at the end of the exchange.

SUMMARY

Understanding the developmental pathways associated with disorganized attachment patterns in adolescence has been limited by the long time line needed for prospective infancy-to-adulthood studies, by the challenges of working with very stressed families, and by the time-intensive nature of developmental attachment assessments. In particular, assessments for the directly observed disorganized or controlling behaviors that have been well documented in infancy and early childhood have not been developed for adolescence. In order to fill this research gap, we designed an observational coding system for disorganized strategies seen among adolescent–parent dyads. The initial validity data presented here reveal that adolescent–parent interactions yield valuable insights into the developmental interactions associated with later adult states of mind on the AAI. Importantly, significant associations were observed between each of the organized categories of interaction on the GPACS and the subsequent organization of attachment narratives seen on the AAI. Equally important was the clear demonstration that Unresolved states of mind on the AAI were preceded by highly unbalanced patterns of interaction with the parent in adolescence. In addition, a robust relation emerged between disorganized/controlling patterns of interaction in adolescence and rare states of mind regarding attachment on the AAI that have not been well understood, including the Cannot Classify, Dismissing/Derogating, and Fearfully Preoccupied classifications. The current results indicate that very unbalanced forms of family interaction around emotionally vulnerable topics in adolescence may be associated in young adulthood with lapses in coherence on the AAI while discussing loss or trauma; derogation of attachment needs; preoccupation with fearful affects regarding attachment; or failure to demonstrate any consistent strategy for dealing with attachment concerns.

Further longitudinal work is now needed to examine the developmental trajectories in infancy and childhood that are associated with these unbalanced and/or role-confused relationships in adolescence. Further work is also needed evaluating how these attachment stances in adolescence are related to adaptation or maladaptation in other realms of development. Attempts to influence another's behavior through punitive or caregiving control, as well as more submissive and disoriented stances, may contribute to the maladaptive outcomes in adolescence and young adulthood already shown to be related to attachment assessments in infancy or adulthood. For example, relations have been shown between disorganized forms of attachment and dissociative symptoms (Carlson, 1998; Dutra, Bureau, Holmes, Lyubchik, & Lyons-Ruth, 2009; Ogawa, Sroufe, Weinfield, Carlson, & Egeland, 1997), borderline personality disorder (Patrick et al., 1994), disruptive behavior disorders (van IJzendoorn, Schuengel, & Bakermans-Kranenburg, 1999), eating disorders (Broberg, Hjalmers, & Nevonen, 2001), and suicidal thoughts or behaviors (Adam, Sheldon-Keller, & West, 1996). A behavioral measure of disorganized attachment interactions in adolescence can augment our understanding of the relational contributions to such disorders and identify useful approaches to family support and clinical intervention.

ACKNOWLEDGMENTS

Work presented in this chapter was funded by National Institutes of Health Grant No. R01 MH062030, a grant from the Milton Fund of Harvard University, and a grant from the Psychoanalytic Research Fund, to Karlen Lyons-Ruth. We dedicate this chapter to the memory of Stuart T. Hauser, a friend, mentor, and influential scholar in the field of adolescent research.

REFERENCES

Adam, K. S., Sheldon-Keller, A. E., & West, M. (1996). Attachment organization and history of suicidal behavior in clinical adolescents. *Journal of Consulting and Clinical Psychology, 64,* 264–272.

Ainsworth, M. D. S., Blehar, M., Waters, E., & Wall, S. (1978). *Patterns of attachment: A psychological study of the Strange Situation.* Hillsdale, NJ: Erlbaum.

Allen, J. P. (2008). The attachment system in adolescence. In J. Cassidy & P. Shaver (Eds.), *Handbook of attachment: Theory, research, and clinical applications* (2nd ed., pp. 419–435). New York: Guilford Press.

Allen, J. P., & Hauser, S. T. (1996). Autonomy and relatedness in adolescent-family interactions as predictors of young adults' states of mind regarding attachment. *Development and Psychopathology, 8,* 793–809.

Allen, J. P., Hauser, S. T., & Borman-Spurrell, E. (1996). Attachment theory as a framework for understanding sequelae of severe adolescent psychopathology: An 11–year follow-up study. *Journal of Consulting and Clinical Psychology, 64,* 254–263.

Allen, J. P., Hauser, S. T., Borman-Spurrell, E., & Worrel, C. M. (1990). *The autonomy and relatedness coding system: A scoring manual.* Unpublished manuscript, University of Virginia at Charlottesville.

American Psychiatric Association (1980). *Diagnostic and statistical manual of mental disorders* (3rd ed.). Washington, DC: American Psychiatric Association.

Baldwin, A. L., Cole, R. E., & Baldwin, C. P. (1982). Parental pathology, family interaction, and the competence of the child in school. *Monographs of the Society for Research in Child Development, 47*(4), 72–80.

Baumrind, D. (1971). Current patterns of parental authority. *Developmental Psychology Monographs, 4*(1), 1–103.

Beebe, B., Jaffe, J., Markese, S., Buck, K., Chen, H., Cohen, P., et al. (2010). The origins of 12-month attachment: A microanalysis of 4–month mother–infant interaction. *Attachment and Human Development, 12*(1–2), 6–141.

Bowlby, J. (1980). *Attachment and Loss: Vol. 3. Loss: Sadness and depression.* New York: Basic Books.

Bowlby, J. (1982). *Attachment and loss: Vol. 1. Attachment.* New York: Basic Books. (Original wotk published 1969)

Bowlby J. (1988). *A secure base: Parent–child attachment and healthy human development.* New York: Basic Books.

Bretherton, I., & Munholland, K. A. (2008). Internal working models in attachment relationships: Elaborating a central construct in attachment theory. In J. Cassidy & P. Shaver (Eds.), *Handbook of attachment: Theory, research, and clinical applications* (2nd ed., pp. 102–129). New York: Guilford Press.

Broberg, A. G., Hjalmers, I., & Nevonen, L. (2001). Eating disorders, attachment and interpersonal difficulties: A comparison between 18- to 24-year-old patients and normal controls. *European Eating Disorders Review, 9,* 381–396.

Bronfman, E., Parsons, E., & Lyons-Ruth, K. (1992). *Atypical Maternal Behavior Instrument for Assessment and Classification (AMBIANCE): Manual for coding disrupted affective communication.* Unpublished manuscript, Harvard

Medical School, Department of Psychiatry, Cambridge Health Alliance, Cambridge, MA.

Bullock, B. M., & Dishion, T. J. (2007). Family processes and adolescent problem behavior: Integrating relationship narratives into understanding development and change. *Journal of the American Academy of Child & Adolescent Psychiatry, 46,* 396–407.

Bureau, J.-F., Easterbrooks, A., Killam, S., Miranda, C., & Lyons-Ruth, K. (2006) *Middle Childhood Disorganization and Controlling Scales.* Unpublished document, University of Ottawa, Department of Psychology, Ottawa, Canada.

Bureau, J. -F., Easterbrooks, A., & Lyons-Ruth, K. (2009). Attachment disorganization and role-reversal in middle childhood: Maternal and child precursors and correlates. *Attachment and Human Development, 11*(3), 265—284.

Carlson, E. A. (1998). A prospective longitudinal study of disorganized/disoriented attachment. *Child Development, 69,* 1970–1979.

Cassidy, J., & Berlin, L. (1994). The insecure/ambivalent pattern of attachment: Theory and research. *Child Development, 65,* 971–991.

Cicchetti, D., & Barnett, D. (1991). Attachment organization in maltreated preschoolers. *Development and Psychopathology, 3,* 397–411.

Chen, E., & Berdan, L. E. (2006). Socioeconomic status and patterns of parent–adolescent interactions. *Journal of Research on Adolescence, 16,* 19–27.

Coplan, J., Andrews, M., Rosenblum, L., Owens, M., Friedman, S., & Gorman, J. (1996). Persistent elevations of cerebrospinal fluid concentrations of corticotrophin-releasing factor in adult nonhuman primates exposed to early life stressors: Implications for the pathophysiology of mood and anxiety disorders. *Proceedings of the National Academy of Sciences, 93,* 1619–1623.

Dodge, K. (2000). Conduct disorder. In A. J. Sameroff, M. Lewis, & S. M. Miller (Eds.), *Handbook of developmental psychopathology* (2nd ed., pp. 447–463). New York: Plenum Press.

Dutra, L., Bureau, J. F., Holmes, B. M., Lyubchik, A., & Lyons-Ruth, K. (2009). Quality of early care and childhood trauma: A prospective study of developmental pathways to dissociation. *Journal of Nervous and Mental Disease, 197,* 383–390.

Finger, B. (2007). *Exploring the intergenerational transmission of attachment disorganization.* Unpublished doctoral dissertation, University of Chicago.

Fraiberg, S., Adelson, E., & Shapiro, V. (1975). Ghosts in the nursery. *Journal of the American Academy of Child Psychiatry, 14,* 387–421.

Francis, D., Diorio, J., Liu, D., & Meaney, M. (1999). Nongenomic transmission across generations of maternal behavior and stress responses in the rat. *Science, 286,* 1155–1158.

Ge, X., Lorenz, F. O., Conger, R. D., Elder, G. H., & Simons, R. L. (1994). Trajectories of stressful life events and depressive symptoms during adolescence. *Developmental Psychology, 30,* 467–483.

George, C., Kaplan, N., & Main, M. (1985). *Adult Attachment Interview.* Unpublished manuscript, University of California at Berkeley.

George, C., & Solomon, J. (1996). Representational models of relationships: Links between caregiving and attachment. *Infant Mental Health Journal, 17,* 198–216.

George, C., & Solomon, J. (2008). The caregiving system: A behavioral systems approach to parenting. In J. Cassidy & P. Shaver (Eds.), *Handbook of attachment: Theory, research, and clinical applications* (2nd ed., pp. 833–856). New York: Guilford Press.

George, C., & West, M. (2001). The development and preliminary validation of a new measure of adult attachment: The Adult Attachment Projective. *Attachment and Human Development, 3,* 30–61.

George, C., & West, M. (in press). *The Adult Attachment Projective Picture System.* New York: Guilford Press.

Grossmann, K., Grossmann, K. E., Fremmer-Bombik, E., Kindler, H., Scheuerer-Englisch, H., & Zimmermann, P. (2002). The uniqueness of the child–father attachment relationship: Fathers' sensitive and challenging play as a pivotal variable in a 16–year longitudinal study. *Social Development, 11,* 307–331.

Hamilton, C. E. (2000). Continuity and discontinuity of attachment from infancy through adolescence. *Child Development, 71,* 690–694.

Hertsgaard, L., Gunnar, M., Erickson, M. F., & Nachmius, M. (1995). Adrenocortical response to the Strange Situation in infants with disorganized/disoriented attachment relationships. *Child Development, 66,* 1100–1106.

Hesse, E. (2008). The Adult Attachment Interview: Protocol, method of analysis, and empirical studies. In J. Cassidy & P. Shaver (Eds.), *Handbook of attachment: Theory, research, and clinical applications* (2nd ed., pp. 552–598). New York: Guilford Press.

Hollingshead, A. B. (1975). *Four-factor index of social status.* Unpublished manuscript, Yale University, New Haven, CT.

Holtzworth-Munroe, A., Stuart, G. L., & Hutchinson, G. (1997). Violent versus nonviolent husbands: Differences in attachment patterns, dependency, and jealousy. *Journal of Family Psychology, 11,* 314–331.

Jimerson, S., Egeland, B., Sroufe, L. A., & Carlson, B. (2000). A prospective, longitudinal study of high-school dropouts: Examining multiple predictors across development. *Journal of School Psychology, 38,* 525–549.

Kobak, R. R. (1993). Attachment and the problem of coherence: Implications for treating disturbed adolescents. *Adolescent Psychiatry, 19,* 137–149.

Kobak, R. R., Cole, H. E., Ferenz-Gillies, R., Fleming, W. S., & Gamble, W. (1993). Attachment and emotion regulation during mother–teen problem solving: A control theory analysis. *Child Development, 64,* 231–245.

Kobak, R., & Duemmler, S. (1994). Attachment and conversation: Toward a discourse analysis of adolescent and adult security. In K. Bartholomew & D. Perlman (Eds.), *Attachment processes in adulthood* (pp. 121–149). London: Jessica Kingsley.

Kobak, R. R., & Sceery, A. (1988). Attachment in late adolescence: Working models, affect regulation, and representations of self and others. *Child Development, 59,* 135–146.

Kraemer, G. W., & Clarke, A. S. (1996). Social attachment, brain function, and aggression. *Annals of the New York Academy of Sciences, 794,* 121–135.

Levine, S., Wiener, S. G., & Coe, C. L. (1993). Temporal and social factors influencing behavioral and hormonal responses to separation in mother and infant squirrel monkeys. *Psychoneuroendocrinology, 4,* 297–306.

Levinson, A., & Fonagy, P. (2004). Offending and attachment: The relationship between interpersonal awareness and offending in a prison population with psychiatric disorder. *Canadian Journal of Psychoanalysis, 12,* 225–251.

Lyons-Ruth, K., Bronfman, E., & Atwood, G. (1999). A relational diathesis model of hostile–helpless states of mind: Expressions in mother–infant interaction. In J. Solomon & C. George (Eds.), *Attachment disorganization* (pp. 33–70). New York: Guilford Press.

Lyons-Ruth, K., Bronfman, E., & Parsons, E. (1999). Maternal disrupted affective communication, maternal frightened or frightening behavior, and disorganized infant attachment strategies. In J. Vondra & D. Barnett (Eds.), Atypical patterns of infant attachment: Theory, research, and current directions. *Monographs of the Society for Research in Child Development, 64*(3), 67–96.

Lyons-Ruth, K., Bureau, J.-F., Hennighausen, K. H., Holmes, B. M., & Easterbrooks, A. (2009, April). Parental helplessness and adolescent role-reversal as correlates of borderline features and self-injury. In J.-F. Bureau & K. Lyons-Ruth (Chairs), *Relational predictors of self-damaging behavior in adolescence: Multiwave longitudinal analyses.* Symposium conducted at the Society for Research in Child Development biennial meeting, Denver, CO.

Lyons-Ruth, K., Hennighausen, K. H., & Holmes, B. M. (2005). *Goal-corrected partnership in adolescence coding system.* Unpublished document, Harvard Medical School, Cambridge Hospital, Department of Psychiatry, Cambridge, MA.

Lyons-Ruth, K., & Jacobvitz, D. (2008). Attachment disorganization: Genetic factors, parenting contexts, and developmental transformation from infancy to adulthood. In J. Cassidy & P. Shaver (Eds.), *Handbook of attachment: Theory, research, and clinical applications* (2nd ed., pp. 666–697). New York: Guilford Press.

Lyons-Ruth, K., Melnick, S., Patrick, M., & Hobson, R. P. (2007). A controlled study of hostile–helpless states of mind among borderline and dysthymic women. *Attachment and Human Development, 9,* 1–16.

Lyons-Ruth, K., Yellin, C., Melnick, S., & Atwood, G. (2003). Childhood experiences of trauma and loss have different relations to maternal unresolved and hostile–helpless states of mind on the AAI. *Attachment and Human Development, 5,* 330–352.

Lyons-Ruth, K., Yellin, C., Melnick, S., & Atwood, G. (2005). Expanding the concept of unresolved mental states: Hostile/helpless states of mind on the Adult Attachment Interview are associated with disrupted mother-infant communication and infant disorganization. *Development and Psychopathology, 17,* 1–23.

Main, M., & Cassidy, J. (1988). Categories of response to reunion with the parent at age 6: Predictable from infant attachment classifications and stable over a 1-month period. *Developmental Psychology, 24,* 415–426.

Main, M., & Goldwyn, R. (1984). *Adult attachment scoring and classification system.* Unpublished manuscript, University of California at Berkeley.

Main, M., & Hesse, E. (1990). Parents' unresolved traumatic experiences are related to infant disorganized attachment status: Is frightened or frightening parental behavior the linking mechanism? In M. T. Greenberg & D. Cicchetti (Eds.),

Attachment in the preschool years (pp. 121–160). Chicago: University of Chicago Press.

Main, M., Hesse, E., & Kaplan, N. (2005). Predictability of attachment behavior and representational processes at 1, 6, and 19 years of age: The Berkeley Longitudinal Study. In K. E. Grossmann, K. Grossmann, & E. Waters (Eds.), *Attachment from infancy to adulthood: The major longitudinal studies* (pp. 245–304). New York: Guilford Press.

Main, M., Kaplan, N., & Cassidy, J. (1985). Security in infancy, childhood, and adulthood: A move to the level of representation. In I. Bretherton & E. Waters (Eds.), Growing points of attachment theory and research. *Monographs of the Society for Research in Child Development, 50*(1–2, Serial No. 209), 66–104.

Main, M., & Solomon, J. (1986). Discovery of a new, insecure–disorganized/disoriented attachment pattern. In T. B. Brazelton & M. W. Yogman (Eds.), *Affective development in infancy* (pp. 95–124). Norwood, NJ: Ablex.

Main, M., & Solomon, J. (1990). Procedures for identifying infants as disorganized/disoriented during the Ainsworth Strange Situation. In M. Greenberg, D. Cicchetti, & E. M. Cummings (Eds.), *Attachment in the preschool years: Theory, research and intervention* (pp. 121–160). Chicago: University of Chicago Press.

Melnick, S., Finger, B., Hans, S., Patrick, M., & Lyons-Ruth, K. (2008). Hostile–helpless states of mind in the Adult Attachment Interview (AAI): A proposed additional AAI category with implications for identifying disorganized infant attachment in high-risk samples. In H. Steele & M. Steele (Eds.), *Clinical applications of the Adult Attachment Interview* (pp. 399–423). New York: Guilford Press.

Miller, B., & Moore, K. (1990). Adolescent sexual behavior, pregnancy, and parenting: Research through the 1980s. *Journal of Marriage and the Family, 52,* 1025–1044.

Moss, E., Cyr, C., & Dubois-Comtois, K. (2004). Attachment at early school age and developmental risk: Examining family contexts and behavior problems of controlling–caregiving, controlling–punitive, and behaviorally disorganized children. *Developmental Psychology, 40,* 519–532.

Nelson, K. (1996). *Language in cognitive development: Emergence of the mediated mind.* New York: Cambridge University Press.

NICHD Early Child Care Research Network. (2001). Child-care and family predictors of preschool attachment and stability from infancy. *Developmental Psychology, 37,* 847–862.

Ogawa, J. R., Sroufe, L. A., Weinfield, N. S., Carlson, E. A., & Egeland, B. (1997). Development and the fragmented self: Longitudinal study of dissociative symptomatology in a nonclinical sample. *Development and Psychopathology, 9,* 855–879.

Patrick, P., Hobson, R. H., Castle, D., Howard, R., & Maughan, B. (1994). Personality disorder and the mental representation of early social experience. *Development and Psychopathology, 6,* 375–388.

Patterson, G. R., & Bank, L. (1989). Some amplifying mechanisms for pathologic processes in families. In M. R. Gunnar & E. Thelen (Eds.), *Systems and devel-*

opment: The Minnesota Symposia on Child Psychology (Vol. 22, pp. 16–20). Hillsdale, NJ: Erlbaum.

Robertson, J., & Robertson, J. (1969). *The response of young children of good previous experience to foster care and residential nursery care.* [Film.] London: Tavistock Institute of Human Relations.

Shelder, J., & Block, J. (1990). Adolescent drug use and psychological health: A longitudinal study. *American Psychologist, 45,* 612–630.

Solomon, J., & George, C. (1996). Defining the caregiving system: Toward a theory of caregiving. *Infant Mental Health Journal, 17,* 183–197.

Solomon, J., & George, C. (1999). The place of disorganization in attachment theory: Linking classic observations with contemporary findings. In J. Solomon & C. George (Eds.), *Attachment disorganization* (pp. 3–32). New York: Guilford Press.

Solomon, J., & George, C. (2006). Intergenerational transmission of dysregulated maternal caregiving: Mothers describe their upbringing and childrearing. In O. Mayseless (Ed.), *Parenting representations: Theory, research, and clinical implications* (pp. 265–295). New York: Cambridge University Press.

Solomon, J., George, C., & DeJong, A. (1995). Children classified as controlling at age six: Evidence of disorganized representational strategies and aggression at home and at school. *Development and Psychopathology, 7,* 447–463.

Spangler, G., & Grossmann, K. E. (1993). Biobehavioral organization in securely and insecurely attached infants. *Child Development, 64,* 1439–1450.

Sroufe, J. (1991). Assessment of parent–adolescent relationships: Implications for adolescent development. *Journal of Family Psychology, 5,* 21–45.

Sroufe, L. A., Egeland, B., Carlson, E. A., & Collins, W. A. (2005). *The development of the person: The Minnesota Study of Risk and Adaptation from Birth through Adulthood.* New York: Guilford Press.

Stalker, C., & Davies, F. (1995). Attachment organization and adaptation in sexually abused women. *Canadian Journal of Psychiatry, 40,* 234–240.

Steinberg, L., & Morris, A. (2001). Adolescent development. *Annual Review of Psychology, 52,* 83–110.

Teti, D. M. (1999). Conceptualizations of disorganization in the preschool years: An integration. In J. Solomon, & C. George (Eds.), *Attachment disorganization* (pp. 213–242). New York: Guilford Press.

van IJzendoorn, M. H., Feldbrugge, J., Derks, F., & de Ruiter, C. (1997). Attachment representations of personality-disordered criminal offenders. *American Journal of Orthopsychiatry, 67,* 449–459.

van IJzendoorn, M. H., Schuengel, C., & Bakermans-Kranenburg, M. J. (1999). Disorganized attachment in early childhood: Meta-analysis of precursors, concomitants, and sequelae. *Development and Psychopathology, 11,* 225–250.

Wakschlag, L. S., Chase-Lansdale, P. L., & Brooks-Gunn, J. (1996). Not just "ghosts in the nursery": Contemporaneous intergenerational relationships and parenting in young African-American families. *Child Development, 67,* 2131–2147.

Wartner, U. G., Grossmann, K., Fremmer-Bombik, E., & Suess, G. (1994). Attachment patterns at age six in south Germany: Predictability from infancy and implications for preschool behavior. *Child Development, 65,* 1014–1027.

Waters, E., & Cummings, E. M. (2000). A secure base from which to explore close relationships. *Child Development, 71,* 164–172.

Waters, E., Merrick, S., Treboux, D., Crowell, J., & Albersheim, L. (2000). Attachment security in infancy and early adulthood: A twenty-year longitudinal study. *Child Development, 71,* 684–689.

Webster, L., & Hackett, R. K. (2005, April). A comparison of unresolved versus resolved status and its relationship to behavior in maltreated adolescents. In J. Wargo Aikins (Chair), *Narrative and discourse approaches towards understanding adolescent adjustment.* Symposium conducted at the Society for Research in Child Development biennial meeting, Atlanta, GA.

Weinfield, N. S., Sroufe, L. A., & Egeland, B. (2000). Attachment from infancy to early adulthood in a high-risk sample: Continuity, discontinuity, and their correlates. *Child Development, 71,* 695–702.

Weinfield, N., Whaley, G. J. L., & Egeland, B. (2004). Continuity, discontinuity, and coherence in attachment from infancy to late adolescence: Sequelae of organization and disorganization. *Attachment and Human Development, 6,* 73–97.

West, M., Rose, S., Spreng, S., & Adam, K. (2000). The Adolescent Unresolved Attachment Questionnaire: The assessment of perceptions of parental abdication of caregiving behavior. *Journal of Genetic Psychology, 161,* 493–503.

Chapter 9

Maternal Solicitousness
and Attachment Disorganization
among Toddlers with a Congenital Anomaly

DOUGLAS BARNETT, MELISSA KAPLAN-ESTRIN,
JULIE BRACISZEWSKI, LESLEY HETTERSCHEIDT,
JACLYN ISSNER, and CHRISTINE M. BUTLER

At the time we planned our study, several investigative teams were reporting relatively high rates of attachment disorganization and unclassifiable attachments among young children with a variety of special needs (see Barnett, Hunt, et al., 1999, for a review). These rates were particularly high among children with neurological disorders such as autism and Down syndrome (Capps, Sigman, & Mundy, 1993; Vaughn et al., 1994). Some speculated that neurological symptoms were being falsely mistaken for signs of attachment disorganization (Ganiban, Barnett, & Cicchetti, 2000; Pipp-Siegel, Siegel, & Dean, 1999). To investigate this hypothesis, we recruited two groups of young children with special needs that would allow us to tease apart the stresses associated with raising a child with a medical condition from the neurological symptoms that accompany conditions such as autism and Down syndrome. Our neurological group was made up primarily of children with cerebral palsy. Children recruited for our comparison group had medical conditions that required special care, but did not have any neurological symptoms. This group was made up primarily of children with cleft lip and palate. Consistent with our hypotheses, we did find significantly more signs of attachment disorganization among the children with neurological disorder. However, removing neurological symptoms from the list of indices of attachment disorganization, particularly those also present at times other than the reunions, eliminated this difference (Barnett, Hunt, et al., 1999). The result was a rate of attachment disorganization of 15.3%, a figure consistent with the rate found in the NICHD Early Child Care Research Network (1997), a national study of 1,300 infants (i.e., 15.4%). Even in an expanded longitudinal sample, we found no evidence that children with special needs, including some neurological disorders, were at elevated risk for attachment disorganization (Barnett et al., 2006).

Instead of being at risk for attachment disorganization, we now believe that many parents adapt quite well to their child's special needs, remain relatively resilient, providing high-quality care to their child with mild-to-moderate special needs (i.e., healthy enough to participate in a Strange Situation). Using the sample reported on in this chapter, our analyses found that based on the Reaction to Diagnosis Interview (RDI; Pianta, Marvin, & Morog, 1999), 47% of parents were classified as resolved concerning their child's diagnosis and nearly 74% of children of resolved mothers were securely attached. While coding signs of disorganization, one of our authors (Butler) made the anecdotal observation that mothers of children classified as disorganized appeared overly involved with their children or solicitous,[1] which the *American Heritage College Dictionary* (2000) defines as "marked by anxious care and often hovering attentiveness." To further examine the anecdotal observation more rigorously, we decided to look for evidence of solicitous outside of the Strange Situation and by observers other than Butler. To this end, we developed a rating scale for solicitousness and then had observers, unaware of our hypothesis and the children's attachment classification, rate the mothers during a play interaction task. This chapter focuses on the rationale for and findings from these analyses.

OVERPROTECTION AND OVERINVOLVEMENT

Raising a child with a special need such as a chronic medical condition, sensory impairment, or pervasive developmental disorder is a major stress for parents (Clements & Barnett, 2002; Lloyd, 2005). Parents of children with special needs report higher levels of stress and psychological symptoms than do parents of children who are developing normally (Britner, Morog, Pianta, & Marvin, 2003; Florian & Findler, 2001). Moreover, parents of children with special needs have more physical manifestations of stress, including premature aging, than parents of normally developing children (Epel et al., 2004). Some of the stress stems from increased demands on parents to attend appointments with professionals involved in the diagnosis, treatment, and education of those children with childhood problems as well as the uncertainty often surrounding their child's prognosis.

Parental stress from a variety of sources including poverty, work, divorce, and child behavioral problems has consistently been found to be associated with decreases in parenting sensitivity as well as increases in parenting hostility, child abuse, and neglect in families with medically healthy children (Grant et al., 2003; Steinberg, Catalano, & Dooley, 1981). As might be expected, some disruptions in parenting, including a very slight increase in risk for child abuse and neglect, have been found in connection with the elevated stress level associated with parenting children with special needs (Clements & Barnett, 2002; Goldson, 1998). However, despite the multitude of stresses related to parenting a child with special needs, these parents primarily demonstrate extraordinary resilience and dedication to their vulnerable children. For instance, unlike other types of parenting stress, raising a child with a special need or disability is not a particularly strong or consistent correlate of child abuse or neglect even as severity of the child's disability increases (Ammerman & Patz, 1996; Benedict, White, Wulff, & Hall, 1990). This, in and of itself, is a remarkable finding, given that children with disabilities have repeatedly been predicted to be at an increased risk for maltreatment because of the demands placed on caregivers of children with special needs.

Attachment theory helps to illuminate some of the reasons why raising a child with special needs, although quite stressful for caregivers, may be more likely to result in considerable parental devotion to vulnerable children than to result in higher instances of child abuse and neglect. From an ethological perspective, Bowlby (1982) theorized that two complimentary behavioral systems—attachment and caregiving—evolved with the goal of protecting children. Behavioral systems are thought to marshal a variety of psychological processes including perception, representation, cognition, and emotion that organize around a goal (e.g., building a nest). The attachment system provides the motivational basis for offspring to monitor the whereabouts of their attachment figure, and to seek proximity and comfort from this specific figure when in danger, distressed, ill, or fatigued (Bowlby, 1982; Sroufe & Waters, 1977). Correspondingly, the caregiving system provides parents with the motivational basis to monitor, protect, and provide comfort to their offspring, ensuring the safety and well-being of their children (Bell & Richard, 2000; George & Solomon, 2008; Solomon & George, 1996). The caregiving system is activated by cues from one's children, including distress, endangerment, and illness.

Under unusual circumstances such as a severe illness or injury, parents may perceive, accurately or not, a child to need a high degree of continuous, intensive care. Theoretically, this perception would result in chronic overactivation of the caregiving system. It follows that researchers have found that parents of a chronically ill child may become overprotective, overinvolved, and solicitous because they perceive their child to be helpless, in constant pain, or in medical danger (Holmbeck et al., 2002). This viewpoint fits our experiences with parents of children with chronic medical conditions. Research like ours may tend to attract parents who are particularly devoted to their child with special needs and who participate in our studies as an extension of their commitment to their child. Anecdotally, some parents expressed this devotion as a motivation for joining our study, saying that they hoped their involvement might provide information to help others.

In addition, we developed and implemented an intervention for parents of young children with special needs. Called "Building New Dreams" (Barnett, Clements, Kaplan-Estrin, & Fialka, 2003), this intervention was designed to help parents resolve their reactions to their child's diagnosis and promote secure attachments within their families. As was the case with this study, we felt that the program attracted parents who were exceedingly devoted to their role as caregivers to their children with special needs. Many of these parents had put aside their own personal goals (e.g., school and careers) in order to be full-time caregivers to their child, taking them to numerous medical appointments and various early interventions such as physical therapy and programs to promote cognitive, social, and emotional development.

How does one determine what is "adaptive" or "healthy" in these situations? Parents have participated in our intervention program whose children have severe and life-threatening conditions such as spina bifida or severe respiratory disorders for which a small cold or infection can have life-threatening consequences. For such disorders, parents have to be constantly vigilant concerning their children's health, making sure their youngsters do not touch or dislodge shunts or tubes that may easily become infected or interfere with vital functions. When acute health risks are present, extreme parental vigilance and involvement is understandable and necessary for the child's immediate survival. As a result, we became aware of the paradox wherein parents' behavior may be vital for their child's physical well-being, but less than ideal, and perhaps disorganizing to their children's attachment.

CAN ATTACHMENT DISORGANIZATION RESULT FROM PARENTAL OVERINVOLVEMENT AND SOLICITOUSNESS?

Theory and research emphasize the role of severe parental psychopathology, unresolved trauma, abuse, neglect, and other fearful, frightening, hostile–helpless parenting behaviors in the etiology of attachment disorganization (Lyons-Ruth, Yellin, Melnick, & Atwood, 2005; Main & Hesse, 1990; Solomon & George, 1999; van IJzendoorn, Schuengel, & Bakermans-Kranenburg, 1999). Chronic overprotection, overinvolvement, and solicitousness may also be frightening by communicating the mother's perception of a high level of danger. Our observations were of parents who appeared so highly attuned to or solicitous of their youngster that they communicated a chronic state of fear. For instance, one parent got a tissue ready for her child before our observers could detect the child was going to sneeze. Other observations included parents who played with toys *for* their child (e.g., narrated a lengthy pretend activity in a highly animated manner). On first encountering these dyads, it would be understandable to predict that these children might be securely attached as a consequence of their mothers' devotion. However, our observations of these dyads in the Strange Situation suggested otherwise (cf. Barnett, Hunt, et al., 1999), and the hypothesis that these maternal behaviors might be alarming to the child led us to the prediction that solicitousness would be associated with attachment disorganization.

We see solicitousness as going considerably beyond parental worry, especially because it involves parental physical infringement on children's autonomy and developmental expectations. We further propose that it involves and communicates intense fear on the part of the parent for the child's well-being. Through the constant hovering and involvement of solicitousness parental behavior children's developing self- and emotion regulation may be disrupted by not providing enough opportunity for children to experience small requisite amounts of experience handling some behavioral and emotional situations autonomously. Biringen, Emde, and Pipp-Siegel (1997) wrote about the positive contributions that moderate levels of dyssynchrony and conflict in the parent–infant relationship make to the development of children's emotion regulation and differentiation of an autonomous self. They theorized that midrange levels of distress and frustration are optimal and perhaps necessary within infant–parent interactions because they facilitate the child's practicing to manage affect. Biringen and colleagues speculated that handling too much or too little emotion would increase the chances children would have emotion regulation problems. Similarly, Winnicott (1965) described the "good enough" parent as not being too perfect, allowing the child to practice handling frustration and learning to delay gratification. Moreover, he also discussed the importance of the young child being able to play in the presence of the mother without her hovering or interfering as a key ingredient for developing the healthy "capacity to be alone." For our sample the implications are that toddlers can handle more physical and emotional space and may require it to stimulate the development of autonomous regulation. Consequently, we wondered whether parental solicitousness might delay the development of requisite regulation skills required for forming an organized attachment pattern.

Research on attachment disorganization has focused primarily on young children who, within their attachment relationship, have experienced intense conflicting emotions or trauma that severely challenge their regulatory capacity and result in disorganization in the presence of their caregiver (Hesse & Main, 2006). Perhaps solicitous parenting fails to provide children with sufficient experience independently managing distress such that they are overwhelmed by more arousal than they can manage when faced with the stress inherent in the Strange Situation. From this perspective, we hypothesized that infants and toddlers whose parents acted solicitously toward them would experience difficulty maintaining a coherent strategy for handling the stresses aroused during the separations and reunions of the Strange Situation, resulting in both attachment disorganization and high levels of separation distress.

To examine these hypotheses we rated the degree of maternal solicitous behavior toward their child during a play activity. In addition, we also wanted to examine for evidence of solicitousness at the representational level. To accomplish these goals, we rated the degree of maternal overinvolvement expressed during a brief speech sample of mothers describing their relationship with their child (Magana et al., 1986). In our analyses, we examined the combined and potential multivariate influences of emotional overinvolvement and solicitousness behavior in predicting attachment disorganization. One hypothesis was that parenting behavior in the form of solicitousness would mediate the relation between overinvolved expressed emotion and attachment disorganization. We also predicted that attachment disorganization among our sample would be associated with heightened distress in the absence of mother.

METHOD

Participants

The participants were 72 toddlers (M = 24.7 months, SD = 5.6, range = 13–33 months) with a congenital anomaly and their mothers. Approximately half of the sample had neurological conditions (n = 39) such as cerebral palsy and the other half had non-neurological conditions (n = 33) such as cleft-lip and palate. There were more boys than girls (n = 45 vs. n = 27). The majority of the sample was Caucasian (n = 49) and the remainder was primarily African American (n = 21), with one Latino family, and one who chose "other." Most mothers were living with a partner or married (n = 57) and of middle-class background. Approximately one-quarter of the sample was receiving welfare (n = 17) and 13 were living in a single-parent household.

Mothers were recruited from local hospitals and specialty clinics for children with handicaps and chronic medical conditions. Codings of attachment, maternal expressed emotion, and parenting behavior were made independent of one another with raters being blind to the participant's status on other relevant variables. For expressed emotion, data were unavailable for three mothers. For the Bayley scales, data were missing for 12 toddlers for motor development, and five toddlers for mental development. Missing data were due to a variety of reasons including equipment failure, the unavailability of a trained examiner, child fatigue, and the assessment being curtailed because of parental concerns of time.

Measures and Procedures

Developmental level was assessed via the Bayley Scales of Infant Development—Second Edition (Bayley, 1993). The Bayley-II yields Mental (MDI) and Psychomotor (PDI) developmental indices that are based on age-referenced items measuring language, nonverbal cognitive skills, gross and fine motor skills. Scorer reliability was examined from videotapes for 30% of the sample and averaged 90% agreement (range: 88–96%).

Attachment patterns were coded from videotapes of the Strange Situation (Ainsworth, Blehar, Waters, & Wall, 1978). Using Ainsworth et al.'s (1978) and Main and Solomon's (1990) systems, the first author observed all videotapes to classify children as either secure (B), or one of three patterns of insecure attachment: avoidant (A), resistant (C), or disorganized (D). In addition, coders utilized a system developed by Pipp-Siegel et al. (1999) to discriminate neurological symptoms from indices of attachment disorganization (see Barnett, Hunt, et al., 1999, for further detail). The purpose of the Pipp et al. coding system is to prevent children with neurological symptoms from being mistakenly assigned to the disorganized classification for reasons of neurological rather than relationship problems. Per convention, all children judged to be disorganized also were assigned to an alternative group based on the classification they would have received had the disorganized category not been an option. To establish reliability, the sixth author coded 18 (25%) randomly selected tapes, obtaining 93% rater agreement, yielding a kappa of .80. Disagreements were resolved through discussion.

Maternal criticism and emotional overinvolvement of the child were assessed via an open-ended 5-minute speech sample for expressed emotion in which the mother was asked to talk about her child and how the two of them got along together (Magana et al., 1986). The monologues were audiotaped and coded from the tape as well as a transcript in order to assess vocal inflection and tone. Criticism was scored as high when the opening statement was negative, the relationship description was negative, or there were numerous critical comments. Emotional overinvolvement was scored high in the presence of tearfulness or excessive emotional display during the interview, a statement indicating excessive self-sacrifice, overprotection of the child, four or more praising comments, or statements of excessive devotion to the child (e.g., "I'll do anything for my child to make him happy"). An expert certified coder at the UCLA Family Center trained a rater from our research team. Interrater reliability for the current sample ranged from 94 to 100% with the established expert.

Maternal behavior was coded from videotaped interactions during a 15-minute play interaction occurring after the Strange Situation. During the first 5 minutes, mothers were asked to play with their child as they normally would. During the next 10 minutes, mothers were placed in a divided-attention situation in which they were asked to complete a lengthy questionnaire while their child continued playing nearby. Dividing attention creates competing demands to attend to the child and to please the researcher and is thought to assist in further revealing individual differences in parenting behavior (Smith & Pederson, 1988). Two types of parental behavior were coded from these videotapes: sensitivity and solicitousness. Two separate teams of raters without knowledge of the hypotheses, attachment classifications, or coding procedures rated these behaviors independently of one another.

Sensitivity was assessed using a 9-point scale (Ainsworth, Bell, & Stayton, 1974) to rate how promptly, sensitively, and contingently mothers responded to their children's cues. A 9 on this scale represented the highest possible sensitivity rating and a 1 represented the lowest possible sensitivity rating. Interrater reliability was examined for 15 randomly selected videotapes. The intraclass correlation between raters was .78 and .64 for the 5- and 10-minute segments, respectively.

Solicitousness was rated on a 7-point scale developed for the current investigation. Solicitous behaviors included the use of excessive or apparently unnecessary praise, playing for the child (e.g., parent puts on a lengthy puppet show for the child), controlling the activity using exaggerated or "overbright" positive affect, and hovering—defined as intense vigilance of the child and his or her reactions. Rater reliability was examined for 20 randomly selected videotapes. The intraclass correlation between raters was .71 and .45 for the 5- and 10-minute segments, respectively. Although reliability was low for the latter segment, it should be noted that exact agreement was 80%, agreement within 1 point was 90%, and agreement within 2 points was 100%.

Separation distress was rated on a 7-point scale for each of the three episodes of the Strange Situation when the mother was absent. During the first separation the child was left with a "stranger." During the second, the child was left alone for 3 minutes, followed by another 3 minutes with the stranger. Scores of 1 indicated no evidence of distress; scores of 7 indicated intense crying for at least 30 seconds. Raters were unaware of the scores given for maternal behavior or the attachment classifications. Rater reliability based on 20 randomly selected videotapes ranged from an interclass correlation of .97 for the first separation to .98 for the second separation with stranger.

RESULTS

Means and standard deviations of study focal variables are presented in Table 9.1. Distribution of attachment classifications were as follows: secure = 39 (54.2%), avoidant = 12 (16.7%); resistant = 10 (13.9%), and disorganized = 11 (15.3%). Alternative classifications for the disorganized toddlers were secure = 2, avoidant = 3, and resistant = 6. Preliminary analyses examined the potential influence of parent (i.e., age, socioeconomic status, and marital status) and child (i.e., age, sex, and race) demographic factors on attachment. Only mothers' age was found to be associated significantly with attachment. Mothers of infants classified as disorganized were older than mothers' of non-D infants ($M = 33.7$, $SD = 7.6$ vs. $M = 29.4$, $SD = 5.3$), $F(1,68) = 5.41$, $p < .03$). Child developmental level, assessed via the Bayley-II, and number of hospitalizations were not significantly related to any of the attachment classifications. Children with nonneurological diagnoses were more likely to be securely attached compared to children with neurological diagnoses (67% vs. 44%, respectively, $\chi^2(1) = 3.83$, $p = .05$).

Table 9.2 presents correlations among focal variables and dichotomous attachment groupings (e.g., D vs. non-D, secure vs. insecure). Although the findings were in the expected direction, maternal expressed emotional overinvolvement was not significantly associated with disorganized attach-

TABLE 9.1. Means, Standard Deviations, and Range for the Focal Parent and Child Variables

Variable	n	Mean	SD	Range
Bayley MDI	67	76.6	38.3	49–118
Bayley PDI	60	68.2	43.6	49–122
Criticism	69	0.217	0.539	0–2
Emotional overinvolvement	69	0.551	0.718	0–2
Expressed emotion—Total	69	0.768	0.987	0–4
Sensitivity—5	72	7.08	1.381	3–9
Sensitivity—10	72	5.44	1.971	1–9
Solicitousness—5	72	2.375	1.674	1–6
Solicitousness—10	72	1.236	0.593	1–4

Note. 5, 5-minute free play; 10, 10-minute divided attention task.

TABLE 9.2. Correlations among Attachment Classification, Expressed Emotion, and Parenting Behavior

Variables	1	2	3	4	5	6	7	8	9	10	11
Disorganized		-.462**	-.190	-.171	.045	.108	.103	-.110	-.096	.253*	.092
Secure			-.486**	-.437**	-.069	-.079	-.095	.198	.237*	.107	.085
Avoidant				-.180	.099	.021	.070	-.081	-.197#	-.235*	-.053
Resistant					-.063	-.026	-.053	-.083	-.030	-.163	-.161
Criticism						.218#	.704**	-.118	-.015	-.091	-.031
Emotional overinvolvement							.846**	-.168	-.004	.105	.327**
Expressed emotion—total								-.187	-.011	.027	.220#
Sensitivity—5									.462**	-.196#	-.248*
Sensitivity—10										-.026	.017
Solicitousness—5											.491**
Solicitousness—10											

Note. 5, 5-minute free play; 10, 10-minute divided attention task. *n* = 72, except for correlations with expressed emotion, where *n* = 69.

**$p < .01$; *$p < .05$; #$p < .10$.

254

ment. However, emotional overinvolvement was significantly associated with maternal solicitousness during the 10-minute divided attention task, supporting the premise that solicitous behavior is an extension of maternal emotional overinvolvement. Maternal solicitousness during the 10-minute divided attention task was significantly negatively associated with sensitivity during that same period, indicating that solicitousness is inconsistent with sensitive parenting. Solicitousness during the 5-minute free play was significantly associated with attachment disorganization and was negatively associated with the avoidant attachment pattern. Figure 9.1 depicts the average solicitousness scores for the different attachment groupings with mothers of disorganized toddlers showing the most, and mothers of avoidant infants the least. Figure 9.2 shows that parental sensitivity was highest among the parents of securely attached children, as would be expected theoretically.

Our multivariate hypothesis was that linkages between maternal emotional overinvolvement and attachment disorganization would be mediated by maternal solicitous behavior. However, the absence of a significant correlation between emotional overinvolvement and attachment disorganization did not support this hypothesis. As an alternative, we examined whether maternal solicitousness combined with maternal emotional overinvolvement would more strongly predict attachment disorganization (i.e., statistical interaction or moderation). We also examined whether the influence of solicitousness was uniquely associated with attachment disorganization over and above the influence of maternal age. Consequently, we conducted a logistic regression predicting attachment disorganization, entering predictors

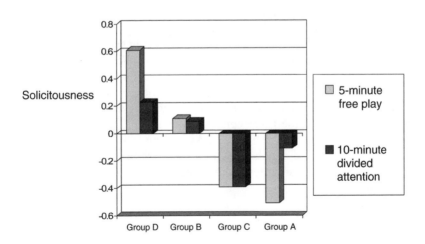

FIGURE 9.1. Average standardized solicitousness ratings for the four attachment groups.

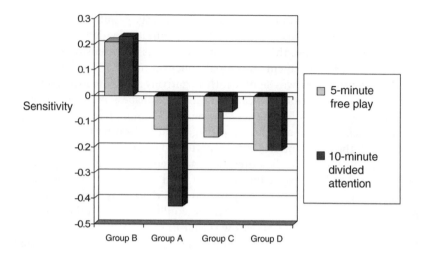

FIGURE 9.2. Average standardized sensitivity ratings for the four attachment groups.

in the following order: maternal age, maternal expressed emotional over-involvement, solicitous parenting during the free play, and the interaction between emotional over-involvement and solicitousness. The overall model was significant (χ^2 = 10.63, df = 4, p <. 04), correctly classifying 85.3% of cases. Only solicitousness significantly predicted attachment disorganization (Wald statistic = 4.12, df = 1, p < .05). The relation between maternal age and attachment disorganization dropped to marginally significant (Wald statistic = 3.47, df = 1, p <. 07). There was not a statistically significant interaction between maternal emotional overinvolvement and solicitousness.

Lastly, we examined our hypothesis that children with attachment disorganization would have difficulty regulating emotion with mother absent from the room. Significant differences were found by attachment group for separation distress in the three episodes without mother ($F(1,68)$ = 4.20, 4.31, and 6.40, respectively, p < .01). As presented in Table 9.3, those in Group D demonstrated significantly more distress than those in Group A, but not significantly less distress than those whose attachment relationship was classified Group C.

DISCUSSION

In this study, we found modest, preliminary evidence linking maternal solicitous behavior with disorganized attachment. Among our sample of toddlers

TABLE 9.3. Separation Distress by Attachment Group

	Group A (n = 12)	Group B (n = 39)	Group C (n = 10)	Group D (n = 11)	Significant post hoc Tukey tests
Mean separation 1 with stranger	1.08	2.36	3.8	2.27	A < C**
SD	0.29	1.87	2.53	1.62	
Range	1–2	1–7	1–7	1–5	
Mean separation 2 alone	3.5	4.5	6.2	5.55	A < C*
SD	2.47	2.00	1.32	1.51	A < D#
Range	1–7	1–7	3–7	3–7	B < C#
Mean separation 2 with stranger	2.25	3.32	5.80	4.55	A < C**
SD	2.30	2.18	1.14	2.07	A < D*
Range	1–7	1–7	4–7	1–7	B < C*

$**p < .01$; $*p < .05$; $\#p < .10$.

with a congenital anomaly, solicitousness (e.g., hovering over the child's play, playing for the child, acting in an overly bright and cheery manner toward the child) during the free play was significantly associated with toddler attachment disorganization. Solicitousness during the divided attention task was in the expected direction; however, this association was not significant. Apparently, the presence of another demand on the parent was enough to weaken the association between solicitousness and disorganization. However, it is noteworthy that solicitousness was significantly correlated across the two interaction contexts, supporting its reliability. The importance of context in detecting meaningful differences in maternal behavior has been noted in other studies. For instance, Madigan, Moran, and Peterson (2006) found that disruptive parent behavior predicted attachment disorganization in a free play without toys but not in a session with toys. Others found that parenting behaviors associated with attachment disorganization were evident specifically during reunions of the Strange Situation (Lyons-Ruth, Bronfman, & Parsons, 1999).

We first observed solicitous behavior during the Strange Situation when attachment patterns were being classified. However, in an effort to develop a stringent test of our hypothesis, we chose to rate solicitousness independent of the Strange Situation where this behavior was initially noticed and independent of the context where attachment patterns were coded.

Maternal emotional overinvolvement assessed during the 5-minute speech sample also was in the expected direction, but was not significantly associated with attachment disorganization. Others have demonstrated significant linkages between maternal expressed emotion assessed via speech sample and child attachment disorganization among children 4 to 9 years old (Green, Stanley, & Peters 2007; Jacobsen, Hibbs, & Ziegenhain, 2000). However, these studies combined overinvolvement with critical and hostile expressed emotion, making it impossible to compare with our findings for just overinvolvement. Researchers have linked critical parental expressed emotion to hostile parenting (McCarty, Lau, Valeri, & Weisz, 2004). However, in their sample of clinically referred children and adolescents, they did not find a predicted relation between emotional overinvolvement and observations of parental fostering of autonomy. Consequently, our study contributes to understanding parental overinvolved expressed emotion by demonstrating its significant linkage with solicitous parenting.

Several research groups have found that frightening behavior by the attachment figure predicts attachment disorganization (Lyons-Ruth et al., 1999; Schuengel, Bakermans-Kranenburg, & van IJzendoorn, 1999). Theoretically this is because it confuses children about whether or not they are safe, making it difficult to form a consistently organized behavioral strategy or representation of the caregiver (Hesse & Main, 2006; Main & Hesse, 1990). Much of what has characterized the frightening and atypical behavior of mothers of children with attachment disorganization has been described as grossly insensitive, hostile, and withdrawn (e.g., laughing while infant is crying, taunting by withholding toy). In many ways this frightening behavior is the converse of the solicitous behavior we observed, in which mothers appeared highly positive and unduly available to their child. Although both frightening and solicitous behavior have some aspects in common (i.e., overly bright maternal affect and an inherent intrusiveness to the child's behavior), solicitous behaviors are particularly different from overtly frightening behavior in their absence of parental hostility. Nonetheless, we believe solicitousness may be frightening by communicating the parents' state of fear with respect to the child's health and safety. The lack of hostility may mean that attachment disorganization in the context of maternal oversolicitousness may have different developmental implications from attachment disorganization resulting from frightening aggressiveness. For instance, this difference in etiology may explain why most of the disorganized attachments in our sample had alternative classifications as ambivalent–resistant in which youngsters are noteworthy for appearing dependent; whereas other samples, especially those high in ecological risk, have tended to find more avoidant alternative insecure classifications (e.g., Lyons-Ruth et al., 1999). As we discuss below, we also wonder whether solicitousness may have both adaptive and maladaptive features for children, and whether the ill effects may be transient.

Not only was solicitous parenting associated with attachment disorganization, it also was significantly negatively associated with the avoidant pattern. Consequently, solicitous parenting appears to be antithetical to forming an organized–avoidant strategy. This suggests that in the context of a parent who behaves in a solicitous manner, children do not appear to anticipate rejection or overstimulation, behaviors that have been associated with the organized–avoidant pattern (Belsky, Rovine, & Taylor, 1984; Main, 1981). Rather, those classified as disorganized in our sample tended to utilize proximity, as evidenced by the preponderance of alternative classifications of secure and dependent, as a strategy for handling activation of their attachment system and regulating the emotions aroused by the Strange Situation.

Several other groups have documented high levels of parental involvement and directiveness among young children with special needs, especially among children with developmental delays (Marfo, 1992; Spiker & Hopmann, 1997). Among these groups, highly directive and involved parenting has been associated with positive cognitive and motor outcomes and is encouraged in early intervention programs (Barnard, 1997). Many young children with developmental delays naturally elicit higher levels of parental involvement by appearing more vulnerable and complacent (Hauser-Cram et al., 1999). Perhaps highly directive and involved parenting may, on the one hand, be important for stimulating early cognitive development among infants and toddlers at developmental risk, but, on the other hand, may have costs to outcomes such as attachment organization and emotion regulation. These costs may balance out during the preschool years as most parents adjust to their children's maturational and developmental gains by giving their children more opportunity and room to direct their own play and free time (Marfo, 1992). These adjustments are important as the benefits of highly directive parenting may be specific to the first year or two of life and are not, for instance, associated with positive cognitive outcomes when they persist into the preschool years (Landry, Smith, Swank, & Miller-Loncar, 2000) or later. Further, Perez-Olivas, Stevenson, and Hadwin (2008) showed that for children 6 to 12 years of age, maternal emotional overinvolvement was associated with greater levels of children's separation anxiety.

Our previous research demonstrated how indices of attachment disorganization and indices of neurological disorder could be confused, as well as how they can be reliably and validly distinguished (Barnett, Hunt, et al., 1999). Our analyses presented herein further suggest that attachment disorganization can be a function of solicitous parenting. We believe this type of parenting can be part of a general pattern of parental overinvolvement that occurs when the caregiving system is highly activated. We believe this is more likely to occur when children are vulnerable because of a medical condition or other health and safety issues. This may be adaptive when children are infants and highly vulnerable and may not be problematic if parents adjust their strategy when appropriate. However, when children's vulnerability is more chronic, parents may become solicitous as a general stylistic approach to their child.

The factors that influence whether a parent becomes solicitous in response to his or her child are currently unknown. The rate of attachment disorganization in our samples of children with relatively mild birth defects was relatively low and comparable (15.3% vs. 15.4%) to those found in low-risk samples (NICHD Early Child Care Research Network, 1997). This raises the question of whether these children would have formed disorganized attachment for other reasons such as unresolved adult attachment pattern or lack of resolution regarding their child's diagnosis. We cannot answer this question with data as we do not have assessments of the parent's attachment pattern. Based on findings from Pianta et al. (1999), we believe that parental reactions to the numerous challenges of having a child with special needs or physical vulnerability override parental attachment organization. Pianta et al. (1999) examined these factors together in the prediction of child attachment among children with cerebral palsy and epilepsy. In the case of these child conditions, parent attachment, including unresolved loss and trauma, was not significantly associated with either parent resolution regarding their child's diagnosis nor their child's attachment disorganization. These findings suggest that when adapting to a child's chronic or severe medical condition, yet to-be-identified factors appear to supersede or disrupt the influence of parental attachment, including parental trauma resolution. Parents' insightfulness about their child's behavior also has not been found to predict parents' resolution of child diagnosis in a sample of children with autism (Oppenheim, Koren-Karie, Dolev, & Yirmiya, 2009). In the case of child disability and chronic medical conditions, aspects of the child's condition and severity may play a yet-to-be understood role (Schuengel et al., 2009). Further study of parent solicitous behavior may lead to identifying the parent-and-child processes that predict parental reactions and behaviors toward their special needs child. Longitudinal research on how parents adapt to their child's special needs over a variety of developmental periods would help to sort out how parents adapt their responses to their child's developmental advances and needs.

Disorganized attachment and solicitous maternal behavior were uncommon in our sample and the exception rather than the rule. The fact that most children in our sample demonstrated organized attachment patterns underscores how well most parents may adapt to their child's condition. Nonetheless, solicitous parent behavior may be a signal of a problem as supported by research on solicitous behavior in the health and pediatric psychology literatures. For instance, solicitousness on the part of parents and spouses in response to a variety of medical conditions (e.g., chronic pain) among their children or partner has been found to predict symptom maintenance and protracted recovery, especially when the patient is exhibiting symptoms of anxiety and depression (Newton-John, 2002; Peterson & Palermo, 2004; Walker, Claar, & Garber, 2002). Within this area of research with child, adolescent, and adult patients, solicitousness has been defined in a variety of ways including frequent attention to pain symptoms, permission to avoid regular activities, and special privileges. Solicitousness also has been measured in a variety of ways including self-report by the patient and researcher observations. Despite the variety of methods, solicitousness in response to a spouse's or child's medical condition tends to be associated with a variety of health and relationship problems. We think understanding the determinants of solicitousness is an important research focus.

Under conditions in which parents are solicitous, children may be prone to disorganization when stressed, perhaps because solicitousness is frightening to children, and perhaps because these youngsters do not receive sufficient practice autonomously managing their emotions (Biringen et al., 1997; Winnicott, 1965). In this latter regard, it is noteworthy that our disorganized group demonstrated quite a bit of separation distress, more so than those classified avoidant and as much as those classified as resistant. Overt expressions are only one index of distress. In other samples, children with disorganized attachment have not been found to be particularly prone to express distress overtly at high levels in the Strange Situation. Instead, they demonstrate it physiologically and become more dysregulated over time (Barnett, Ganiban, & Cicchetti, 1999; Van IJzendoorn et al., 1999).

Taken as a whole, we believe our findings tentatively demonstrate that parental solicitousness may have (hopefully short-term) costs to other developmental domains such as attachment and emotion regulation. On the other hand, these parental tendencies may be an adaptive reaction to raising a highly vulnerable child. They may have positive implications for maintaining child physical health as well as promoting child cognitive and motor development. We consider these to be tentative hypotheses that require further investigation.

ACKNOWLEGMENTS

This study was supported by grants from the National Institute of Mental Health, the March of Dimes Birth Defects Foundation, and Wayne State University. We also wish to thank the numerous individuals who were so dedicated and generous in their contributions to data collection and coding: Josee Blais, Cindy Bui, Melissa Clements, Meliksah Demir, Deanna Dotterer, Sheila Harris Hicks, Kelli Hill Hunt, Heather Janisse, Katherine Lovell, John McCaskill, Barbara Perrone, Sandra Pipp-Siegel, Margaret Rea, Kimberly Rogers, Karen Schieferstein, Jill Schram, Raymond Small, Rebecca Thompson, Miriam Walton, Shannon Waroway, and Sibyl Zaden.

Additional thanks goes to Jill Meade and Judith Solomon for helpful questions and comments on the manuscript. Finally, we especially want to express our thanks to the participating families who so generously shared their time and lives with us.

NOTE

1. We thank Judith Solomon for suggesting the term *solicitous*.

REFERENCES

Ainsworth, M. D. S., Bell, S. M., & Stayton, D. J. (1974). Infant–mother attachment and social development: "Socialization" as a product of reciprocal responsiveness to signals. In M. P. Richards (Ed.), *The integration of a child into a social world* (pp. 99–135). London: Cambridge University Press.

Ainsworth, M. D. S., Blehar, M. C., Waters, E., & Wall, S. (1978). *Patterns of attachment: A psychological study of the Strange Situation.* Hillsdale, NJ: Erlbaum.

Ammerman, R. T., & Patz, R. J. (1996). Determinants of child abuse potential: Contribution of parent and child factors. *Journal of Clinical Child Psychology, 25,* 300–307.

Barnard, K. (1997). Influencing parent–child interactions for children at risk. In M.J. Guralnick (Ed.), *The effectiveness of early intervention* (pp. 249–268). Baltimore: Brookes.

Barnett, D., Clements, M., Kaplan-Estrin, M., & Fialka, J. (2003). Building new dreams: Supporting parents' adaptation to special needs. *Infants and Young Children, 16,* 184–200.

Barnett, D., Clements, M., Kaplan-Estrin, M., McCaskill, J. W., Hill Hunt, K., Butler, C., et al. (2006). Maternal resolution of child diagnosis: Stability and relations with child attachment across the toddler to preschooler transition. *Journal of Family Psychology, 20,* 100–107.

Barnett, D., Ganiban, J., & Cicchetti, D. (1999). Maltreatment, negative expressivity and the development of Type D attachments from 12 to 24 months of age. *Monographs for the Society for Research in Child Development, 64*(Serial No. 258), 97–118.

Barnett, D., Hunt, K. H., Butler, C. M., McCaskill, J. W., Kaplan-Estrin, M., & Pipp-Siegel, S. (1999). Indices of attachment disorganization among toddlers with neurological problems. In J. Solomon & C. George (Eds.), *Attachment disorganization* (pp. 189–212). New York: Guilford Press.

Bayley, N. (1993). *Bayley Scales of Infant Development—Second edition.* New York: Psychological Corporation.

Bell, D. C., & Richard, A. J. (2000). Caregiving, the forgotten element in attachment. *Psychological Inquiry, 11,* 69–83.

Belsky, J., Rovine, M. J., & Taylor, D. G. (1984). The Pennsylvania Infant and Family Development Project: III. The origins of individual differences in infant–mother attachment. *Child Development, 55,* 718–728.

Benedict, M. I., White, R. B., Wulff, L. M., & Hall, B. J. (1990). Reported mal-treatment in children with multiple disabilities. *Child Abuse and Neglect, 14,* 207–217.

Biringen, Z., Emde, R. E., & Pipp-Siegel, S. (1997). Dyssynchrony, conflict, and resolution: Positive contributions to infant development. *American Journal of Orthopsychiatry, 67,* 4–19.

Bowlby, J. (1982). *Attachment and loss: Vol. 1. Attachment.* New York: Basic Books. (Original work published 1969)

Britner, P. A., Morog, M. C., Pianta, R. C., & Marvin, R. S. (2003). Stress and cop-ing: A comparison of self-report measures of functioning in families of young children with cerebral palsy or no medical diagnosis. *Journal of Child and Family Studies, 12,* 335–348.

Capps, L., Sigman, M., & Mundy, P. (1994). Attachment security in children with autism. *Development and Psychopathology, 6,* 249–261.

Clements, M., & Barnett, D. (2002). Parenting and attachment among toddlers with congenital anomalies: Examining the Strange Situation and attachment Q-sort. *Infant Mental Health Journal, 23,* 625–642.

Epel, E. S., Blackburn, E. H., Lin, J., Dhabhar, F. S., Adler, N. E., Morrow, J. D., et al. (2004). Accelerated telomere shortening in response to life stress. *Proceed-ings of the National Academy of Sciences of the United States of America, 101,* 17312–17315.

Florian, V., & Findler, L. (2001). Mental health and marital adaptation among mothers of children with cerebral palsy. *American Journal of Orthopsychiatry, 71,* 358–367.

Ganiban, J., Barnett, D., & Cicchetti, D. (2000). Negative reactivity and attach-ment: Down syndrome's contribution to the attachment–temperament debate. *Development and Psychopathology, 12,* 1–21.

George, C., & Solomon, J. (2008). The caregiving system: A behavioral systems approach to parenting. In J. Cassidy & P. R. Shaver (Eds.), *Handbook of attachment: Theory, research, and clinical applications* (2nd ed., pp. 833–856). New York: Guilford Press.

Goldson, E. (1998). Children with disabilities and child maltreatment. *Child Abuse and Neglect, 22,* 663–667.

Grant, K. E., Compas, B. E., Stunlmacher, A. F., Thurm, A. E., McMahon, S. D., & Halpert, J. A. (2003). Stressors and child and adolescent psychopathology: Moving from markers to mechanisms of risk. *Psychological Bulletin, 129,* 447–466.

Green, J., Stanley, C., & Peters, S. (2007). Disorganized attachment representation and atypical parenting in young school age children with externalizing disor-der. *Attachment and Human Development, 9,* 207–222.

Hauser-Cram, P., Warfield, M. E., Shonkoff, J. P., Krauss, M. W., Upshur, C. C., & Sayer, A. (1999). Family influences on adaptive development in young children with Down syndrome. *Child Development, 70,* 979–989.

Hesse, E., & Main, M. (2006). Frightened, threatening, and dissociative parental behavior in low-risk samples: Description, discussion, and interpretations. *Development and Psychopathology, 18,* 309–343.

Holmbeck, G.N., Johnson, S. Z., Wills, K. E., McKernon, W., Rose, B., Erklin,

S., et al., (2002). Observed and perceived parental overprotection in relation to psychosocial adjustment in preadolescents with a physical disability: The mediational role of behavioral autonomy. *Journal of Consulting and Clinical Psychology, 70,* 96–110.

Jacobsen, T., Hibbs, E., & Ziegenhain, U. (2000). Maternal expressed emotion related to attachment disorganization in early childhood: A preliminary report. *Journal of Child Psychology and Psychiatry, 41,* 899–906.

Landry, S. H., Smith, K. E., Swank, P. R., & Miller-Loncar, C. L. (2000). Early maternal and child influences on children's later independent cognitive and social functioning. *Child Development, 71,* 358–375.

Lloyd, C. M. (2005). Exploring mental health outcomes for low-income mothers of children with special needs: Implications for policy and practice. *Infants and Young Children, 18,* 186–199.

Lyons-Ruth, K., Bronfman, E., & Parsons, E. (1999). Maternal frightened, frightening, or atypical behavior and disorganized infant attachment patterns. *Monographs of the Society for Research in Child Development, 64*(Serial No. 258), 67–96.

Lyons-Ruth, K., Yellin, C., Melnick, S., & Atwood, G. (2005). Expanding the concept of unresolved mental states: Hostile/Helpless states of mind on the Adult Attachment Interview are associated with disrupted mother–infant communication and infant disorganization. *Development and Psychopathology, 17,* 1–23.

Madigan, S., Moran, G., & Pederson, D. R. (2006). Unresolved states of mind, disorganized attachment relationships, and disrupted interactions of adolescent mothers and their infants. *Developmental Psychology, 42,* 293–304.

Magana, A. B., Goldstein, M. J., Karno, M., Milkowitz, D. J., Jenkins, J., & Falloon, R. H. (1986). A brief method for assessing expressed emotion in relatives of psychiatric patients. *Psychiatry Research, 17,* 203–212.

Main, M. (1981). Avoidance in service of attachment: A working paper. In K. Immelmann, G. Barlow, L. Petrinovich, & M. Main (Eds.), *Behavioral development: The Bielefeld Interdisciplinary Project* (pp. 651–693). New York: Cambridge University Press.

Main, M., & Hesse, E. (1990). Parents' unresolved traumatic experiences are related to infant disorganized attachment status: Is frightened and/or frightening parental behavior the linking mechanism? In M. Greenberg, D. Cicchetti, & M. Cummings (Eds.), *Attachment during the preschool years* (pp. 161–182). Chicago: University of Chicago Press.

Main, M., & Solomon, J. (1990). Procedures for classifying infants as disorganized/disoriented during the Ainsworth Strange Situation. In M. Greenberg, D. Cicchetti, & E. Cummings (Eds.), *Attachment in the preschool years* (pp. 120–160). Chicago: University of Chicago Press.

Marfo, K. (1992). Correlates of maternal directiveness with children who are developmentally delayed. *American Journal of Orthopsychiatry, 62,* 219–233.

McCarty, C. A., Lau, A. S., Valeri, S. M., & Weisz, J. R. (2004). Parent–child interactions in relation to critical and emotionally over-involved expressed emotion (EE): Is EE a proxy for behavior? *Journal of Abnormal Child Psychology, 32,* 83–93.

Newton-John, T. R. O. (2002). Solicitousness and chronic pain: A critical review. *Pain Reviews, 9,* 7–27.

NICHD Early Child Care Research Network. (1997). The effects of infant child care on infant–mother attachment security: Results of the NICHD Study of Early Child Care. *Child Development, 68,* 860–879.

Oppenheim, D., Koren-Karie, N., Dolev, S., & Yirmiya, N. (2009). Maternal insightfulness and resolution of the diagnosis are associated with secure attachment in preschoolers with autism spectrum disorders. *Child Development, 80,* 519–527.

Perez-Olivas, G., Stevenson, J., & Hadwin, J. A. (2008). Do anxiety-related attentional biases mediate the link between maternal overinvolvement and separation anxiety in children? *Cognition and Emotion, 22,* 509–521.

Peterson, C. C., & Palermo, T. M. (2004). Parental reinforcement of recurrent pain: The moderating impact of child depression and anxiety on functional disability. *Journal of Pediatric Psychology, 29,* 331–341.

Pianta, R. C., Marvin, R. S., & Morog, M. C. (1999). Resolving the past and present: Relations with attachment organization. In J. Solomon & C. George (Eds.), *Attachment disorganization* (pp. 379–398). New York: Guilford Press.

Pipp-Siegel, S., Siegel, C. H., & Dean, J. (1999). Neurological aspects of the disorganized/disoriented attachment classification system: Differentiating quality of the attachment relationship from neurological impairment. *Monographs of the Society for Research in Child Development, 64*(Serial No. 258), 25–44.

Schuengel, C., Bakermans-Kranenburg, M. J., & van IJzendoorn, M. H. (1999). Attachment and loss: Frightening maternal behavior linking unresolved loss and disorganized infant attachment. *Journal of Consulting and Clinical Psychology, 67,* 54–63.

Schuengel, C., Rentinck, I. C. M., Stolk, S. J., Voorman, J. M., Loots, G. M. P., Ketelaar, M., et al. (2009). Parents' reactions to the diagnosis of cerebral palsy: Associations between resolution, age and severity of disability. *Child: Care, Health, and Development, 35,* 673–680.

Smith, P. B., & Pederson, D. R. (1988). Maternal sensitivity and patterns of infant–mother attachment. *Child Development, 59,* 1097–1101.

Solomon, J., & George, C. (1996). Defining the caregiving system: Toward a theory of caregiving. *Infant Mental Health Journal, 17,* 183–197.

Solomon, J., & George, C. (1999). The place of disorganization in attachment theory: Linking classic observations with contemporary findings. In J. Solomon & C. George (Eds.), *Attachment disorganization* (pp. 3–32). New York: Guilford Press.

Spiker, D., & Hopmann, M. R. (1997). The effectiveness of early intervention for children with Down syndrome. In M.J. Guralnick (Ed.), *The effectiveness of early intervention* (pp. 271–305). Baltimore: Brookes.

Sroufe, L. A., & Waters, E. (1977). Attachment as an organizational construct. *Child Development, 48,* 1184–1199.

Steinberg, L. D., Catalano, R., & Dooley, D. (1981). Economic antecedents of child abuse and neglect. *Child Development, 52,* 975–985.

van IJzendoorn, M. H., Schuengel, C., & Bakermans-Kranenburg, M. H. (1999).

Disorganized attachment in early childhood: Meta-analysis of precursors, concomitants, and sequelae. *Development and Psychopathology, 11,* 225–249.

Vaughn, B. E., Goldberg, S., Atkinson, L., Marcovitch, S., MacGregor, D., & Seifer, R. (1994). Quality of toddler–mother attachment in children with Down syndrome: Limits to interpretation of Strange Situation behavior. *Child Development, 65,* 95–108.

Walker, L. S., Claar, R. L., & Garber, J. (2002). Social consequences of children's pain: When do they encourage symptom maintenance? *Journal of Pediatric Psychology, 27,* 689–698.

Winnicott, D. W. (1965). *The maturational process and the facilitating environment: Studies in the theory of emotional development.* New York: International Universities Press.

PART III

CLINICAL APPLICATIONS

Chapter 10

Viewing Young Foster Children's Responses to Visits through the Lens of Maternal Containment

Implications for Attachment Disorganization

TERESA OSTLER and WENDY HAIGHT

This chapter focuses on the interactions of mothers and young children in the context of visitation during foster care. We give special attention to the relation between mothers' containment of children's separation-related feelings and the quality of children's attachment behaviors, especially disorganized behaviors. Attachment theory (Ainsworth, Blehar, Waters, & Wall, 1978; Bowlby, 1973) has underscored the central role of the primary attachment figure (parent) in alleviating stress in young children. "Containment" is a clinical concept that refers to caregivers' ability to know, tolerate and support their young children in understanding and alleviating their distress (Bion, 1962). The concept has clear links to Ainsworth's concept of maternal sensitivity (Ainsworth et al., 1978) and to the notion of a secure base (Bowlby, 1982), yet it has conceptual differences as well in that it focuses on maternal processes involved in young children's internalization of a self-soothing reflective capacity. We draw on this concept to elucidate the critical role that maternal toleration, understanding, and coping may play in supporting or hindering young children's internalization of ways to self-soothe and assuage intense distress. We propose that the quality of maternal containment is a central component of the interpersonal context in which variation in attachment relationships emerge, from secure to extremely disorganized, and may contribute to young children's abilities to tolerate, know, and learn from their experiences.

Foster children's visits with their biological parents provide a unique context for studying maternal containment, child disorganized attachment behavior, and processes involved in young children's internalization of a self-soothing reflective capacity. The primary goal of visits is to support the parent-child relationship while the child is in care. What parents say during visits and how they respond to their children's distress are likely to influence children's developing abilities to assuage distress and to understand their feelings. Yet evidence indicates that parents struggle in this supporting role for a variety of reasons. Visits are highly stressful and elicit intense attachment behavior and feelings on the part of parents and children alike due both to the actual separation itself and to current events and circumstances. The visits themselves may occur in new and often confusing conditions for mother and child (Haight, Kagle, & Black, 2003). The visitation context is not only stressful and disruptive for mother–child attachment, it is likely that the attachment relationships of some parents and their children prior to foster care placement included disorganized features (Carlson, 1998; Lyons-Ruth, Connell, Grunebaum, & Botein, 1990). Furthermore, parents and children often have unmet mental health and attachment needs that predate separation and foster care (Jacobsen, & Miller, 1999; Lyons-Ruth et al.,1990). It is not surprising, therefore, that in the course of two studies of families with child protective service involvement, we observed a wide variety of maternal responses to visits and an equally wide range of attachment patterns from secure to disorganized (Haight et al., 2003; Jacobsen & Miller, 1999). In our view, understanding the essentially disorganized nature of the attachment behavior of some children in these circumstances and mothers' difficulties with containment could expand our understanding of what young children with attachment disorganization may internalize during the transition to representational thought and may elucidate maternal processes that contribute to the difficulties these children may have in tolerating, understanding, and regulating their own intense feelings.

In what follows, we describe the visitation context more fully, review the literature on children's extreme responses to separation and attachment disorganization, and explore the relevance of the construct of containment for understanding variations in children's responses to visitation and processes involved in young children's internalization of a self-soothing reflective capacity. We then illustrate with case examples the relation between mothers' containment and young children's attachment behaviors during visits. We conclude by considering the implications of these observations for attachment disorganization and clinical interventions.

VISITATION AND THE EXPERIENCE OF FOSTER CARE

When children are taken into custody following allegations of child maltreatment, both parents and children experience high levels of stress. Children experience multiple new caretaking contexts, often in rapid succession, including a medical checkup, a stay in a transitional home until a foster family becomes available, and sometimes one or more shifts in foster families. There may be little communication with children about why they have been removed from their homes or when they will see their parents again. In addition, since foster care homes vary widely in quality, children may experience further stress or even maltreatment as a result of problems within foster families. Even in the best foster care settings, children often have to contend with new homes, neighborhoods and schools (or daycare), new caregivers and siblings, and new routines. These life-altering changes are faced without their parents, that is, the people who typically are most able to alleviate children's distress.

Parents also face profound stress. They are without children and have lost, at least temporarily, basic power over their ability to control their children's lives. Control over their own lives is also diminished as parents may be asked by courts to make significant and emotionally difficult life changes, such as entering treatment and abstaining from substance misuse or giving up a relationship that was violent, in order to regain custody of their children. In this context, visits become an essential venue for parents and children to reaffirm and maintain their relationships until a decision about permanency is made.

Visits may occur in an office with no toys or other amenities and under the watchful eyes of "outsiders" with whom parents and children may not be comfortable. While visits are usually scheduled weekly, they are often brief (an hour or two duration), and may require the parent to divide attention among several children. Perhaps most important from the perspective of attachment, every visit contains a reunion between mother and child that may be eagerly awaited, feared, or both, as well as a separation that may be involuntary and abrupt. It is not surprising, then, that naturalistic observations of visits reveal high levels of child and parent distress, especially surrounding leave taking when the visit ends (Haight et al., 2003).

EXTREME RESPONSES TO SEPARATIONS: RELATION TO ATTACHMENT DISORGANIZATION

Separations, including those that occur when a child is placed in foster care, exert a powerful effect on the behavior of children and may alter the quality of the parent–child attachment bond (Bowlby, 1973). Young children respond initially to separation from their primary caregiver with intense shock (Robertson & Robertson, 1989), distress, sadness, and anger (Bowlby, 1973). Extreme defensive ways of responding may develop if the separation is prolonged and if young children are cared for by a series of adults with whom they are unfamiliar (Robertson & Robertson, 1989). When young children are finally reunited with their parents, they may evidence extreme disorganized or disoriented behavior. They may fail to recognize the parent, reject him or her, or show highly contradictory behavior (Robertson & Robertson, 1989). Parents often respond to such behaviors with anguish.

Bowlby (1973, 1980) underscored the view that children respond in extreme defensive ways to separation when they are chronically faced with intense, painful emotions to which they are developmentally unready to respond independently (Bowlby, 1973, 1980). If parents are not available or able to comfort children and if the distress is chronic and remains unassuaged, young children resort to the only means available to deal with their distress by inhibiting such feelings (not showing them outwardly) or by displacing them elsewhere (e.g., a child may show avid interest in candy, but fails to recognize the parent). Bowlby (1980) used the term "segregated systems" to describe such extreme defensive responses. These responses protect young children from the overwhelming pain of separation, but they also come at a high emotional cost as children become cut off from vital attachment feelings, memories, and thoughts.

Solomon and George (1999) have highlighted the parallels between extreme defensive responses shown by young children undergoing major separation as described in the early, "classic" observations upon which Bowlby's attachment theory is founded and the disorganized attachment behavior shown by infants and young children who are classified as disorganized–disoriented in Ainsworth's Strange Situation. Following brief separation from their parent, children with disorganized attachment also evidence strongly inhibited (e.g., freezing) or disoriented and disorganized behavior toward the parent (Main & Solomon, 1990).

Young children's extreme responses to separation and disorganized attachment behavior both involve key features of segregated systems: a marked absence of attachment behavior in situations in which it is expected and/or the presence of out-of-context or out-of-control attachment behavior, affect, and thought. Solomon and George (1999) proposed that in many cases nonseparated children classified as disorganized also have experienced chronic failure of the attachment system to be assuaged by the presence and comforting behavior of the attachment figure and that other aspects of maternal behavior that have been linked to disorganized attachment, such as frightened and frightening maternal behavior (Main & Hesse, 1990; van

IJzendoorn, Schuengel, & Bakermans-Kranenburg, 1999), role confusion, withdrawal, and negative intrusive behavior (Goldberg, Benoit, Blokland, & Madigan, 2003; Lyons-Ruth, Yellin, Melnick, & Atwood, 2005) may also be understood as failures to assuage the child's attachment needs.

In her pioneering study of the development of attachment, Ainsworth (Ainsworth et al., 1978) emphasized the primacy of maternal *behavioral* sensitivity, especially prompt and appropriate response to infant attachment signals, in the development of secure attachment. More recently, and building upon British object relations theory (Bion, 1962; Klein, 1964; Winnicott, 1965), investigators have begun to examine whether mothers' capacity to reflect on their own and on their infant's feelings and thoughts (also called "mentalization") are an important mechanism underlying behavioral sensitivity (Allen, Fonagy, & Bateman, 2008; Fonagy, Gergely, Jurist, & Target, 2002; Schechter et al., 2008; Slade, Grienenberger, Bernbach, Levy, & Locker, 2006) and mother–infant attachment quality (Dozier, Stoval, Albus, & Bates, 2001). We find Bion's concept of containment, which contains elements of behavioral response and internal reflective processes within the mother, to be helpful in thinking about the ways in which mothers respond to their children's distress during foster care visits and how mothers may assist young children in internalizing ways to self-soothe and understand intense emotional experiences and feelings.

Bion (1962) defined *containment* as the process of attempting to know and comprehend the reality of oneself or another. A parent who has the ability to contain tries to understand the child by taking the child's emotions in. The parent tolerates these feelings, makes sense of them, and gives them back to the child in a way that they can be tolerated and known by the child. According to Bion (1962), children need repeated experiences of containment to internalize the parent's way of soothing, understanding, and coping with distress.

Failure to contain, by contrast, describes a situation in which the parent is not available to receive, tolerate, and interpret her child's anxieties in a way that the child can manage and understand. A mother may fail to recognize the child's anxiety, for instance, or ignore, distort, or exaggerate it. In such instances, a child experiences a sense of "nameless dread" as the child's anxiety remains unnamed and not understood, and therefore unassuaged (Bion, 1962). Children who do not experience maternal containment have difficulties in internalizing a self-soothing reflective capacity and in knowing what they feel. Such children may express feelings physically, but remain distressed because they cannot think about and make sense of their feelings.

The concept of containment includes notions of the container and the contained (Symington & Symington, 1999). The container is the process that a parent undertakes to hold, tolerate, and interpret feelings in herself and with her child. This process occurs in a state of "reverie," meaning that the parent's state of mind is calm and open to the reception of any emotions from the child whether they are felt by the child as good or bad (Bion, 1962).

Beta elements are what a parent contains. Defined as the most elemental of feelings, beta elements are feelings that are expressed physically (Bion, 1962). They are not yet understood or thought. Over the course of development, a parent helps his or her young child transform beta elements into emotional experiences that the child can render meaningful, that is, know as part of the self (Ogden, 2004). A parent helps his or her child to create meaningful experiences (also called alpha elements) through the alpha function, that is, the parent tolerates and accepts intense and unpleasant emotions in the child, and then helps the child to consider and understand his or her own feeling states (Bion, 1962).

While parents play a primary role in containing their young children's anxiety, in Bion's (1962) view, containment is also a fundamentally transactive process. Young children contribute to the process of containment by taking in their parents' meaning in their own way and by giving their renderings of understanding back to parents. Parents' ability to contain their children's feelings is influenced in turn by parents' ability to tolerate their own intense feelings of anxiety (Ogden, 2004). It follows that parents who have not experienced containment in their own childhoods may be frightened or overwhelmed by their children's feelings, especially if they themselves are traumatized or distressed, as are many parents during visits.

RATIONALE

We draw on the concept of containment to explore maternal processes that might facilitate or impede the ability of young children in foster care to internalize a self-soothing and reflective function. Recent research has examined maternal processes that contribute to young children's developing capacity to represent and understand mental states (Fonagy et al., 2002; Meins et al., 2003; Slade, 2005), but research on these processes in mothers and young children who have been traumatized (see, however, Schechter et al., 2008) and who are undergoing separation is largely lacking. Yet it is an internalized ability to self-soothe and to contemplate experience that could help mothers and young children to better regulate intense anxiety and to make sense of experiences of trauma and separation.

The early years of development are a critical period in which to study the contribution of containment to young foster children's responses to visits, as children are still highly dependent on the parent for regulating their feelings and alleviating distress (Bowlby, 1982). Young children are just beginning to internalize their parent's ability to soothe and make sense of feelings, processes greatly facilitated by the emergence of the symbolic function and language (Piaget, 1951). How mothers soothe and comfort their children during visits and what they say to them, that is, how they symbolize the soothing process, are likely to be internalized as integral aspects of young children's internal models of self and other (Lieberman, 1999; Lieberman, Padron, Van Horn, & Harris, 2005; Slade, 2005). We therefore focused on how mothers took in, made sense of, and tolerated their young children's responses to visits. We also explored children's responses and how they affected their mothers and looked at possible intergenerational influences.

In the sections that follow, we look at the relation between mothers' failure to *contain* their children's separation-related feelings and the varieties of disorganized attachment behavior shown by children undergoing such visits in order to elucidate how failure to contain might impede young children's ability to internalize a self-soothing and reflective function. We also explore brief examples of successful containment so as to illustrate positive processes that assuage children's distress and that may facilitate their internalization of a self-soothing reflective capacity. We then consider how the concept of containment may expand understanding of attachment disorganization followed by an examination of implications for clinical interventions.

CASE VIGNETTES

The vignettes below are drawn from two studies of families with child protective service involvement (Haight et al., 2003; Jacobsen & Miller, 1999). The studies focused on ethnically and socioeconomically diverse samples of children (ages 18 months to 4 years), who were placed in foster care because of neglect or abuse. Their mothers had multiple risk factors, including mental illness, substance abuse, criminal behavior, intimate partner violence, and homelessness and poverty. We selected dyads demonstrating a wide range of emotional functioning to better understand the process of containment. The visits we observed involved only the mother and child. Thus, they were not always typical of visits that often included siblings and, at times, fathers or partners.

Information on containment and on children's responses to reunion was obtained from videotapes and records of mother–child interactions during a 1-hour visit. We also reviewed available case records of each family and notes taken by observers on the transport of the child to the visit and on interviews with parents. All examples were modified to protect confidentiality.

When Containment Is Lacking

The first four vignettes illustrate profound difficulties that mothers had in containing and the extreme disorganized responses shown by their young children to visits.

Vignette 1: A Young Child Who Feigned Sleep

Ana, a 24-month-old child with a Hispanic background, had been removed from her mother's care 4 months prior after she tried to cross a busy street on her own. She was subsequently placed in a traditional foster home where she had been able to see her mother, Mrs. O, regularly during 2-hour visits each week.

When Mrs. O arrived for the observed visit, she stood in the doorway but did not look at Ana. After a few minutes, Ana initiated contact by holding a magic wand toy out to her mother. Mrs. O, who remained in the door looking tense and stiff, did not note this. Later on Mrs. O made a brief attempt to interact with Ana, who still clutched the wand firmly in her hand, but the attempt was not successful. The two then were silent, standing motionless by each other. Ana finally sat down with her back to her mother for a long period of time. Later on, Ana and Mrs. O each shook bells separately. Ana then rubbed her stomach and touched her head as if she was in pain. Mrs. O shook her bells, failing to note that Ana's stomach and head hurt.

Long silences ensued, interrupted by fleeting attempts to interact. Sometimes when Mrs. O spoke, her words did not match what Ana's behavior suggested and contained vocabulary and syntax not appropriate to a toddler. For instance, she told Ana "You give me the impression you want to talk" even though Ana was not looking at her. She also told Ana, "You give me a headache." There also were some positive interactions, suggesting the complexity of this mother–child relationship. Mrs. O, for instance, whispered, "Mommy loves you," in Ana's ear at which point Ana laid her head on her mom's shoulder.

Toward the end of the visit, Ana looked miserable. When Mrs. O told her to "smile" and give her a hug, Ana cried inconsolably. Surprised at Ana's response, Mrs. O asked Ana what was wrong. She then told Ana that she was stubborn and tired. Ana responded by rubbing her eyes and feigning sleep for the next 20 minutes. During this time, Mrs. O repeatedly said "Wake up" and "Keep me company." Ana's eyes remained tightly closed, but her sleep was feigned. In the time she "slept" she also opened her eyes a few times furtively to glance at her mother. When the visit ended, Ana clung to her mother's legs and sobbed.

COMMENTS

Mrs. O had clearly looked forward to the visit with Ana, but once there she struggled to contain her daughter's distress. When Ana gave clear bodily signs that she was in pain (e.g., by rubbing her stomach, touching her head, and wincing), Mrs. O missed Ana's cues and continued to shake the bells. On other occasions, Mrs. O failed to grasp where Ana was at emotionally. For instance, she told Ana to "smile" when Ana was crying. Mrs. O later told Ana that she was stubborn and "tired" when Ana cried. Moreover, Mrs. O gave Ana contradictory feedback, telling her in quick succession that she (Ana) gave Mrs. O a headache, but that she loved her. It is possible that Mrs. O herself was too distressed and could therefore not tolerate Ana's intense feelings. Ana responded by shutting down the intense feelings of distress she was experiencing in her mother's presence. She did this by feigning sleep. Ana thus appeared to have segregated systems. One system, which emerged when she pretended to be asleep, allowed Ana some physical closeness with her mother. But she could only achieve this closeness in a feigned state of sleep, that is, by suppressing any outward expression of her intense feelings of distress. Ana's other system was evident when Ana cried and clung to her mother. It was these intense feelings that Ana suppressed when it became clear that her mother could not tolerate or assuage them.

Mrs. O did not have a calm and open state of mind and could not be receptive to Ana's emotional needs, an important condition for containment. Except for brief unsustained moments, Mrs. O could not talk about Ana's feelings, nor could she comfort her. She commented instead on Ana's physical states or wanted Ana to meet her own needs ("Keep me company"). Ana was not delayed in her language, but spoke only three utterances during the visit. None described an inner state, although such language is typically part of the vocabulary of young children in this age group (Bretherton & Beeghly, 1982).

Vignette 2: An Extreme Example of a Child Who Feigned Sleep

Victoria, an 18-month-old child of Caucasian background, had been removed from her mother's care after her mother had left her unattended in a bathtub with the water running and had covered her mouth to prevent her from crying. An ensuing evaluation revealed bruises and scars on Victoria's legs and arms. Since her placement with relatives 1 year prior, Victoria had seen her mother regularly during weekly 2-hour visits as well as on weekends.

When Victoria arrived for the visit, Mrs. R called her name and asked her to come to her. But when Victoria approached, Mrs. R stated in rapid succession, "Why did you come? I didn't want you to come." Victoria looked confused and whimpered. When the whimpers changed to tears, Mrs. R told her, "You'll make me kill myself if you keep acting up." During the visit, Mrs. R also told Victoria she was "stinky" and asked Victoria why she was "so mad" at her. Mrs. R also glared at Victoria in an angry manner and said that she wished she had never had her as Victoria had "too many" needs. The pair was otherwise silent.

After a brief separation, Victoria approached her mother, but Mrs. R taunted her: she bid Victoria to come to her by extending her arms to her, but then Mrs. R simultaneously walked backward away from Victoria. As Victoria tried to follow her mother, Mrs. R sped up, but continued calling Victoria to her. When Victoria began sobbing, Mrs. R placed her on a chair. She then said she was leaving and walked toward the door to make good on her promise. At that point Victoria screamed inconsolably. Mrs. R subsequently picked Victoria up by her arms and sat down with her on the floor. Victoria immediately became limp and feigned sleep in her mother's arms. The feigned sleep was evident in Victoria's opening her eyes briefly and furtively to glance over at her mother. Mrs. R held Victoria on her lap only briefly. She soon placed her on the floor, but Victoria again screamed inconsolably. This sequence of picking up, feigning sleep, and screaming repeated itself numerous times before the visit ended.

COMMENTS

Mrs. R appeared fragile and distressed during the visit. Although she had looked forward to the visit, seeing Victoria appeared to trigger intense feelings. As a result, Mrs. R could not tolerate or make sense of Victoria's distress and so could not alleviate her daughter's intense feelings. Her behaviors with Victoria in fact became increasingly hostile.[1] When Victoria reached a point where her anxiety became intolerable, she, like Ana, shut off her feelings by feigning sleep.

Mrs. R's actions and words appeared to place Victoria in an irresolvable bind. They activated Victoria's attachment system at a high level, propelling her to seek out her mother for comfort. However, Mrs. R's actions and words simultaneously forbade Victoria to come, making it impossible for her to seek out her mother for comfort. With her mothers' profound difficulties in containing, it seemed unlikely that Victoria would be able to internalize a soothing, reflective capacity. It was more likely that she would internalize the belief that asking for comfort was forbidden or even unthinkable and that it was better to be silent. Under these conditions, she might also identify with her mother's belief that she (Victoria) was bad and intolerable.

Vignette 3: A Boy Who Pretended to Kill

Henry, a 30-month-old child of mixed African American and Caucasian background, had been removed from his mother's care 10 months prior following founded claims of neglect. Since that time, Henry had being living with relatives. At the time of the observed visit, his mother, Mrs. S, was about to serve a sentence for drug-related activities. Up to this time, the pair had had weekly, 2-hour visits with each other.

Henry was active the minute he arrived for the visit. The door flew open and Henry stomped into the room making loud noises. His mother greeted him by telling him what not to do. When she subsequently pulled out a punching bag, Henry kicked it, shouting "Dooh! Dooh!" in an aggressive manner. On several occasions, Mrs. S provoked Henry's behavior through hostile behaviors. For instance, when the two hammered wooden pegs into a peg board, Mrs. S grabbed Henry's hammer and aimed it as if to hit him. He immediately kicked her and she screamed "Ahhghh." She again acted as if she would hit him. Henry laughed at this. Later on, when Henry picked up a play bat, Mrs. S egged him on, stating "You'd better not hit me with that." She then patted her bottom, screaming "Whoop me, whoop me!" When he hit her, she laughed.

Mrs. S's behaviors incited fear in Henry. When Mrs. S picked up a leopard puppet and held it out to Henry, his face showed clear signs of apprehension. When she moved the leopard toward him while growling, Henry ran away and wailed as Mrs. S smiled. Mrs. S then made the puppet bite Henry's hand. Henry could barely tolerate this and ran away as Mrs. S laughed.

At times, Henry's anxiety turned into aggression: when Mrs. S picked up a pair of play handcuffs and handcuffed Henry, he whined and pulled away. She then called him to her and laughed, telling him she would take him to jail. When he approached walking backward, she grabbed him and shot him with a play gun. Her face had a frightening expression. When Henry jumped, she shouted that he should "break out" (of jail). She then aimed the toy gun at his head. Henry pleaded "No, no" as she fired. Henry only laughed after Mrs. S "stabbed" him with a toy knife and made a vomiting sound. He then picked up a toy gun, pointed it to his mother's head, firing several times. He then "stabbed" his mother with the toy knife.

There also were positive exchanges during the visit: Mrs. S taught Henry how to hug a toy bear and how to hold and feed a baby doll. These sequences, however, seemed motivated by Mrs. S's own desires. Mrs. S, for instance, fed her own doll before engaging Henry in feeding. More often, the predominant theme was one of control. If Henry didn't comply with his mother's commands, Mrs. S threatened to end the visit. Henry in turn cried for an extended period of time.

COMMENTS

Although the visit included brief positive interactions, we noted profound difficulties in containing. Mrs. S's behaviors were often hostile in nature.

She threatened Henry repeatedly, engaged him in adult themes, incited him to extreme aggression, laughed at his fears, and failed to hear his pleas to stop. Her behaviors escalated over time. In some instances, the escalation may have been in response to Henry's lack of compliance. More frequently, however, they appeared to be a response to Henry's distress, which Ms. S could not tolerate. In turn, Henry's anxiety appeared to be triggered by his mother's actions and words. Rather than containing his feelings and helping Henry to make sense of them, Mrs. S's words exacerbated his anxiety. The segregated systems become noticeable when Henry's anxiety became intolerable. At this point, he shut off these feelings by identifying with his mother's behavior and turning it into aggression (Lieberman, 1999). Identifying with his mothers' aggression may have allowed Henry to not know or feel (Miller, 1997) the fear he experienced in his mother's presence.

Mrs. S could not think or talk much with Henry about feelings. The two emotions she talked about were Henry's fear and craziness, feelings that appeared to describe her own anxieties probably about her upcoming jail sentence which was frightening to contemplate.

Although Henry's language was developmentally appropriate, he too did not use words to describe any inner states during the visit. Rather, he used emotional sounds ("Dooh! Aggghhh") to express feelings. These sounds appeared to be "beta elements," that is emotions expressed physically (Bion, 1962). Like Henry, Mrs. S's language contained some beta elements, seen, for instance, in the vomiting sounds she made following the stabbing.

Vignette 4: The Girl Who Did Not Feel

Abra, a 4-year-old child of African American and Caucasian background, had been in foster care for 1 year when she was observed during a regular visit. Prior to that she had stayed briefly in four temporary homes before being placed in her current foster home. Mrs. T, her mother, had lost custody of Abra and her younger sister, Mae, when she failed to feed her children and change their clothes. Mrs. T also became violent and once caused bruising to Abra's thighs. She had also scratched her husband's arms with her nails and punched herself in the jaw. Abra's father had serious problems with alcohol abuse and had been violent toward Mrs. T on numerous occasions. Since her removal, Abra had been able to see her mother regularly in weekly 2-hour visits.

When Abra saw her mother for the observed visit, she was initially silent for a long period of time. Her mother also did not talk and averted her eyes. Later on, however, Abra talked incessantly, but her stories were hard to follow. Mrs. T appeared lost in her own thoughts and did not seem to hear or even know what Abra said. Mrs. T also had marked difficulties in paying attention to both Abra and Mae when they were together. When

Mae cried, for instance, Mrs. T did not seem to notice. When Mae persisted, Mrs. T glanced toward Abra for cues about what to do. Abra's father could not tolerate the strong emotions evoked during the visit either. He blamed others for the family's problems. If Abra even whimpered, he would put a stop to it with a glare.

Abra's face and arms were covered with scratches. According to her foster mother, Abra inflicted these scratches on herself. In addition, she had recently stabbed her breast with a tack and placed tape over it. Mrs. N, Abra's foster mother, also noted that Abra did not seem to feel any pain when she hurt herself. According to Ms. N, Abra never talked about her own mother and if she was asked about her, Abra would exhibit a flat "who cares" attitude. A few weeks prior, for instance, Mrs. N had shown Abra a photo of her mother along with other adults. Abra would not say who her mother was, although she readily recognized her father. Mrs. N did not believe that Abra had developed an attachment to any members in her home. When she was recently taken to a respite home for a week, for instance, Abra showed no outward emotion.

COMMENTS

Mrs. N failed to contain in the sense that she struggled to focus on Abra's needs. While Mrs. N had looked forward to the visit, she had little energy to reach out to her daughter emotionally and to help Abra make sense of what she was going through. Instead, Abra needed to be alert to tend to her mother's needs. Abra's constant talking suggested that she was trying to maintain some connection with her often absent mother.

As with the other children we observed, Abra evidenced segregated systems. On the one hand, we observed Abra, the girl who felt no pain and one who outwardly did not feel or care. On the other hand, we became aware of Ruby, an imaginary child, who embodied most of Abra's attachment feelings. According to Abra, Ruby loved her mom and her mom loved her. Ruby also had negative feelings that Abra did not feel. For instance, Abra told us that it was Ruby who had scratched Abra on her cheeks and arms. Ruby had also jumped on Abra's back and bit her fingers.[2] Children often suppress anger so as to not further alienate a parent on whom they depend (Bowlby, 1973). Inflicting anger on the self is less frightening than putting it on a parent (Lieberman, 1999). By putting anger on the self, a child may gain some measure of control over these feelings and may also forget what he or she is actually angry about (Lieberman, 1999).

The observations of the visit suggested that Abra's parents could not tolerate vulnerable feelings. For instance, when Abra whimpered, her father responded by glaring at her. He also blamed her mother and others for the family's problems. While we do not know what he precisely blamed others for, it is possible that he let Abra know that her feelings had led to her mother's mental illness and to child protective involvement. While Abra's mother was eager to regain custody, she too could not contain. She failed to recognize and interpret Abra's feelings with her. Rather than calmly taking in Abra's feelings and helping her to find a way to understand and deal with them, Mrs. T turned to Abra for feedback about her own uncertainties in parenting. This lack of calm, coupled with her lack of response, increased Abra's anxiety as evidenced in Abra's nonstop talking, which consisted in unintelligible and unconnected phrases (beta elements).

Maternal Containment of Child's Distress

The last two vignettes are briefly presented to illustrate cases where mothers contain their children's distress. The containment in Vignette 5 occurred in favorable conditions. In Vignette 6, the conditions for maternal containment were less favorable.

Vignette 5: Containment under Favorable Conditions

Milly, a 3-year-old African American child, had been in foster care for 1 month when we observed a visit with her mother. Milly had been taken into custody after the police found a cache of drugs at her father's home. Since this time, Milly and her mother had seen each other each week during scheduled 2-hour visits.

Milly and her mother looked at each other at the moment of reunion and smiled. Mrs. B then scooped Milly up in her arms and hugged her. She also reassured her that she missed her and loved her. Milly responded in kind, telling her mother, "I miss you." Mrs. B then talked with Milly about feelings related to the separation and oriented her to future events. For instance, she reminded Milly which lady would take her back to her foster home. When the visit ended, Milly cried and clung to her mother's leg. This visibly affected Mrs. B, but she was able to remain calm and reassure Milly that they would see each other again soon.

COMMENTS

Mrs. B struck us as having a calm, open state of mind that allowed her to be receptive to what Milly was feeling (reverie). She remained calm and emotionally available, despite the fact that she was likely under considerable stress. During the visit, she prioritized Milly's needs and was open to whatever emotions Milly had. Mrs. B was affected when Millie cried, for instance, but was able to accept this and to address Milly's separation fears. Mrs. B also appeared to help her child to tolerate intense and unpleasant emotions so they could be understood by Milly. This was evident when Mrs. B scooped Milly up and contained her physically. Mrs. B also reached out to reassure Milly and to reaffirm their relationship. She let Milly know how important she was to her; that she was missed; and that they would see each other again. Mrs. B also prepared Milly for what was to come, by telling her who would take her home. Mrs. B's physical containment, her sizing up Milly's feelings, and her use of language to address Milly's distress all appeared to be components of the alpha function in that they helped Milly to calm, to understand, and to regulate her distress. Repeated experiences of this type could facilitate Milly's ability to internalize her mother's ability to remain calm, open, and emotionally sensitive and to use language to understand intense emotional feelings and experiences.

Conditions for containment were largely favorable for Mrs. B, who had a small, but solid support network and a good working alliance with her therapist. Mrs. B also noted that her relationship with her own mother was a strength and that her mother had helped her in developing coping strategies for dealing with anxiety. Milly had only been in foster care for a month. She was able to signal her needs clearly to her mother and reciprocated when her mother told her she loved her by telling her she loved her too.

Vignette 6: Containment under Unfavorable Conditions

Zusana, a 3-year-old girl of European background, had been removed from her mother's care 1 year prior following her mother's difficulties in meeting her daughter's basic needs for food and housing. Zusana was sexually abused by a foster uncle in her first foster home. When the current visit was observed, she had been living in her second home for 2 months. During her time in foster care, Mrs. K had maintained weekly 2-hour visits with Zusana.

Zusana screamed when her mother arrived for the visit. She then hit and bit her mother before pushing her decidedly away. Mrs. K showed anguish at this response and paused. She then knelt down on the floor so that she could hold Zusana in her arms. Zusana again pulled herself away and banged her head on the wall repeatedly. Mrs. K remained near Zusana and looked at her for a brief while. When she spoke, she was calm and affirmed that she loved Zusana. She added that they were together now and she would help. Zusana sobbed in her mother's arms for some time before calming.

COMMENTS

As with Mrs. B, Mrs. K remained calm and made clear attempts to understand what Zusana might be feeling. She contained her daughter behaviorally by holding Zusana in her arms. She also tolerated and accepted Zusana's angry, out-of-control behavior and reassured her, thus helping Zusana to know that the relationship would not be lost through her angry behavior. As a result of the containment, Zusana was able to calm and the dyad could use the visit to maintain and develop their relationship.

The conditions for containment were not as favorable as they were for Milly's mother. Zusana had been in foster care for 1 year, where she experienced sexual abuse and multiple foster placements. As a result, she rejected her mother's attempts to reach out to her. Mrs. K herself had had several relapses of depression. Despite these odds, Mrs. K had had a stable childhood. She was also in therapy, responded well to feedback, and could rely on others in crisis. It may be noteworthy to underscore that, though highly distraught, Zusana eventually gave her mother clear attachment signals, by allowing her to hold and soothe her.

SUMMARY AND DISCUSSION

The mothers that we observed varied greatly in their ability to contain their children's emotional responses to visits. Mothers who successfully soothed their children had a quiet, composed state of mind that allowed them to be receptive to what their children were feeling. Under the stress of the visit, these mothers maintained a calm, open state of mind and were receptive to what their young children were experiencing and feeling. They also used actions and words to make sense of their children's feelings and to help their children to understand what they were going through emotionally. They helped the children to understand and cope by affirming their love through gestures and words, by reassuring their children that they would see each other, and by picking their distressed children up and comforting them. Moreover, mothers had a calm, open state of mind that was receptive (reverie) to whatever their children were feeling—positive or negative.

Mothers who failed to contain were not calm and open and could not be receptive to where their children were emotionally. Seeing their children in the context of visitation appeared to trigger intense feelings that the mothers could not tolerate. As a result, these mothers did not grasp where their young children were emotionally. They failed to note, pay attention to, tolerate and understand their children's feelings. Some misunderstood or distorted their children's feelings (e.g., telling a sad and distraught child that she was "tired"). In the place of understanding, mothers enacted their own anxieties with their children. One mother, for instance, threatened to abandon her child and blamed her child for her own distress and anxiety. She also blocked her child's access to her and glared at her child. Another became aggressive and threatening. What is interesting with regard to attachment theory is that mothers' behaviors simultaneously exacerbated children's attachment behaviors and exacerbated their distress. The children's attachment systems were thus being chronically activated at high levels by their attachment figures, important prerequisites for the emergence and maintenance of segregated systems.

How mothers contained appeared to be closely linked to children's responses to visits. When mothers successfully contained, children were ultimately able to calm down. The pairs were then able to utilize the visit to strengthen their relationship. A failure to contain, by contrast, was linked to extreme defensive responses in children who responded by feigning sleep, transforming their anxiety into aggression, and inflicting anger on the self.

Children's extreme defensive responses to visits involved similar elements to those observed in nonseparated children with disorganized attachment in that they had characteristic hallmarks of segregated systems: a marked absence of attachment behavior in situations in which it would be expected or out-of-context and out-of-control behavior, affect, and thought (Bowlby, 1980). At the same time, the segregated systems we observed in children appeared to fall at a more extreme end of the continuum of defenses than those described for children with attachment disorganization (Solomon & George, 1999). They were more extreme in their length (e.g., child feigning sleep for prolonged period), intensity (e.g., child's aggressive shooting), and complexity (incorporation of pretense and fantasy).

While mothers' failure to contain evoked extreme defensive responses in children, children also contributed to interactions. Children's behaviors during the visit appeared to overwhelm or threaten mothers, possibly because these responses reminded them of feelings that mothers could not tolerate. In the closed feedback loops we observed, then, children's and mothers' behaviors each inadvertently triggered defensive responses in the other. These reactive, defensive responses, then, were such that they may have maintained and/or exacerbated segregated attachment systems in the other. The communications essentially led to escalating anxiety and not knowing rather than to security and understanding.

The extreme defensive responses we observed in young children may have retraumatized mothers, triggering more extreme defenses that aimed to preserve and protect mothers' already fragile self-structures. Under such circumstances mothers' own attachment needs may be so highly activated that they eclipse the emergence of the caregiving system and impede mothers' ability to step in to meet their children's needs. Future research is needed to explore whether retraumatization (Banyard, 2001) also occurs with attachment disorganization, that is, whether extreme defensive responses inadvertently trigger unresolved trauma in a parent.

Mothers who could not contain had extreme difficulties in talking about attachment feelings and experiences from childhood. Some responded in physical ways to questions about their childhoods, for example, by running out of the room, yawning constantly, or talking about their blood pressure. One mother recalled that in childhood no one had ever talked with her about her feelings. Three of the four mothers who could not contain, however, also recalled their caregivers screaming at them or glaring at them for no reason. As with refusal to talk, these behaviors suggest that, in childhood, mothers' own feelings were not contained. As a result, mothers may not have learned to use thought to understand and know experiences and feelings. The inability to integrate attachment memories and thoughts and to use language to reflect on childhood experiences has also been observed in mothers of children with disorganized attachment (Solomon & George, 1999).

The construct of containment extends understanding of attachment disorganization in several ways. For one, it focuses attention on a larger maternal regulatory ability as a main contributor to attachment disorganization. In this view, containment comprises individual maternal behaviors (e.g., frightening, mocking, misperceiving) and functions (failure to recognize, tolerate, and assuage distress) that have been specifically linked to the disorganized attachment pattern (Lyons-Ruth et al., 2005). The regulatory ability that is lacking, containment, involves at its essence security regulation and is hence closely linked to Bowlby's (1988) notion of a secure base and to Ainsworth's (Ainsworth et al., 1978) concept of behavioral sensitivity. However, the concept of containment combines this ability with the process of knowing. Mothers who contain have a calm, open state of mind that allows them to try to know what their young children experience and feel. They also help their young children to internalize this self-soothing reflective capability so that their children can understand their feelings and can learn from them.

More importantly, perhaps, the concept of containment focuses attention on important maternal interactions involved in young children's internalization of a self-soothing reflective capacity. Specifically, the concept of containment emphasizes the critical role that tolerating, understanding, and symbolizing play in supporting or hindering children as they *internalize* ways to assuage distress and to make sense of intense feelings. Having a calm, open state of mind that is receptive to where the child was emotionally, a part of containment, emerged, for instance, as an important precondition for young children to internalize a self-soothing and reflective function. As such, this view of early internalizing processes shares important similarities to Werner and Kaplan's (1984) work on symbolic developments in young children.

Like Bion, Werner and Kaplan viewed internalizing processes as emerging out of a sharing relationship, where the parent comments on and shares experiences with the child. By examining and sharing experiences with a safe parent, the child is helped to give names to feelings and thoughts. As a child's feelings and thoughts are given form, structure, and meaning in dialogue with the parent, the child moves from acting on experience to using symbols to contemplate experience. In this way, the child can gradually use thought to know and regulate his or her intense emotions internally. The notion of containment also shares similarity to Vygotsky's (1962) concept of "scaffolding" in cognitive development, underscoring the critical role that a safe and more experienced parent plays in facilitating the child's ability to interpret and respond to intense attachment feelings, important to an emerging sense of self.

Finally, the concept of containment expands understanding of what young children with attachment disorganization may internalize as they construct internal working models of attachment in the transition to representational thought. On the one hand, children with disorganized attachment may identify with negative attributions conveyed to them by their mothers. For instance, they may accept their mother's belief that they are bad or intolerable (see also Lieberman, 1999). At the same time, young children with disorganized attachment may also be finding out that their attempts to know and be known and understood are ignored, distorted, or received in hostile ways. Children in these circumstances may learn that it is best not to think about attachment experiences and that knowing may be "off limits." What these children may be internalizing, then, is a negative self-structure that fails to understand and know, and one that may attack and misunderstand endeavors by others to understand them (Symington & Symington, 1999).

Attempts at knowing and at being known that are misunderstood, ignored, and rejected come at a high cost since they can carry with them a loss of a sense of self (Fordham, 1974) and difficulties in learning from experience, which is central to growth in selfhood (Bion, 1962). Since mother and children may reinforce defensive and extreme reactions in the other, early interventions are critical to avert unfavorable pathways. Maternal processes that suppress thought may take a particular toll on children's thinking about attachment, especially if they occur in early childhood, the period when internal working models of self and other are being internalized.

This study focused on *maternal* processes that hinder or support children's early internalizations of a self-soothing reflection capacity. Children's internalizations will also be influenced, however, by the ability of alternate attachment figures to contain, including fathers (Steele & Steele, 2005) and foster parents (Dozier et al., 2001). To some extent, young children may also choose what they internalize (Beiser, 1996). More research is needed on the contribution of such processes to the internalization of a self-soothing reflective capacity.

The construct of containment has important implications for clinical services aimed at supporting mothers and children during visitation. Professionals who supervise visits must be sensitive to processes of containment in both parents and children. When parents and children show behaviors indicative of difficulties with containment, professional mental health intervention could be helpful if visits are to meet their goals of supporting parent–child relationships. For skilled mental health clinicians, problems with containment could become a "port of entry" to address in therapy (Lieberman, Compton, Van Horn, & Ippen, 2003). Since visits are the one opportunity for mothers to reconnect with their children, mothers could learn to contain their child's feelings by acknowledging them and by helping their child to accept and interpret these responses. By holding a child's anxiety at a manageable level, then, containment during visits could strengthen a child's ability to internalize healthy ways of dealing with intense stress, thus curtailing the development of extreme defenses.

For parents who fail to contain, then the therapeutic pathway is clear (Lieberman et al., 2003; Lieberman & Van Horn, 2005; Slade, 2006; Schechter & Willheim, 2009). Rather than teaching mothers concrete parenting skills, therapeutic interventions would focus on the underlying regulatory mechanism from which such deficits stem. The therapist's primary role in the intervention is to provide containment to the mother in the context of a trusting relationship (Bowlby, 1988). This would involve being available, listening, and tolerating whatever the mother says, including her silences and anger. With repeated experiences of containment, the therapist would help a mother to contain, that is, to bear to put words to her feelings. A related task is to help a mother connect feelings of anger and helplessness to childhood experiences of trauma or abuse (Lieberman et al., 2003; Lieberman & Van Horn, 2005) and to the relationship she has established with the therapist. For mothers who do not understand what they feel and why they feel as they do, the groundwork for interpreting such feelings and experiences will need to be laid.

A next step would be to help a mother contain her child's feelings and to connect the child's feelings to situations that have triggered them. A trusted therapist could do this by being available to tolerate the powerful feelings that the visit engenders in mother and child. However, this could also be facilitated through video feedback aimed at helping a mother to regulate her young children's intense feeling states (Schechter & Willheim, 2009). If a mother struggles to contain her own feelings during visits, the therapist could help her to do this so as to curtail positive feedback loops, whereby the child's distress triggers extreme responses in the mother and the mother's triggers extreme responses in the child. In this way, a therapist may set the stage for mothers to internalize healthier ways of dealing with their own and their child's distress. With this ability, the potential will be created for mother and child to strengthen their relationship. Over time, the relationship itself could become a protective mechanism that could help a young child assuage distress and make sense of experience (Lieberman & Van Horn, 2005).

ACKNOWLEDGMENTS

We wish to extend a special thanks to Linda Miller and to Ernst Luerssen and Elizabeth Feldman.

NOTES

1. Lyons-Ruth and colleagues (Lyons-Ruth et al., 2005) has described similar hostile maternal behaviors. These hostile behaviors apparently alternate with more helpless maternal behaviors. Both the hostile and helpless behaviors are associated with infant attachment disorganization.
2. Abra's foster mother also confirmed that Ruby was an imaginary, not a real, child.

REFERENCES

Ainsworth, M. D. S., Blehar, M., Waters, E., & Wall, S. (1978). *Patterns of attachment: A psychological study of the Strange Situation.* Hillsdale, NJ: Erlbaum.

Allen, J. G., Fonagy, P., & Bateman, A. W. (2008). *Mentalizing in clinical practice.* Washington, DC: American Psychiatric Publishing.

Banyard, V. L. (2001). Retraumatization among adult women sexually abused in childhood: Exploratory analyses in a prospective study. *Journal of Child Sexual Abuse, 11*, 19–48.

Beiser, H. R. (1996). A fifty year follow-up of an abandoned child: A personal commentary. *Child Psychiatry and Human Development, 26*, 211–220.

Bion, W. R. (1962). *Learning from experience.* London: Heinemann.

Bowlby, J. (1973). *Attachment and loss: Vol. 2. Separation.* New York: Basic Books.

Bowlby, J. (1980). *Attachment and loss: Vol. 3. Loss.* New York: Basic Books.

Bowlby, J. (1982). *Attachment and loss: Vol. 1. Attachment* (2nd ed.). New York: Basic Books. (Original work published 1969)

Bowlby, J. (1988). *A secure base: Clinical applications of attachment theory.* London: Routledge.

Bretherton, I., & Beeghly, M. (1982). Talking about internal states: The acquisition of an explicit theory of mind. *Developmental Psychology, 18*, 906–921.

Carlson, E. A. (1998). A prospective longitudinal study of attachment disorganization/disorientation. *Child Development, 69*, 1107–1128.

Dozier, M., Stoval, K. C., Albus, K. E., & Bates, B. (2001). Attachment for infants in foster care: The role of caregiver state of mind. *Child Development, 72,* 1467–1477.

Fonagy, P., Gergely, G., Jurist, E., & Target, M. (2002). *Affect regulation, mentalization, and the development of the self.* New York: Other Books.

Fordham, M. (1974). Defenses of the self. *Journal of Analytic Psychology, 19,* 192–199.

Goldberg, S., Benoit, D., Blokland, K., & Madigan, S. (2003). Atypical maternal behavior, maternal representations, and infant disorganized attachment. *Development and Psychopathology, 15,* 239–257.

Haight, W., Kagle, J., & Black, J. (2003). Understanding and supporting parent–child relationships during foster care visits: Implications of attachment theory and research. *Social Work, 48,* 195–208.

Jacobsen, T., & Miller, L. J. (1999). The caregiving contexts of young children who have been removed from the care of a mentally ill mother: Relations to mother–child attachment quality. In J. Solomon & C. George (Eds.), *Attachment disorganization* (pp. 347–378). New York: Guilford Press.

Klein, M. (1964). The importance of symbol-formation in the development of the ego. In *Contributions to Psychoanalysis, 1921–1945.* New York: McGraw-Hill. (Original work published 1930)

Lieberman, A. F. (1999). Negative maternal attributions: Effects on toddlers' sense of self. *Psychoanalytic Inquiry, 19,* 737–757.

Lieberman, A. F., Compton, N. C., Van Horn, P., & Ippen, C. G. (2003). *Losing a parent to death in the early years: Guidelines for the treatment of traumatic bereavement in infancy and early childhood.* Washington, DC: Zero to Three Press.

Lieberman, A. F., Padron, E., Van Horn, P., & Harris, W. W. (2005). Angels in the nursery: The intergenerational transmission of benevolent parental influences. *Infant Mental Health Journal, 26,* 504–520.

Lieberman, A. F., & Van Horn, P. (2005). *Don't hit my mommy!: A manual for child–parent psychotherapy with young witnesses of family violence.* Washington, DC: Zero to Three Press.

Lyons-Ruth, K., Connell, D. B., Grunebaum, H. U., & Botein, S. (1990). Infants at social risk: Maternal depression and family support services as mediators of infant development and security of attachment. *Child Development, 61,* 85–98.

Lyons-Ruth, K., Yellin, C., Melnick, S., & Atwood, G. (2005). Expanding the concept of unresolved mental states: Hostile/helpless states of mind on the Adult Attachment Interview are associated with disrupted mother–infant communication and infant disorganization. *Development and Psychopathology, 17,* 1–23.

Main, M., & Hesse, E. (1990). Parents' unresolved traumatic experiences are related to infant disorganized status: Is frightened and/or frightening parental behavior the linking mechanism? In M. T. Greenberg, D. Cicchetti, & E. M. Cummings (Eds.), *Attachment in the preschool years* (pp. 161–182). Chicago: University of Chicago Press.

Main, M., & Solomon, J. (1990). Procedures for identifying infants as disorganized/disoriented during the Ainsworth Strange Situation. In M. T. Greenberg, D.

Cicchetti, & E. M. Cummings (Eds.), *Attachment in the preschool years* (pp. 121–160). Chicago: University of Chicago Press.

Meins, E., Fernyhough, C., Wainwright, R., Clark-Carter, D., Das Gupta, M., Fradley, E., et al. (2003). Pathways to understanding mind: Construct validity and predictive validity of maternal mind-mindedness. *Child Development, 74,* 1194–1211.

Miller, A. (1997). *The drama of the gifted child: The search for the true self* (rev. ed.). New York: Basic Books. (Original work published 1981)

Ogden, T. H. (2004). An introduction to the reading of Bion. *International Journal of Psychoanalysis, 85,* 285–300.

Piaget, J. (1951). *Play, dreams, and imitation in childhood.* London: Heinemann.

Robertson, J., & Robertson, J. (1989). *Separation and the very young child.* London: Free Association Books.

Schechter, D. S., Coates, S. W., Kaminer, T., Coots, T., Zeanah, C. H., Davies, M., et al. (2008). Distorted maternal mental representations and atypical behavior in a clinical sample of violence-exposed mothers and their toddlers. *Journal of Trauma and Dissociation, 9,* 123–147.

Schechter, D. S., & Willheim, E. (2009). When parenting becomes unthinkable: Intervening with traumatized parents and their toddlers. *Journal of the American Academy of Child and Adolescent Psychiatry, 48,* 249–253.

Slade, A. (2005). Parental reflective functioning: An introduction. *Attachment and Human Development, 7,* 269–281.

Slade, A. (2006). Reflective parenting programs: Theory and development. *Psychoanalytic Inquiry, 26,* 640–657.

Slade, A., Grienenberger, J., Bernbach, E., Levy, D., & Locker, A. (2006). Maternal reflective functioning, attachment, and the transmission gap: A preliminary study. *Attachment and Human Development, 7,* 283–298.

Solomon, J., & George, C. (1999). The place of disorganization in attachment theory: Linking classic observations with contemporary findings. In J. Solomon & C. George (Eds.), *Attachment disorganization* (pp. 3–32). New York: Guilford Press.

Steele, H., & Steele, M. (2005). The construct of coherence as an indicator of attachment security in middle childhood: The Friends and Family Interview. In K. Kerns & R. Richardson (Eds.), *Attachment in middle childhood* (pp. 137–160). New York: Guilford Press.

Symington, J., & Symington, N. (1999). *The clinical thinking of Wilfred Bion.* New York: Brunner-Routledge.

van IJzendoorn, M. H., Schuengel, C., & Bakermans-Kranenburg, M. J. (1999). Disorganized attachment in early childhood: Meta-analysis of precursors, concomitants, and sequelae. *Development and Psychopathology, 11,* 225–250.

Vygotsky, L. S. (1962). *Thought and language.* Cambridge, MA: MIT Press.

Werner, H., & Kaplan, B. (1984). *Symbol formation: An organismic–developmental approach to the psychology of language.* Hillsdale, NJ: Erlbaum. (Original work published 1963)

Winnicott, D. W. (1965). *Maturational processes and the facilitating environment.* New York: International Universities Press.

Chapter 11

An Exploratory Investigation of the Relationships among Representational Security, Disorganization, and Behavior Ratings in Maltreated Children

LINDA WEBSTER and RACHELLE KISST HACKETT

Bowlby (1982) hypothesized that individuals construct mental representations of relationships based upon their actual experiences with a primary caregiver. These "internal working models" organize behavior, thought, memory, and defenses with regard to activation of the attachment system. Under optimal conditions of responsive and sensitive caregiving, the child's attachment system is flexibly integrated and organized in such a way that it allows the child to seek comfort when he or she needs it, and to pursue exploration of the environment when threats in the environment are minimal. Under conditions associated with neglect, rejection, and abuse, the child may develop defensive processes that serve to keep painful feelings, thoughts, and memories from consciousness. Bowlby (1980) conceptualized three distinct forms of defensive processes that he termed defensive exclusion–deactivation, cognitive disconnection, and segregated systems. It wasn't until recently, however, that these defensive processes were delineated and measured (George & Solomon, 1996; Solomon, George, & De Jong, 1995; George & West, 2001, in press; Solomon & George, 1996). "Deactivation" is defined as a process of reducing awareness of or the intensity of cues that might activate the attachment system. The child is thus able to effectively reduce the intensity of activation of attachment—in an attempt to avoid the possibility of experiencing rejection or disappointment. It might be conceived of as the defensive pattern that modulates patterns of behavior that Main (1990) describes as "minimizing" attachment. "Cognitive disconnection" similarly functions to transform attachment distress, but by splitting or "disconnecting" attachment-related affect from its source. The child becomes intermittently aware of attachment-related distress, often becoming consumed with sadness and the desire to be close to attachment figures. Cognitive disconnection might be conceived of as the defensive pattern that modulates patterns of behavior that Main describes as "maximizing" attachment. Finally, Bowlby (1980) postulated a more extreme form of defensive exclusion, the "segregated system." Segregated systems develop as a form of defensive exclusion to block trauma-related attachment memories and emotions and store them, so to speak, in a separate organized mental model—the function of this defense is to attempt to keep these painful memories from consciousness, but this cannot occur indefinitely (George, West, & Pettem, 1997). The child is especially sensitive to environmental and internal attachment cues; when activated, attachment distress can become overpowering. In these moments, the segregated system fails and the child's defensive structure is at risk for breaking down (Solomon & George, 2008). Segregated systems failure (producing flooding) or hyperactivation (producing representational and behavioral constriction) is associated with children and adults whose attachments are disorganized or unresolved (Solomon et al., 1995).

Bowlby (1988) predicted that early attachment experiences and the representations of those experiences affect relationships, self-esteem, and self-regulation of emotion and behavior. There is evidence that disorganized attachment is associated with significant risk for maladaptive outcomes in infants, children, and adolescents (Carlson, 1998; Fish, 2004; Granot & Mayseless, 2001; Jacobsen, Huss, Fendrich, Kruesi, & Ziegenhein, 1997; Lyons-Ruth, Alpern, & Rapacholi, 1993; Lyons-Ruth, Connell, Grunebaum, & Botein, 1990; Moss, Bureau, Cyr, Mongeau, & St-Laurent, 2004; Moss, Cyr, & Dubois-Comtois, 2004; Moss, Rousseau, Parent, St-Laurent, & Saintonge, 1998; Solomon et al., 1995; Ogawa, Sroufe, Weinfield, Carlson, & Egeland, 1997; Stams, Juffer, & van IJzendoorn, 2002; van IJzendoorn, Schuengel, & Bakersman-Kranenburg, 1999). Child maltreatment has been consistently associated in the research literature with disorganized attachment (Cichetti & Toth, 1995; van IJzendoorn et al., 1999; Weinfeld, Whaley, & Egeland, 2004). These findings highlight the importance of gaining a better understanding of how to move maltreated children toward greater organization and ultimately security.

Doll play story stem techniques and narrative assessments have been increasingly used to understand the mental representation, or generalized scripts, of attachment relationships of preschool- and latency-age children (e.g., Bretherton, Ridgeway, & Cassidy, 1990; Gloger-Tippelt & Konig, 2007; Granot & Mayseless, 2001; Green, Stanley, Smith, & Goldwyn, 2000; Hodges, Steele, Hillman, Henderson, & Marta, 2000; Moss & St-Laurent, 2001; Solomon et al., 1995; Stacks, 2007). Although methods and story stems vary, the essential procedure involves an adult introducing a story, and asking the child to "show and tell" what happens next. Both verbal and nonverbal content are recorded and transcribed for analysis. In addition to increased use of these methods with older children, some research has begun to use such methods with maltreated populations. For example, Katsurada (2007) used the George and Solomon (1990/1996/2000) doll play story stem technique and coding system to investigate the mental representations of Japanese children living in institutions as compared to children living with their biological parents. No secure attachment was found for the institutionalized children, and there were more institutional children classified as disorganized than the comparison group of children.

Steele and colleagues (e.g., Hodges, Steele, Hillman, Henderson, & Kaniuk, 2003; Steele, Hodges, Kaniuk, Hillman, & Henderson, 2003) developed a story stem assessment technique that incorporated five stems developed from their work with abused children (known as the "Little Pig" stories), as well as some of the stems from the MacArthur Story Stem Battery (MSSB; Bretherton & Oppenheim, 2003). Their coding system includes a global "Security" composite, as well as "Insecurity" and "Disorganization" composites, although the stories were not classified into attachment categories. Steele et al. (2003; Hodges et al., 2003) used this story stem technique to investigate change in attachment representations among a sample of high-risk maltreated children who had been in multiple placements and recently adopted. Not surprisingly, they found increased markers, or indicators of disorganization, in the children's narratives, including dysregulated aggression and catastrophes in the stories. One of the most interesting findings was that, over time in the adoptive placement, indicators of security increased, and indicators of avoidance decreased, while indicators of disorganization and insecurity remained fairly constant—thus suggesting that, while security may increase, it does not transform the remaining representations, and the disorganized representations remain in existence alongside the newly developed secure representations.

In the first study to use George and Solomon's (1990/1996/2000) doll play story stem technique with foster children, Russell (2005) investigated the attachment representations of 12 children in the foster care system. She examined markers of disorganization (using the George & Solomon, 1998, procedure for disorganization), as well as pathological mourning (as measured by an autobiographical interview adapted from Main, 1991, and Hamilton-Oravetz, 1993). Although she worked with a small sample, she found strong associations between the amount of frightening and violent content in the doll play and clinical scales on the Child Behavior Checklist (Achenbach & Edelbrock, 1983). In addition, 92% of the children showed pathological mourning. She hypothesized that the underlying disorganization contributed to risk status regardless of the child's attachment classification, and that the uncertainty inherent in the foster care system prevents foster children from being able to process their loss and grief in an integrative fashion.

Venet, Bureau, Gosselin, & Capuana (2007) also used the George and Solomon (1990/1996/2000) technique and the George and Solomon (1998) procedure for coding disorganization to investigate mental representations in a group of neglected and non-neglected preschoolers. They found a significantly higher proportion of avoidant attachment in the neglected group; these children also had more frightening material and depicted the mother as being less available than the normative group.

Both Steele et al.'s (2003) and Russell's (2005), and to some extent Venet et al.'s (2007), research represent a movement away from an investigation of classification alone, and toward an investigation of indicators of disorganization as explanatory constructs of maltreated children's mental representation of attachment relationships and associated behavior. Given that knowledge of the child's attachment classification alone may not provide optimal explanatory power for individual differences in children's behavior—particularly for high-risk populations such as maltreated children—as this population may represent a restricted range of variance, the present investigation also sought to move beyond the use of classification, and explore the presence of *markers* of security and disorganization as explanatory constructs for reported behavioral differences in maltreated children. If it is assumed that these representations at least partially mediate subsequent development, then such an exploration might provide a better understanding for the development of interventions that promote organization and security in this population. It is also anticipated that this study will contribute to the knowledge base examining the relationship between this method of analysis and theoretically relevant variables. We hypothesized that markers of security would be associated with more positive reports of children's behavior, and that markers of disorganization would be associated with more negative reports of children's behavior.

METHODS

Participants

Subjects were 57 children with a history of maltreatment who were referred for a psychological evaluation. The reasons for the referral varied, but most were referred for diagnostic clarification and to make treatment and place-ment recommendations. As such, these children cannot be said to reflect the larger population of maltreated children in general, but may reflect the population of referred maltreated children. All evaluations were conducted by the primary investigator over a 5-year period. The mean age was 8.55 years (SD = 1.67), with a range of 5.16 to 11.91. Forty-two percent (n = 24) were female and 58% (n = 33) were male. The sample consisted of 47% African American (n = 27); 23% Caucasian (n = 13); 12% Hispanic (n = 7); and 17% biracial (n = 10). The majority of the children (60%, n = 32) had experienced neglect, 4% had experienced physical abuse (n = 2), 4% had experienced sexual abuse (n = 2), 23% had experienced neglect and physi-cal abuse (n = 12), 2% had experienced neglect and sexual abuse (n = 1), and 4% had experienced neglect, physical abuse, and sexual abuse (n = 2). Two cases were missing information regarding the reason for referral to the child welfare system. Sixty-eight percent (n = 38) of the children were placed in regular foster homes; 8% (n = 5) were placed in designated therapeutic foster homes; another 8% (n = 4) were in group home placements; and the remaining 16% (n = 10) were placed in adoptive homes (the length of time in the adoptive placement ranged from 2 to 15 months). The mean age at time of removal from their biological parents was 5.02 years (SD = 2.96), and the mean number of placements was 2.64 (SD = 1.17), with a range of one to five placements. Eleven children had been in only one placement, 11 had been in two, 15 had been in three, 11 had been in four, and two children had been in five placements. The average length of time that these children had been in their current placement was 18 months (SD = 24 months), with a range from 1 month to 8.5 years. It should be mentioned here that 1 month could be considered too brief a period of time for attachment to be orga-nized around a new caregiver. The focus of our investigation, however, was on the generalized mental representation of attachment, which is assumed to have developed from repeated experiences with previous caregivers, and its relationship to behavior as reported by the current caregiver.

Classification Procedure

The children were administered the doll play attachment technique devel-oped by George and Solomon (1990/1996/2000), as one part of a larger psychological evaluation. (Permission was obtained from the child welfare worker to use this procedure as a component of the larger assessment in order to provide useful information regarding the child's attachment sta-tus.) This classification system has been validated with children's laboratory reunion behavior, with overall classification agreement at 79% (kappa = .79, p < .001). The primary author had achieved reliability with George and Solomon, following training on the procedure and coding of 50 cases. A random set of 14 cases from this study's sample were double-coded by Carol George, who was blind to all information regarding the participants, with overall interjudge, four-way attachment classification agreement at 88.7% (kappa = .88, *p* < .001).

Administration

The child was presented with an attractive doll platform resembling a dollhouse, but without walls so that the play can be easily observed and recorded. The child was asked to *choose a doll to represent him- or herself* and then to select members of a *pretend* family. The administrator then administered a "warm-up" story stem about lost pets who need a home, followed by the story stems that are actually coded. All doll play was transcribed from videotape, and included all verbal behavior as well as the child's and the dolls' behaviors.

Four story stems are administered and coded in this system, and are based on the Bretherton et al. (1990) stories: *Hurt Knee* (the child falls off a rock and hurts his or her knee), *Monster* (the child sees a monster in the bedroom), *Separation* (parents leave the child with a babysitter for an overnight trip), and *Reunion* (parents return from their trip). Each story is introduced separately, and in sequence, with the administrator introducing the story, and then asking the child, "Show me and tell me what happens next."

Coding

The transcripts were coded using the George and Solomon system (1990/1996/2000). Of particular interest in the system is how the child responds to the activation of the attachment system and how, or whether, the attachment system is successfully "terminated." This approach to attachment representation classification emphasizes understanding children's symbolic representations in terms of underlying differences in information processing or what Bowlby (1980) called "defensive exclusion." It is assumed that the content of doll play narratives will reflect the child's age, the testing circumstances, and the nature of projective stimuli. Key to classification, however, is the identification of the underlying commonalities in information processing and defense associated with each of the attachment groups. These information-processing and defensive strategies are demonstrated by the organization of the narratives; the kind of information that is used or discarded, emphasized or glossed over; and how attachment-related aspects of the story stems are integrated, distorted, or transformed (Solomon et al., 1995; George & West, 2001, in press; Solomon & George, 1996). The system identifies key features of information processing and defense for each of the four attachment classification groups (A, B, C, D). Secure children show little evidence of defensive exclusion of information. The attachment "dilemma" presented by each story and the associated feelings are integrated straightforwardly into the narrative. The stories show evidence of one of four "markers":

1. *Haven of safety.* Caregivers provide prompt, effective care; for example, Mother calls the doctor and makes him come to their house to fix the child's knee; the knee is better and the doctor leaves.
2. *Internalized secure base.* The child is able to engage successfully in exploration or autonomous activities; for example, Once Mother has cared for his knee, the child climbs the rock again.
3. *Danger and rescue and/or genuine reintegration of the family.* Coded only for the Separation–Reunion story; for example, the babysitter is irresponsible and the children get lost; Father finds them when he returns home and the babysitter is punished.
4. *Thematic integration.* The child recognizes and addresses the complexity of feelings and relationships; for example. Father effectively demonstrates to the child that the monster is a shadow; the child is satisfied with his explanation and says she will call him if there is a real monster.

Avoidant children use the defensive strategy of deactivation to "transform" the situation so that care and protection are essentially not necessary (i.e., the child is not hurt or in need; the child can take care of him- or herself). *Ambivalent children* use "cognitive disconnection," most often played out with themes of uncertainty, confusion, diversion, and delay as to the nature of the attachment problem and its resolution (e.g., Father injures himself when he returns home someone has to go to the store for more Band-Aids).

Dysregulation of defensive processes characterizes the doll play of *disorganized children*, such that the stories themselves are dysregulated (i.e., chaotic, destructive, or violent without constructive resolution or protection) or *constricted* (i.e., they refuse to engage in the doll play story in an attempt to maintain tight control over their attachment fears). Although each story is coded and assigned a classification, the child's overall attachment classification is determined by the response to the Separation–Reunion story. In this study, there were an insufficient number of cases coded as "secure" ($n = 8$) for a robust analysis (power < .50). We chose to investigate markers of security and dysregulation in each story, as it was thought that these markers would provide the most explained variance for the population of maltreated children. Haven of safety is arguably of importance for children who have been dysregulated by maltreatment. Markers of cognitive disconnection and deactivation were not investigated, although future studies may find these defenses to make important contributions to development.

Security Markers

Due to an insufficient number of secure base, reintegration, and integrative markers in the story responses of these children, these markers were not included in the analyses. (Interestingly, the one child who did demonstrate secure base and reintegration also demonstrated haven of safety). The lack of secure markers such as secure base, reintegration, and integrative is not surprising given this population. Mental representations regarding haven of safety could arguably be of primary salience for children who have been maltreated, who may have limited opportunities to develop mental representations for elements connected to exploration capacities and integration. This is consistent with Hodges, Steele, Hillman, Henderson, and Kaniuck's (2005) findings that, over time, children who had been adopted showed an increase in mental representations of caregiving figures as being responsive, providing more help, and providing more emotional comfort and affection, that is, representations associated with haven of safety. Only those stories that contained haven-of-safety markers were included in subsequent analyses. Haven of safety was coded as present versus absent for each story. Interjudge reliability for each story stem was calculated based on a random set of 14 cases. Classification agreement was 80% for Hurt Knee; 100% for Monster in the Bedroom, and 100% for Separation–Reunion.

Dysregulation Markers

In addition to the indices of dysregulation that are used to identify the stories of disorganized and controlling children, George and Solomon (1998) further delineated an additional set of content codes typically associated with dysregulation. This coding system provided the "dysregulation markers" for the present study. These codes include whether the mother doll figure is physically or psychological absent; a story is frightening and depicts out-of-control behavior; the child is constricted and unable to respond to the story, or actively avoids it; and behavioral signs that the child is experiencing anxiety or fear during the task and/or the child is exhibiting controlling behavior. In our sample, there was insufficient variance in the behavioral indices of fear and control; only the markers of mother absence, frightening material, and constriction were included in analyses.

Mother Absence

In the case of mother absence, children's stories were categorized as to whether the mother was present in all stories versus whether the mother was absent in one or more stories.

Frightening Material

Each story stem was rated from 0–3, with a score of 0 indicating no markers or frightening material; a score of 1 indicating only one or two low-level markers (e.g., dolls trip and fall); a score of 2 indicating that there are frightening events, but that they do not overwhelm or dominate the story (e.g., a ghost opens and closes a cabinet door); and a score of 3 when the story is pervasively frightening and/or out of control (e.g., Dad kills everyone and self, then they all rise up from the dead and fight each other). Most of the doll play stories exhibited a pattern where the frightening material was either contained versus a pattern where the frightening material was dysregulated. Based upon the observed patterns present in the data, as well as the rational that children who were able to contain their dysregulation would differ on important behavioral indictors from those who were clearly dysregulated, we chose to dichotomize the groups where scores of 0, 1, or 2 were combined into a single category (contained) against which scores of 3 were contrasted (dysregulated).

Constriction

Constriction as coded in the George and Solomon (1998) system was also rated according to three levels. A score of 1 was assigned when the story contained no constriction; a score of 2 was assigned when the story was somewhat constricted; and a score of 3 was assigned when the child was constricted to the extent that he or she was unable to tell a story. The Constriction codes were dichotomized into those stories in which there was no constriction (score = 1; no constriction) versus those rated 2 or 3 (high constriction) (code = 2–3).

Behavior Rating Scale

The Behavior Assessment System for Children (BASC; Reynolds & Kamphaus, 1998), is a multimethod, multidimensional system used to evaluate the behavior and self-perceptions of children and young adults ages 2 through 25 years. It includes rating scales for parents and teachers, and a self-report scale on which children age 8 and older can rate their own emotions and behavior. The reliabilities for all scales are reported to be .85 or higher for test–retest, and in the mid- to upper .70s on the internal consistency measures. The primary caregivers of these children (the foster mother) completed the Parent Rating Scales of the BASC and the child's teacher was asked to complete the Teacher Rating Scale. It should be noted that teachers completed BASCs for only 31 children out of a sample of 57.

In some cases, the assessments were conducted in the summer when school was not in session and teachers were unavailable, and this is the reason for the disparity.

Cronbach reliabilities were calculated for all of the subscales for the Teacher and Parent Rating Scales (n = 23). Of these, two subscales had relatively low internal consistency compared with those reported in the literature and by conventional standards (e.g., $p > .70$). These subscales were the Somatization scale on the Teacher rating form (.522) and the Social Skills scale on the Parent rating form (.526). The remainder of the scales had acceptable internal consistency, with over half above .80. The low alphas on the two aforementioned subscales may limit the ability to detect potential differences between the groups.

RESULTS

Analyses of Security and Dysregulation

For the main analyses reported below, one-tailed tests using alpha = .05 were employed, as we expected the differences to favor one particular subgroup over the other. No correction of alpha for multiple tests was employed in order to avoid overlooking promising trends that might be confirmed in future studies utilizing larger samples. We hypothesized that more positive behavioral outcomes would be associated with stories including haven of safety, and that more negative outcomes would be associated with higher levels of frightening material and mother absence. Since constriction, in the George and Solomon system, is associated with the controlling–caregiving group, we anticipated that higher ratings of constriction would be associated with more positive behavioral ratings, as these children in some studies are less prone to acting out.

Haven of Safety

The comparison was conducted as a planned contrast using an independent samples t-test with doll play that contained a marker of haven of safety compared to doll play that had no such indication across stories. Results indicated that there were significant differences between children who had haven-of-safety markers in their attachment stories and those who did not for the BASC Parent Rating Form for Aggression ($t = 2.163$, $p < .05$) and Conduct Problems ($t = 2.323$, $p < .05$); and for the BASC Teacher Rating Form for Aggression ($t = 2.193$, $p < .05$) Conduct Problems ($t = 2.329$, $p < .05$), and Hyperactivity ($t = 2.438$, $p < .01$). These differences favored the group of children who had haven-of-safety markers in their attachment stories. (See Table 11.1.)

TABLE 11.1. Comparison of Mean Differences on the BASC for Children with at Least One Indication of Haven of Safety Present versus No Haven of Safety Present across All Three Stories

	No HOS present			Some HOS present			
BASC scale	n	M	SD	n	M	SD	t
PRS Aggression	37	71.11	20.586	14	59.50	15.590	2.163*
PRS Conduct Problems	34	72.82	19.914	13	61.23	13.113	2.323*
TRS Aggression	20	63.30	13.929	11	53.00	9.230	2.193*
TRS Conduct Problems	19	63.11	12.380	10	52.80	8.664	2.329*
TRS Hyperactivity	20	60.60	14.21	11	50.64	8.524	2.438**

Note. PRS, Parent Rating Scale; TRS, Teacher Rating Scale; HOS, haven of safety.
*$p < .05$ (one-tailed); **$p < .01$ (one-tailed).

Dysregulation

The comparison was conducted using independent samples t-tests for the variables of interest. Results for the variable of "mother absence" indicated that there were significant differences only for the BASC Parent Rating Form for Conduct Problems ($t = -1.837$, $p < .05$). The mean difference was 13.55, with children who had the mother absent from one or more stories scoring significantly higher on conduct problems.

Results for the "constriction" variable indicated that there were significant differences only for the BASC Teacher Rating Form for Conduct Problems ($t = 2.224$, $p < .01$). The mean difference was 11.4, with children who evidenced some constriction in their stories obtaining lower ratings on conduct problems.

Consistent with our prediction, results for the "frightening" variable indicated that there were significant differences for the BASC Parent Rating Form for Adaptability ($t = 1.684$, $p < .05$), Social Skills ($t = 1.644$, $p < .05$), and Leadership ($t = 1.902$, $p < .05$), with children who were dysregulated scoring lower (poorer) on these adaptive outcomes. (See Table 11.2.)

DISCUSSION

This study found that representations of haven of safety were associated with lower scores on both parent and teacher ratings of aggression and conduct disorder. In addition, teachers rated these children lower on hyperactivity. These behavioral problems can be viewed as difficulties with affect regulation, which has been tied to insecure attachment (Cassidy, 1994;

TABLE 11.2. Comparison of Mean Differences on the BASC for Children with Contained versus Dysregulated Frightening Ratings across All Stories

BASC scale[a]	Contained fright rating			Dysregulated fright rating			
	n	*M*	*SD*	*n*	*M*	*SD*	*t*
PRS Adaptability	38	38.92	11.714	12	32.33	12.131	1.684*
PRS Social Skills	38	39.37	11.068	12	33.67	8.150	1.644*
PRS Leadership	37	42.41	9.628	10	36.00	8.692	1.902*

[a]For these positive outcomes, we hypothesized that the group with contained frightening ratings would score higher, on average.

*$p < .05$ (one-tailed).

Magai, 1999). Of particular interest is that the average parent ratings of aggression and conduct problems were in the "clinically significant" range, that is, above two standard deviations from the mean, for children who did not have any haven of safety in their stories. The average scores for children who did have some haven of safety present in their stories were only mildly elevated (approximately one standard deviation from the mean). The average teacher ratings for aggression, conduct problems, and hyperactivity were mildly elevated for children who did not have any haven of safety in their stories, and not elevated for children who did have some haven of safety present in their stories. This suggests that representations of haven of safety may serve to guide children's behavior in appropriate ways—perhaps toward using adult caregiving figures more effectively to regulate negative affect (vs. acting out). The finding that teachers in general rated children lower on the behavior rating scale may suggest that acting-out behavior is intensified toward the mother—as being in the primary caregiving role. Bowlby (1973) argued that anger is a normative response to the unavailability of the caregiver, and the externalizing nature of conduct problems could be seen as an attempt to gain the caregiver's attention. The findings from this study are consistent with some of the research with teen populations (e.g., Allen & Land, 1999; Holland, Moretti, Verlaan, & Peterson, 1993; Moretti, Holland, & Peterson, 1994; Obsuth, Moretti, Holland, Braber, & Cross, 2006) that suggest that conduct-disordered behavior is an active attempt to gain the caregiver's attention.

In regards to dysregulation, the results of this study found that parent ratings on the BASC subscale of conduct problems were found to differ between groups of children for whom the mother was absent versus present in their stories. Children who portrayed the mother as being absent in one or more stories on average evidenced clinically significant levels of conduct problems. Indeed, the average score of these children was extremely high ($M = 79.69$)—almost three standard deviations from the mean. Of the children who had the mother absent in their attachment story, 61.5% had scores above 70, while only 42% of the children who had the mother present in their stories had scores above 70. The fact that this difference was not found in the teacher ratings may indicate that the mental representation is particularly salient for the home environment. The absence of the mother as an attachment and protective figure has been noted in previous research (Solomon et al., 1995; George & Solomon, 1996) as a marker associated with disorganized mental representations of attachment, and "mother absence" is considered in the George and Solomon (1998) system to be a form of failed protection. The lack of a mother at the representational level could be interpreted to mean that these children have never experienced protection from a mother caregiving figure, and thus have not developed a mental representation that informs them that mothers are persons to whom you turn in times of fear and/or stress.

This study also found that children who evidenced more constriction had lower teacher ratings on the conduct problems scale, with average scores having essentially no elevation ($M = 51.75$). "Constriction" is defined by George and Solomon (1998) as an inability of the child to respond to the attachment story. It is thought that constriction is a means to block or shut down the feelings associated with attachment experiences that have been segregated from consciousness. These results suggest that children who are prone to the use of constriction as a defensive process evidence fewer conduct problems as observed by teachers. It may be that the inhibitory function inherent in the use of constriction also serves to inhibit the externalizing, acting-out behavior associated with conduct problems. This would be consistent with Solomon et al.'s (1995) finding that the children in response to the Separation–Reunion story sequence during doll play were predominantly controlling–caregiving with their mothers on reunion in the Strange Situation. Children who are controlling-caregiving attempt to control the caregiver by behaving compliantly, and attempting to please and gain approval so as not to upset the caregiver and thus evoke frightening behavior from her (Jacobvitz & Hazen, 1999). George and Solomon (Chapter 6, this volume, and Solomon and George, Chapter 2, this volume) propose that the caregiving strategy is a mechanism that the child has developed to nurture the mother back into the role of being a responsible caregiver. Arguably, teachers may find children with these characteristics much easier to manage in the classroom than children with disruptive behavior problems.

George and Solomon (Chapter 6, this volume) reported that mothers whose caregiving representations depicted their children as having both dysregulated and constricted characteristics reported the highest number of externalizing behavior problems on the Child Behavior Checklist (CBCL; Achenbach & Rescorla, 2001), a measure comparable to the BASC used in the present study. They explained this pattern as the child being placed in a double bind in which the soothing and nurturing strategies are not working to control the mother's caregiving system and the mother is nevertheless scary or frightened herself. Their sample was comprised of mothers of low-risk, family-reared children. It may be the case in this maltreated sample, a sample in which children's biological parents have not only "abdicated the caregiving system" (Solomon & George, 1996) but also may have been in the role of abuse perpetrator, that whatever caregiving strategies the child developed were not working to control the mother's caregiving behavior. Thus, the children in our maltreatment sample may be especially poised to be in this double-bind situation, explaining why in the presence of the attachment figure and not teachers (who are not attachment figures) the mother reports such extremely high levels of behavior problems.

Finally, this study found that parent ratings of positive behaviors of adaptability, social skills, and leadership were significantly lower for children who had dysregulated levels of frightening material in their doll play. These children had average scores corresponding to a mild deficit, although adaptability and social skills were nearing the clinically significant range. In contrast, children whose frightening material was contained had scores much closer to average, although adaptability and social skills were slightly depressed. This finding suggests that children who are dysregulated by being overwhelmed and flooded with frightening material are especially at risk for not developing appropriate prosocial and adaptive skills. This is consistent with research on child maltreatment that has shown that children who have experienced maltreatment manifest significantly poorer outcomes on measures of affect regulation, peer relationships, and school functioning, in addition to developing behavior problems (Cicchetti, 1989; Cicchetti & Lynch, 1995; Cicchetti & Manly, 2001; Cicchetti & Toth, 1995). The results of this study suggest, however, that these negative outcomes can be mitigated, in part, by the development of a mental representation of safety and protection—presumably formed as a function of caregiving provided. As mentioned previously, mental representations regarding haven of safety may be especially important for children who have experienced maltreatment.

Although not a primary focus of this study, we found that the majority of the children had ambivalent mental representations in regards to attachment, 51% ($n = 29$). Only 14% ($n = 8$) had secure representations, and both disorganized and avoidant representations had proportions of 17.5% ($n = 10$). This is consistent with Russell's (2005) foster care sample that also had a large proportion (42%) of children classified as ambivalent in her study—it should be noted that her sample was not a referred sample. This suggests that the majority of the children were either already insecure–ambivalent (prior to placement), or that their attachment systems reorganized around the care being provided in the foster home. Dozier and colleagues' research (Bates & Dozier, 2002; Dozier, Stovall, Albus, & Bates, 2001; Stovall & Dozier, 2000) found that insecure infants were eventually able to reorganize their attachment system and develop secure attachments to their secure foster mothers, while infants placed with dismissing caregivers often developed a disorganized attachment. The present sample, however, is not an infant sample, and Dozier's findings with infants may or may not apply to older children who have experienced multiple placements. Russell (2005) argued that the transient and precarious nature of foster care itself left foster children in a state of uncertainty—a state that is associated with ambivalent attachment (Solomon & George, 2008). It is thus not surprising to find a large proportion of ambivalent children in this population, although more study is needed to investigate this hypothesis.

CLINICAL IMPLICATIONS

The findings from this study suggest the possibility that the existence of some sense of haven of safety is associated with less acting-out behavior in maltreated children, and may have clinical implications in the treatment of these children. For example, interventions may be focused on helping these children attain a sense of haven of safety through consultation with primary caregivers that emphasizes the importance of providing contingent, prompt, and effective care. George and Solomon (1989, 2008; Solomon & George, 2008) believe that the behavioral goal of the caregiving system is to provide protection for the child. The mother's caregiving representation is thought to derive from her own internal working model of relationships, and mirrors the concept of interrelated "self" and "other" components described in the child's attachment representation (Sroufe & Fleeson, 1988). The caregiving system, however, is distinct from the mother's own attachment system in that the caregiving system appears to mediate between the mother's own attachment system and the infant's. The caregiving system thus has a separate representational model that influences the quality of care an infant receives (Solomon & George, 2008).

Solomon and George argue that the caregiving representation should logically include a willingness to respond to the child, an ability to read and understand the child's signals, and an evaluation of the potential effectiveness of care. In their studies of separated and divorced families, Solomon and George (1999a, 1999b) found that some mothers were unwilling or unable to comfort or reassure the infant (i.e., provide psychological protection) during transitions in visitation with the father, and these infants were at higher risk for having a disorganized attachment. In contrast, divorced mothers of secure infants described themselves as taking specific, active measures to avoid or mitigate the child's distress—despite whatever stress they themselves might be experiencing. In the dysregulated caregiving system mothers see themselves as helpless and unable to protect their children, while in the secure caregiving system the mothers were confident about their ability to comfort and reassure their infants, and to adjust their behavior flexibly and appropriately. George (1996) thus argues that interventions should take place at the level of the caregiving system, and not only at the level of reworking the childhood experiences of the foster mother.

The results of this study also suggest that children who exhibit high levels of frightening material in their play have impaired ability to adjust to changes in routine, to shift from one task to another, and to share toys or possessions. They are also rated lower on friendship-making skills, concern for others, and empathy, as well as decision making and social problem solving. Bowlby (1980) thought that the underlying cause or source of segregated systems was failure to terminate the attachment system. Obviously, separation from the mother—such as that experienced by children in foster care—could be one source of chronic activation without termination. In addition, Bowlby argued that strong parental rejection, and direct and implied threats to abandon the child, might also serve to create and maintain segregated systems. We argue that many foster children in long-term care, who have been in multiple placements, have experienced chronic rejection and abandonment, and must segregate the anxiety, fear, and anger associated with this abandonment. The chronic state of uncertainty that many foster children experience may thus result in an impairment of resiliency, and associated impairments in self-esteem, self-reliance, and empathy.

In sum, the results of this study, combined with previous research, suggest that interventions should be targeted toward developing a mental representation of protection in children, and toward improving the ability of the caregiver to recognize, accurately interpret, and appropriately respond to signals of need and distress that may be distorted or transformed in maltreated children.

CASE ILLUSTRATION

The following case description depicts the disorganized classification that Solomon et al. (1995) refer to as "Disorganized Frightened," which is associated with the punitive–controlling group (D1 attachment classification subgroup).

Sam is a 10-year-old boy who is the third child of five born to their mother who had a long history of drug and alcohol abuse. The youngest three children were removed from her care when Sam was approximately 4 years old due to general neglect and reports of abuse by the mother's boyfriends. One sister was approximately 2 years of age, while the youngest was an infant. The two older sisters (4 and 6 years older than Sam) had been removed some time prior (records were not clear), but Sam reported that he had never lived with them. Sam and his two younger sisters were initially placed with maternal grandparents for approximately 2 years until the grandparents could no longer care for them due to their own medical concerns. Sam and his sisters then went through a series of five foster home placements until he was placed in his current foster home placement at about age 6 with the older of his two sisters. The youngest sister was placed in a nearby home, and Sam had regular visitation. There were reports of food being withheld in one placement, and reports that a foster sibling may have molested Sam and his sister in another home. Sam had been in his current placement for approximately 4 years when plans were introduced to move Sam and his younger sisters to a relative in another distant state who had expressed an interest in adopting the children. All accounts at that time indicated that Sam had established a positive relationship and attachment to his long-term foster mother, and he began acting out by becoming increasingly argumentative in response to the possibility that he might be separated from her. In addition to this stressor, over the 4 years, the grandparents had repeatedly demanded that Sam and his sister be placed in a racially congruent foster home (his current foster mother was of a different race), and were quite intrusive and intimidating with the children in their attempts to coerce them into stating that they wanted to leave their current placement. On one occasion, the grandfather had grabbed Sam's jacket and inadvertently choked him in an attempt to gain Sam's full attention. Although Sam was not seriously harmed, it was a frightening experience for him. Sam's therapist, whom he had been seeing since his placement in his current home, reported that Sam's play in the therapy sessions was often filled with aggression, violence, and chaos. Sam was afraid of his grandparents, but also loved them and wished to continue visitation. He was vocal with his therapist that he wanted to remain in his current home until "I grow up."

Sam's response to the doll play story stems was one of increasing chaos and frightening material as each successive story stem was introduced. For example, in the Monster in the Bedroom story, he began his response with what initially appeared to be a "secure" response. The father came into the bedroom and immediately attacked the monster, but then was overcome by the monster, and eventually told the child that there was no monster. The child in the story responded with the following statement, "Ooh, you don't believe me," while the father went back to reading the newspaper. The child was thus left feeling vulnerable and unprotected, and the attachment theme appeared to be that adults may try to offer protection, but it is ultimately ineffective. In the Separation–Reunion story stem, the babysitter was actively frightening and physically abusive. When the parents came home from their trip, they and the sitter were immediately embroiled in violence, and the parents were ineffective in stopping it. It was hypothesized that Sam did not ultimately believe that his foster mother could protect him from the uncertainty of his situation in the foster care system—including the intrusiveness of his grandparents and a move to unknown relatives out of state.

Based upon the results of the assessment, and, in particular, the doll play responses, the first author recommended that Sam's therapist introduce concepts of safety and protection in his play, particularly when it was aggressive and frightening, and that the therapist help support the foster mother in setting appropriate limits with the grandparents, while also actively advocating for protection with the child's welfare worker and attorney. Whenever Sam's play in therapy became chaotic and frightening, the therapist would interject questions such as, "Who can help protect this character?" In the event that Sam was not able to respond to these suggestions with protection, the therapist would introduce a protective character, or would transform one of the characters into a protective character. Based upon his response to the doll play, particular attention was paid to "believing" the signals of distress from the characters. The focus on "believing" the signals of distress is consistent with sensitive and responsive caregiving, and the emphasis on protection, which is at the heart of attachment theory, was intended to help develop a mental representation of haven of safety. Theory predicts that this emphasis would help to establish a blueprint that children can and do turn to adult caregiving figures to signal distress and expect comfort.

At the same time, the therapist worked with the foster mother, through consultation, and some sessions involving her and Sam, to help focus her caregiving on correctly interpreting Sam's signals, and then evaluating the effectiveness of the care provided. For example, if Sam became argumentative, she was asked to consider whether this might be a signal that he was feeling anxious about potential loss and abandonment, and thus to provide him with reassurance that she would do everything possible to protect him and remain in his life, while supporting him in the transition to the adoptive home of his relatives. Particular attention was paid to believing, accepting, and acknowledging how frightening and upsetting it was to him that his grandparents did not believe or accept his love for and desire to stay with his foster mother. She was then instructed to consider whether this intervention appeared to help reduce his anxiety and corresponding arguing. In addition, the therapist addressed whether the foster mother's caregiving system might be dysregulated by her own fears regarding the grandparents. She admitted that she was intimidated by them, and the therapist worked with her to strengthen her ability to provide a buffer for her foster children while also protecting herself from their psychological threat.

The therapist attempted an intervention with the grandparents, but the grandmother clung rigidly to her views that her grandson could not possibly be happy in a racially incongruent home. The therapist next approached the child welfare worker and the child's attorney and enlisted their aid in protecting Sam by setting limits on the grandparents (directing them not to discuss changing placements with him). As it turned out, the relatives withdrew their bid for adoption, and Sam remained in his placement with his sister and foster mother. The therapist saw a change in Sam's behavior in the therapy session such that Sam responded to the introduction of the concept of protection, and the themes of chaos and violence diminished and eventually disappeared. One year later, Sam's behavior problems were reduced to occasional arguments.

Approximately 2 years after the first evaluation, Sam began having difficulty at school in December of his first year at middle school with two of his teachers who complained that he was lazy, and he had four failing grades. Sam told his therapist and foster mother that his teachers were "mean" and "yelled a lot." The school held a meeting, and informed the foster mother that she needed to have him put on medication. At about the same time, Sam's foster family agency social worker threatened Sam that if he did not improve his grades, he would move his placement away from his current foster mother. Sam was understandably quite frightened with this threat, and reported it immediately to his therapist, who admonished the worker. The worker withdrew the threat at the time, but made it again in February (2 months later), and added that Sam was "lazy" and only went to therapy to "snivel." Sam again reported this to his therapist, and the worker was removed from the case. At about this same time, Sam's grandmother brought a petition to the court to have Sam removed from the care of his foster mother. The petition was denied by the judge, but the experience was nevertheless quite frightening and upsetting for Sam. He was not able to recover academically for the rest of the school year, and his therapist requested another evaluation to aid in the case conceptualization and help with intervention recommendations. As a part of this evaluation, Sam—now age 12—was administered the Adult Attachment Projective Picture System (AAP). The AAP is a relatively new measure of mental representation of attachment classification based on the analysis of a set of projective stimuli designed to systematically activate the attachment system (George et al., 1999; George & West, in press), and in many ways parallels the coding process and markers in the doll play. Interestingly, Sam's classification on the AAP was secure, with a large number of instances of internalized secure base. Internalized secure base (ISB) refers specifically to that state in which the sense of security is derived largely from the individual's internal relationship to the attachment figure. Story characters typically demonstrate an integrative or reflective inner strength to solve problems or to resolve feelings. For example, in Sam's stories, when characters were confronted with difficulties, loss, or potential loss, they thought about the situation and/or relationships, and then determined an appropriate course of action. It was hypothesized, however, that although his mental representation of attachment was now secure, he could still potentially become easily dysregulated by unsupportive and threatening relationships (e.g., teachers, foster family agency worker, and his grandmother). This interpretation is consistent with Steele and colleagues' (e.g., Hodges et al., 2003) findings that security does not transform the remaining disorganized representations. Despite the presence of this dysregulation, Sam was nevertheless able to appeal to the caregiving adults in his life for help, and to use their help effectively in resolving problems. Consistent with his development of representational exploration (in the form of ISB), his therapist reports that Sam now comes to therapy and sits on the couch talking about the events, issues, or relationship problems that are troubling him, and engaging in a problem-solving process to resolve them. It appears that the steady work on introducing Sam to the haven of safety during therapy as a child had become internalized as a strength of personal agency. He is able to reflect on his own, as well as others', behavior, and has come to understand and accept his grandparents' behavior, as well as that as his biological mother. This allowed him to be separate from them so that he did not have to agree with their behavior, but could continue to have a relationship with them.

This case illustrates the importance of providing emotional protection to foster children—despite the constraints and realities of the foster care system. The foster mother was helped to see the attachment function of Sam's behavior and to respond therapeutically to his signals of distress. She subsequently obtained legal guardianship of Sam and his sister, which allowed for even more protection against the intrusiveness of the grandparents. Themes of protection were introduced into the play therapy, and limits were set on frightening, intrusive behavior from the grandparents. Over time, with permanency and the sense of availability from the foster mother and the therapist, Sam was able to turn to representational exploration and problem solving. The result was a diminishing of symptoms and a return to a normal developmental trajectory.

CONCLUSION

The results of this exploratory investigation have provided support for the use of the George and Solomon methodologies and for the use of this measure with older, school-age children. This case represents how knowing specific information about a child's representational attachment constructs (e.g., ISB) and problems (e.g., dysregulated frightened behavior, inability to count on attachment figures as a haven of safety) can provide for the development of specific attachment intervention strategies. The articulation and measurement of defensive processes can provide additional explanatory variance for understanding children's adaptation to aversive circumstances, as well as provide a window into understanding a possible pathway toward security and healthy adaptation. The finding that defensive processes are related to theoretically relevant variables provides additional support for the constructs as well as this methodology. In addition, the finding that representational markers of security and dysregulation were systematically related to children's behavior in the home and at school is an indication of the importance and robust nature of mental representation. It should be noted, however, that the conclusions that can be drawn from these data are constrained by the fact that they are not longitudinal, and thus it cannot be determined whether these children already possessed the mental representation measured in this study *prior* to placement, or whether they developed one as a result of the caregiving they were receiving at the time of the testing. The findings are nevertheless consistent with the findings from Steele and colleagues' (e.g., Hodges et al., 2003; Steele et al., 2003) longitudinal research with maltreated children who had been adopted. In particular, the findings from this study and from Steele et al.'s research converge to direct future research and clinical interventions toward an investigation of defensive processes and indicators or markers of security, and away from global classifications of attachment.

Future research may wish to focus on investigations of how children's representations vary according to perceived permanence, ongoing connection to birth mother, or placement with relatives; and how representations vary with the quality of caregiving. In addition, researchers and clinicians may wish to use this method to document change in representations, measure intervention effects, and investigate whether representational change precedes behavioral change.

REFERENCES

Achenbach, T. M., & Edelbrock, C. (1983). *Manual for the Child Behavior Checklist and revised Child Behavior Profile.* Burlington, VT: Queen City Printers.

Achenbach, T. M., & Rescola, L. A. (2001). *Manual for the ASEBA school-age forms and profiles.* Burlington, VT: University of Vermont, Research Center for Children, Youth, and Families.

Allen, J. P., & Land, D. (2008). Attachment in adolescence. In J. Cassidy & P. R. Shaver (Eds.), *Handbook of attachment* (2nd ed., pp. 419–435). New York: Guilford Press.

Bates, B. C., & Dozier, M. (2002). The importance of maternal state of mind regarding attachment and infant age of placement to foster mothers' representations of their foster infants. *Infant Mental Health Journal, 23,* 417–431.

Bowlby, J. (1973). *Attachment and loss: Vol. 2. Separation, anxiety, and anger.* New York: Basic Books.

Bowlby, J. (1980). *Attachment and loss: Vol. 3. Loss.* New York: Basic Books.

Bowlby, J. (1982). *Attachment and loss: Vol. 1. Attachment.* New York: Basic Books. (Original work published 1969)

Bowlby, J. (1988). *A secure base.* New York: Basic Books.

Bretherton, I., & Oppenheim, D. (2003). The MacArthur Story Stem Battery: Development, directions for administration, reliability, validity and reflections about meaning. In R. N. Emde, D. P. Wolf, & D. Bretherton (Eds.), *Revealing the inner worlds of young children: The MacArthur Story Stem Battery and parent–child narratives* (pp. 55–80). New York: Oxford University Press.

Bretherton, I., Rigeway, D., & Cassidy, J. (1990). Assessing internal working models of attachment relationships: An attachment story completion task for 3-year-olds. In M. T. Greenberg, D. Cicchetti, & E. M. Cummings (Eds.), *Attachment in the preschool years* (pp. 273–308). Chicago: University of Chicago Press.

Carlson, E. A. (1998). A prospective longitudinal study of attachment disorganization/disorientation. *Child Development, 69,* 1107–1128.

Cassidy, J. (1994). Emotion regulation: Influences of attachment relationships. In N. A. Fox (Ed.), *The development of emotion regulation: Biological and behavioral considerations* (pp. 228–249). Chicago: University of Chicago Press.

Cicchetti, D. (1989). How research on child maltreatment has informed the study of child development: Perspectives from developmental psychopathology. In D. Cicchetti & V. Calrson (Eds.), *Child maltreatment: Theory and research on the causes and consequences of child abuse and neglect* (pp. 377–431). New York: Cambridge University Press.

Cicchetti, D., & Lynch, M. (1995). Failures in the expectable environment and their impact on individual development: The case of child maltreatment. In D. Cicchetti & D. J. Cohen (Eds.), *Developmental psychopathology: Vol. 2. Risk, disorder, and adaptation* (pp. 32–71). New York: Wiley.

Cicchetti, D., & Manly, J. T. (Eds.). (2001). Operationalizing child maltreatment: Developmental processes and outcomes [Special issue]. *Development and Psychopathology, 13.*

Cichetti, D., & Toth, S. L. (1995) A developmental psychopathology perspective on child abuse and neglect. *Journal of the American Academy of Child and Adolescent Psychiatry, 34,* 1067–1091.

Dozier, M., Stovall, K. C., Albus, K. E., & Bates, B. (2001). Attachment for infants in foster care: The role of caregiver state of mind. *Child Development, 72,* 1467–1477.

Fish, B. (2004). Attachment in infancy and preschool in low socioeconomic status rural Appalachian children: Stability and change and relations to preschool and kindergarten competence. *Development and Psychopathology, 16,* 293–312.

George, C. (1996). A representational perspective of child abuse and prevention: Internal working models of attachment and caregiving. *Child Abuse and Neglect, 20,* 411–424.

George, C., & Solomon, J. (1989). Internal working models of caregiving and security of attachment at age six. *Infant Mental Health Journal [Special issue]. Internal Representations and Parent–Infant Relationships, 10*(3), 222–237.

George, C., & Solomon, J. (1996). Representational models of relationships: Links between caregiving and representation. *Infant Mental Health Journal, 17,* 198–216.

George, C., & Solomon, J. (1998). *Six-year doll play classification system supplement attachment disorganization coding.* Unpublished classification manual, Mills College, Oakland, CA.

George, C., & Solomon, J. (1990/1996/2000). *Six-year attachment doll play classification system.* Unpublished classification manual, Mills College, Oakland, CA.

George, C., & Solomon, J. (2008). The caregiving system: A behavioral systems approach to caregiving. In J. Cassidy & P. R. Shaver (Eds.), *Handbook of attachment: Theory, research, and clinical implications* (2nd ed., pp. 333–356). New York: Guilford Press.

George, C., & West, M. (2001). The development and preliminary validation of a new measure of adult attachment: The Adult Attachment Projective. *Attachment and Human Development, 3,* 30–61.

George, C., & West, M. (in press). *The Adult Attachment Projective Picture System.* New York: Guilford Press.

George, C., West, M., & Pettem, O. (1997). *The Adult Attachment Projective.* Unpublished attachment measure and coding manual, Mills College, Oakland, CA.

Gloger-Tippelt, G., & Konig, L. (2007). Attachment representations in 6-year-old children from one and two parent families in Germany. *School Psychology International, 28,* 313–330.

Granot, D., & Mayseless, O. (2001). Attachment security and adjustment to school in middle childhood. *Attachment and Human Development, 25,* 530–541.

Green, J., Stanley, C., Smith, V., & Goldwyn, R. (2000). A new method of evaluating attachment representations in young school-age children: The Manchester Child Attachment Story Task (MCAST). *Attachment and Human Development, 2,* 48–70.

Hamilton-Oravetz, S. (1993). *Patterns of attachment and grief in primary care medicine patients.* Unpublished dissertation, California School of Professional Psychology, Alameda.

Hodges, J., Steele, M., Hillman, S., Henderson, K., & Kaniuk, J. (2003). Changes in attachment representations over the first year of adoptive placement: Narratives of maltreated children. *Clinical Child Psychology and Psychiatry, 8,* 351–367.

Hodges, J., Steele, M., Hillman, S., Henderson, K., & Kaniuk, J. (2005). Change and continuity in mental representations of attachment after adoption. In D. M. Brodzinsky & J. Palacios (Eds.), *Psychological issues in adoption: Research and practice. Advances in applied developmental psychology* (pp. 93–116). Westport, CT: Praeger/Greenwood Press.

Hodges, J., Steele, M., Hillman, S., Henderson, K., & Marta, N. (2000). Effects of abuse on attachment representations: Narrative assessments of abused children. *Journal of Child Psychotherapy, 26,* 433–455.

Holland, R., Moretti, M. M., Verlaan, V., & Peterson, S. (1993). Attachment and conduct disorder: The response program. *Canadian Journal of Psychiatry, 38,* 420–431.

Jacobsen, T., Huss, M., Fendrich, M., Kruesi, M. J. P., & Ziegenhain, U. (1997). Children's ability to delay gratification: Longitudinal relations to mother–child attachment. *Journal of Genetic Psychology, 158,* 411–426.

Jacobvitz, D., & Hazen, N. (1999). Developmental pathways from infant disorganization to childhood peer relationships. In J. Solomon & C. George (Eds.), *Attachment disorganization* (pp. 127–159). New York: Guilford Press.

Katsurada, E. (2007). Attachment representation of institutionalized children in Japan. *School Psychology International, 28,* 331–345.

Lyons-Ruth, K., Alpern, L., & Repacholi, B. (1993). Disorganized infant attachment classification and maternal psychosocial problems as predictors of hostile–aggressive behavior in the preschool classroom. *Child Development, 64,* 572–585.

Lyons-Ruth, K., Connell, D. B., Grunebaum, H. U., & Botein, S. (1990). Infants at social risk: Maternal depression and family support services as mediators of infant development and security of attachment. *Child Development, 61,* 85–98.

Main, M. (1990). Parental aversion to infant-initiated contact is correlated with the parent's own rejection during childhood: The effects of experience on signals of security with respect to attachment. In K. E. Barnard & T. B. Brazelton (Eds.), *Touch: The foundation of experience* (pp. 461–495). Madison, CT: International Universities Press.

Main, M. (1991). Metacognitive knowledge, metacognitive monitoring, and singular (coherent) vs. multiple (incoherent) models of attachment: Findings and directions for future research. In C. M. Parkes, J. Stevenson-Hinde, & D. Marris (Eds.), *Attachment across the life cycle* (pp. 127–159). New York: NY, Tavistock/Routledge.

Magai, C. (1999). Affect, imagery, and attachment: Working models of interpersonal affect and the socialization of emotion. In J. Cassidy & P. R. Shaver (Eds.), *Handbook of attachment* (pp. 787–802). New York: Guilford Press.

Moretti, M. M., Holland, R., & Peterson, S. (1994). Long term outcome of an attachment-based program for conduct disorder. *Canadian Journal of Psychiatry, 39,* 360–370.

Moss, E., Bureau, J. F., Cyr, C., Mongeau, C., & St-Laurent, D. (2004). Correlates of attachment at age 3: Construct validity of the preschool attachment classification system. *Developmental Psychology, 40,* 323–334.

Moss, E., Cyr, C., & Dubois-Comtois, K. (2004). Attachment at early school age and developmental risk: Examining family contexts and behavior problems of controlling–caregiving, controlling–punitive, and behaviorally disorganized children. *Developmental Psychology, 40,* 519–532.

Moss, E., Rousseau, D., Parent, S., St-Laurent, D., & Saintonge, J. (1998). Correlates of attachment at school age: Maternal reported stress, mother–child interaction, and behavior problems. *Child Development, 69,* 1390–1405.

Moss, E., & St-Laurent, D. (2001). Attachment at school age and academic performance. *Developmental Psychology, 37,* 863–874.

Obsuth, I., Moretti, M. M., Holland, R., Braber, K., & Cross, S. (2006). Conduct disorder: New directions in promoting effective parenting and strengthening parent–adolescent relationships. *Journal of the Canadian Academy of Child and Adolescent Psychiatry, 15,* 6–15.

Ogawa, J. R., Sroufe, L. A., Weinfield, N. S., Carlson, E. A., & Egeland, B. (1997). Development of the fragmented self: Longitudinal study of dissociative symptomatology in a non-clinical sample. *Development and Psychopathology, 9,* 855–879.

Reynolds, C. R., & Kamphaus, R. W. (1998). *Behavioral assessment system for children: Technical manual.* Circle Pines, MN: American Guidance Service.

Russell, P. (2005). *Attachment and grief in foster children.* Paper presented at the annual meeting of the Society for Research in Child Development, Atlanta, GA.

Solomon, J., & George, C. (1996). Defining the caregiving system: Toward a theory of caregiving. *Infant Mental Health Journal, 17,* 183–197.

Solomon, J., & George, C. (1999a). The development of attachment in separated and divorced families. *Attachment and Human Development, 1*(1), 2–33.

Solomon, J., & George, C. (1999b). The caregiving system in mothers of infants: A comparison of divorcing and married mothers. *Attachment and Human Development, 1*(2), 171–190.

Solomon, J., & George, C. (2008). The measurement of attachment security in infancy and childhood. In J. Cassidy & P. R. Shaver (Eds.), *Handbook of attachment* (2nd ed., pp. 383–416). New York: Guilford Press.

Solomon, J., George, C., & DeJong, A. (1995). Children classified as controlling at age six: Evidence of disorganized representational strategies and aggression at home and at school. *Development and Psychopathology, 7,* 447–463.

Sroufe, L. A., & Fleeson, J. (1988). The coherence of individual relationships. In R. A. Hinde & J. Stevenson-Hinde (Eds.), *Relationships within families: Mutual influences* (pp. 27–47). Oxford, UK: Oxford University Press.

Stacks, A. (2007). Defensive dysregulation in preschool children's attachment story narratives and its relation to attachment classification and externalizing behavior. *School Psychology International, 28,* 294–312.

Stams, G. J. M., Juffer, F., & van IJzendoorn, M. H. (2002). Maternal sensitivity, infant attachment, and temperament in early childhood predict adjustment in middle childhood: The case of adopted children and their biologically unrelated parents. *Developmental Psychology, 38,* 806–821.

Steele, M., Hodges, J., Kaniuk, J., Hillman, S., & Henderson, K. (2003). Attachment representations and adoption: Associations between maternal states of mind and emotion narratives in previously maltreated children. *Journal of Child Psychotherapy, 29,* 187–205.

Stovall, K. C., & Dozier, M. (2000). The development of attachment in new relationships: Single subject analyses for 10 foster infants. *Development and Psychopathology, 12,* 133–156.

van IJzendoorn, M. H., Schuengel, C., & Bakermanns-Kranenburg, M. J. (1999). Disorganized attachment in early childhood: Meta-analysis of precursors, concommittants, and sequelae. *Development and Psychopathology, 11,* 225–249.

Venet, M., Bureau, J., Gosselin, C., & Capuana, F. (2007). Attachment representations in a sample of neglected preschool-age children. *School Psychology International, 28,* 264–293.

Weinfield, N. S., Whaley, G. J. L., & Egeland, B. (2004). Continuity, discontinuity, and coherence in attachment from infancy to late adolescence: Sequelae of organization and disorganization. *Attachment and Human Development, 6,* 73–97.

Chapter 12

The Circle of Security Intervention
Using the Therapeutic Relationship to Ameliorate Attachment Security in Disorganized Dyads

CAROLINE A. ZANETTI, BERT POWELL,
GLEN COOPER, and KENT HOFFMAN

> Although initiated in adolescence, the caregiving
> representational system probably undergoes its greatest growth
> during the transition to parenthood.... This period, often
> accompanied by intense emotion and emotional swings, has
> the potential for both psychological disorganization and a new
> reorganization of the self.
> —SOLOMON AND GEORGE (1996, p. 191)

The Circle of Security (COS; Cooper, Hoffman, Powell, & Marvin, 2005; Powell, Cooper, Hoffman, & Marvin, 2009) is a model encompassing the three behavioral control systems that make up a child's world. Two of these belong to the child himself: the exploration system and the attachment system. The third, the caregiving system, belongs to his parent. These three systems work together toward the same goal of keeping the child safe while he grows and learns how to function autonomously.

In this chapter, we describe the way in which the COS model encompasses some of the theoretical tenets of attachment theory and object relations theory, and show how these ideas can inform therapy with disorganized dyads, using a case illustration.

Because there are a number of possible ways of using the COS concepts with parents, we would like to make clear some terms relating to it: the COS Project was a therapeutic intervention, evaluated with pre- and post-program measures (including Strange Situation Procedures) with families from a high-risk population attending the Head Start program in Spokane, Washington (Hoffman, Marvin, Cooper, & Powell, 2006; Marvin, Cooper, Hoffman, & Powell, 2002; Powell, Cooper, Hoffman, & Marvin, 2007); the COS Protocol is the therapeutic program itself (Cooper et al., 2005); the term *Circle of Security* refers to the COS graphic and the attachment concepts it depicts (see Figure 12.1). Throughout this chapter, we refer to the child as "he" and the parent as "she."

The parent is visible on the COS in the form of a pair of hands, holding the child's world together. Holding is an essential function that parents provide for their children (Winnicott, 1978a, 1978b). At the beginning, the mother's love, care, and protection is conveyed in a concrete physical way, through her hands. As their relationship develops, their bond, and the mother's understanding of her child's needs and feelings, extend his sense of her support.

If the hands that held the parent's world together when she herself was little were too harsh, or too shaky, or perhaps barely there at all, it may be difficult for her to be sure of her own capacity to provide strong, wise, and loving care for her child, with dire consequences for them both. When a parent has her Hands on the Circle, she is taking a Bigger, Stronger, Wiser, and Kind stance that allows her to see and respond to her child's needs, whether the child is exploring or requiring closeness and protection. The COS model takes a broad view of the range of children's needs that might activate the parent's caregiving system (after Ainsworth, 1972; Sroufe & Waters, 1977). If the overarching goal of the caregiving system is protection of the young (Bowlby, 1969) *within* an environmental context (Bowlby, 1969, 1988; George & Solomon, 1996), then it makes sense that caregiving will be activated not only to protect the child from danger, but also to support his adaptation to the world. As the primary environment of human beings tends to be a social one, the experience of delight in one another seems to be a primary indicator of successful adaptation. The child's legitimate need for delight, and the expectation that a healthy caregiver should be able to provide it, puts this need on both the top half of the Circle of Security and the bottom half.

Each half of the Circle of Security relates to a particular caregiving function. The top half represents the child's needs when his exploration system is activated, complemented by the caregiver's availability and readiness to support him (see Figure. 12.1, "Support My Exploration"). As a child puts his focus on something of interest, he needs to know that his caregiver is available to watch over, and to provide protection—perhaps at a distance, or maybe up close to scaffold his approach to the object or task. Emotional

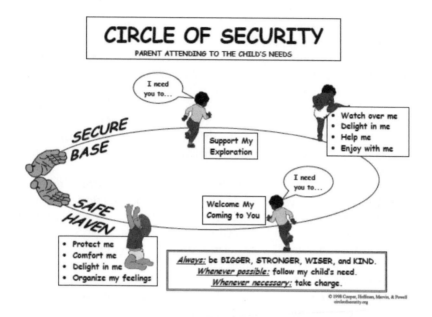

FIGURE 12.1. The Circle of Security and formula. Copyright 1998 by Glen Cooper, Kent Hoffman, Robert Marvin, and Bert Powell. Reprinted by permission.

connection can also be considered an important component of support for exploration as it builds on the child's capacity to develop his skills and self-confidence. On the top half of the Circle of Security the parent's overall task is to provide a secure base for exploration and developing mastery.

The bottom half represents the attachment system. When a child's attachment needs are activated, exploration ceases, and his overarching need is for his caregiver to signal that she is available and competent, and it is safe for him to approach her (Figure 12.1, "Welcome My Coming to You") for protection or comfort. A child needs to know that his caregiver is not resentful, overburdened, or critical of his need for protection and comfort. The COS model also recognizes two other needs that may be present when children's attachment needs are activated—when a parent feels delight in being close to her child it allows him to enjoy her strength and availability, and establishes a sense of self-worth in him that will later form part of his representations of self in relationship, and as caregiver. " Organize My Feelings" is a further essential need, relating to the caregiver's capacity to help the child with emotional regulation, so he can think and learn from experience. From his caregiver being with him in this way, a child also learns both to regulate his own emotions and to bring his emotions into relationships.

Organizing feelings can sometimes be seen in terms of *scaffolding*—an important caregiving function that helps children to regulate emotions like anxiety or frustration when they are exploring, or fear, anger, disappointment, or physical pain activating the attachment system. Sometimes parents must scaffold the transition between exploration and attachment—for example, when the parent calls an end to play, or asks a child to perform a chore. For a parent to do this successfully, she must attune herself to her child's state, and use her wisdom and strength to build a platform for him to step up to what is required in the moment. Bowlby (1969) remarked that parents need to be stronger and wiser, but parental warmth has also been shown to be strongly associated with infant security (Sroufe, 1997), as has the parent's capacity to see him or herself as bigger than the child (Bowlby, 1988; Lyons-Ruth & Jacobvitz, 2008; Main & Solomon, 1990).

The COS makes explicit that children cannot move from their attachment needs to exploration until they have "filled their cup" in the safe haven provided by attuned connection with their caregiver. The Circle of Security has placed a unique emphasis on providing a safe haven as a separate and equal function to secure base provision (Powell et al., 2009; Hoffman et al., 2006; Cooper et al., 2005). It is only when a person has reached a safe haven offering renewal that he or she can use it as a secure base for further exploration. This distinction is helpful for parents, as it makes the child's need explicit, and provides a framework for response. Most parents are more comfortable with meeting their child's needs on one half of the Circle of Security than the other. Some tend to feel more pleasure in meeting exploration needs and supporting autonomy, and others favor having the child in close connection, supporting dependence.

Solomon and George (1996) noted that the balance a caregiver can achieve between her preference for providing distant or close protection correlates with the attachment classifications described by Mary Ainsworth and colleagues (Ainsworth, Blehar, Waters, & Wall, 1978). Parents of secure children are able to balance their responses to the child's feelings, situation, and developmental capacity. Insecure children tend to have parents who favor distant protection (classified as Avoidant) or close protection (classified as Resistant). Children were observed to have adapted the expression of their need, particularly when distressed, to the parent's preference—despite having an insecure attachment, they had developed an *organized* strategy to maximize the parent's capacity to provide a secure base (Sroufe & Waters, 1977).

Some children appear to lack an organized strategy for ensuring adequate proximity to their caregiver when anxious—in fact, they seem disorganized or disoriented when their attachment needs are activated in the parent's presence (Main & Solomon, 1990). The antecedents of attachment disorganization are considered to reside in the caregiving environment, through internal or external impingements on the mother's capacity to provide adequate care and protection (Cyr, Euser, Bakermans-Kranenburg, & van IJzendoorn, 2010; George & Solomon, 1996, 2008; this volume, Chapter 6; Lyons-Ruth, Bronfman, & Atwood, 1999; Main & Hesse, 1990; Sroufe, Egeland, Carlson, & Collins, 2005). Disorganized attachment in the child correlates with disorganized maternal caregiving representations (George & Solomon, 2008) associated with maternal helplessness, hostility, and role-reversal (George & Solomon, 2008; Lyons-Ruth & Jacobvitz, 2008; Main & Hesse, 1990). From preschool-age, children with attachment disorganization tend to adopt a predominantly caregiving or punitive approach towards their parent, which is understood to be an attempt to manage the fear associated with an unreliably available secure base/safe haven (Main & Hesse, 1990). These children have been found to be at higher risk for disturbed psychosocial adjustment during childhood, adolescence, and adulthood (Sroufe et al., 2005; van IJzendoorn, Schuengel, & Bakermans-Kranenburg, 1999).

Solomon and George (1999) have suggested that disorganized attachment results from repeated moments in which the parent behaves in such a way that she frightens the child, eliciting his attachment behavior, and fails to terminate it by providing adequate proximity, protection, and reassurance. This is an important idea, emphasizing the crucial nature of repair after relationship rupture. In COS terms, the relationship is ruptured when the parent fails to take a bigger, stronger, wiser, and kind stance, and repaired once she resumes it, acknowledging the rupture.

The COS provides a "formula" for parenting: "*Always* be Bigger, Stronger, Wiser, and Kind. Whenever possible follow your child's need. Whenever necessary, take charge." It is important that parents strive to maintain all four qualities simultaneously, but many struggle to do so in moments of high affective arousal. Being "Bigger and Stronger" can come readily when dealing with a smaller person, especially when angry, but if not tempered with wisdom and kindness, the parent is experienced as mean, rather than as a secure base or safe haven. Similarly, if a parent tries to be "Kind" at the expense of strength, she will seem weak. Some parents, particularly those who are prone to dissociation, or substance abuse, may simply be experienced as "gone," with no Hands on the Circle of Security at all. The parent's Hands also disappear from the Circle when the parent is overwhelmed by her own internal experience, and thus unable to see and respond to her child's need. When these three forms of disturbed caregiving: "Mean," "Weak," and "Gone," occur repeatedly, without repair, the parent can be said to have abdicated the caregiving role (Solomon & George, 1996). Children feel fear when their attachment figure is unavailable. If the caregiver is herself a source of fear, the child is disorganized by the paradox of being frightened by his safe haven. George and Solomon

(1996, 2008) have also described abdication as "suspended" or "disabled" caregiving. The implication is that the underlying capacity for a bigger, wiser, stronger, and kind stance is present, but too often disused. The COS intervention capitalizes on the parent's positive intentions to be competent and protective toward her child, to help her recognize and build on her underutilized capacity.

Bowlby suggested that an infant builds up mental models based on his experiences of being with his attachment figure, which can be used to predict and guide the course of subsequent interactions. He referred to these increasingly influential structures as "internal working models" (Bowlby, 1969, 1988). An *internal working model* is a more or less integrated set of memories, feelings, and beliefs about the self in relation to various aspects of the world, including important others. Originating in actual interpersonal exchanges between the growing self and others, internal working models are dynamic in nature, and open to modification or confirmation, according to subsequent experience. It is important to understand that in a relationship with a significant other, such as a caregiver, the developing model encompasses a complementary view of self and other. Thus, if a caregiver is perceived as loving, the child will perceive him- or herself as lovable (Bowlby, 1988) and vice versa.

It can be very difficult for a small child to take in feelings of being unworthy of care and protection without becoming dysregulated, or falling apart. Bowlby (1980, 1988) suggested that adverse experiences with parents could have a powerful effect on the child's developing cognitive structures through the formation of defensive processes designed to exclude such experiences from thought, feeling, or memory. It is important to recognize that the attachment system provides a compelling force on a child to stay close to his attachment figure. Where the relationship contains consistently painful interactions, the child must nevertheless find a way of staying close, and getting what support he can from his parent. Thus, through driving painful information from consciousness, defensive exclusion contributes to maintenance of a steady representational state (Bowlby, 1998; see also George & Solomon, Chapter 6, this volume).

All parents fail to provide protection and care sometimes, and all people develop some degree of defensive exclusion. However, when attachment trauma is intense and/or persistent, a child may attempt to completely block painful or threatening memories and their associated affects from consciousness, resulting in "segregated systems" (Bowlby, 1980; see also George & Solomon, Chapter 6, this volume). Thus, the contents of unbearable experiences might remain, but as a separate representational model, coexisting with a contradictory, more comfortable model. For example, a child may see his parent as both loving and affectionate (and thus himself as lovable and worthy of affection), yet also have a separate representation of the same parent as terrifying and maltreating (and himself as frightened and annihilated). Bowlby (1988, p.106) referred to a patient who asked herself "Have I two fathers?" when memories of a segregated representation of abuse surfaced after the birth of her child. Although maintained separately, segregated systems remain extremely influential in their effects on thought, feeling, and behavior (Bowlby, 1988). George and Solomon (2008; Chapter 6, this volume) have proposed that caregiving disorganization results from the parent's efforts to keep segregated systems related to early attachment trauma out of awareness through maintenance of a hypervigilant defensive stance toward the child.

The COS model uses the term "Shark Music" for talking with parents about the way that unconscious forces related to unintegrated affects from their own past attachment assaults may interfere with their capacity to see and respond to their children's needs (see Powell et al., 2009). One of the tasks of the COS intervention is to help parents recognize this process within themselves—to see that specific needs or behaviors in their children tend to make them uncomfortable because pain related to buried memories of their own unmet childhood needs threatens to break through. Automatically going to defense, the parent will protect herself from something that *is* safe but *feels* frightening by finding a way to deflect the child away from the specific need/s evoking her discomfort and threatening dysregulation. As the parent learns to recognize the presence of Shark Music through observing and reflecting on the way she and her child miscue each other when the child has particular needs, she is able to make a choice to meet the child's need, instead of attending to past phantoms.

The parent's traumatic attachment representations form segregated representations of a good self and other, and a bad self and other. Defensive strategies to maintain connection with the good other and protect from the bad other are used in habitual ways. The COS program pays particular attention to defensive processes, informed by James Masterson's description of three defensive styles: borderline, narcissistic, and schizoid (Masterson, 1976, 1988; Masterson & Lieberman, 2004; Masterson & Klein, 1995). These styles form an integral and stable part of personality structure, developing out of unspoken rules and requirements that the individual's early attachment figures imposed as a condition of relationship. All people use some measure of these strategies. When a person utilizes them in a pervasive and rigid way, they constitute personality disorder. In lesser degrees of expression, they simply reflect the person's innermost concerns about preserving a coherent sense of self within relationship. Cooper and colleagues (2005) have reconceptualized Masterson's work in terms of sensitivity to specific sorts of assault on one's sense of self in relationship. Viewing defensive working models as a way of managing sensitivity to a specific form of emotional distress is an important reframing, as it supports a therapeutic stance characterized by empathy and compassion for the parent, as well as the child.

These three core sensitivities are named to reflect the central concern of the individual about being in relationship. Individuals with borderline disorders fear that being separate from the other will lead to abandonment (Buchheim & George, Chapter 13, this volume). So they focus on what the other needs, wants, feels, and thinks while disavowing their own sense of self as a way to avoid being separate—in other words, they are "separation-sensitive." Parents who rely heavily on this defensive strategy find it difficult to tolerate the child's moves toward individuation—it is painful for them, so they tend to discourage exploration. Also, conflict, setting limits, and/or enforcing expectations, or in any way being in charge may be experienced as being separate from the other. This failure of executive functioning (dropping their Hands from the Circle) may lead to disorganization of the attachment relationship.

Individuals with narcissistic personalities believe that being held in high esteem for their performance and achievements is what makes them worthy of attachment—that is, they are "esteem-sensitive." Believing themselves to be essentially unlovable, with no real sense of self-worth, they project a veneer of success and perfection, bolstered by efforts to have others recognize them as special and flawless. Eliciting esteem from others keeps their true doubts about themselves (and annihilating memories of unmet childhood need) at bay. Keeping others oblivious to their vulnerability can interfere with their capacity for empathy with their children's attachment needs because when the child shows the world a lack of distress and a capacity for success, it demonstrates the parent's caregiving competency. Masterson described two forms of narcissistic personality functioning: the exhibitionist (marked by grandiose demands for attention and mirroring) and the closet narcissist, whose self-worth is drawn from being associated with another idealized figure.

Individuals with schizoid defensive strategies are particularly sensitive to the dangers that can be experienced in close relationships—such people are "safety-sensitive." Although desiring closeness, they fear being overtaken by the demands of the other, with no space for their own self. They respond by stepping back from intimacy, into isolation, which can feel just as unbearable. Neither choice offers a safe haven in relationship. A safety-sensitive parent will often focus on maintaining a distance that is comfortable for him or her, but sometimes too much for the child. The parent may attempt a compromise by encouraging the child to dampen the intensity of expressed emotion, so that closeness is more comfortable.

Identifying the parent's core sensitivity allows a better understanding of the problems within each particular dyad. Struggles can be presented in a way that lessens the activation of defenses, allowing more insight and reflection. Careful following of the parent's affect and discourse in their moment-by-moment interaction during tape reviews allows the therapist to notice and to support the parent at moments when she opens herself to a more accurate view of child or self, discarding her habitual defense.

Masterson (1995) described such moments as self-activation: an individual momentarily takes the risk of stepping outside the constraints of his or her usual defensive representations of self and other by opening up to the possibilities new perceptions and behaviors might afford (i.e., activates the "true," rather than the defensive "false" self). Self-activation opens access to the painful memories and longings the defense was designed to avoid, the person experiences a dreadful emotional state related to infantile experiences of abandonment, then quickly resumes the old defense. In the case illustration we will show how tracking this defensive process allows the therapist to monitor and maintain the parent's reflective capacity during tape reviews.

The COS protocol is a manualized 20-week group program for six participants—mothers (and occasionally, fathers) of children ages 11 months to 5 years. A detailed description of the COS protocol can be found in Cooper et al. (2005), Hoffman et al. (2006), and Powell et al. (2009). The initial assessment involves filming a Strange Situation Procedure (SSP). The Ainsworth system (Ainsworth et al., 1978; Main & Solomon, 1990) is used with children younger than 24 months, and the Pre-school (Cassidy & Marvin, 2000) system for older children. Two extra episodes are added to the SSP: a 5-minute episode in which the parent is asked to read a story to the child, and a 3-minute episode in which the parent is asked to organize the child to clean up the toys. The SSP is used as for clinical assessment, and is not usually formally scored prior to the program. Instead, the therapist examines the interaction throughout each episode in the procedure, looking for moments when the child feels comfortable to cue the parent directly to have his need met, and those where he "miscues" by disguising the real need, to avoid the pain of having it go unmet or worse, rejected. For example, a child who is anxious, and wants to come closer to the parent (a bottom-half attachment need) may miscue by asking for help with a toy (a top-half exploration need) because his history with this parent has taught him that she is more comfortable with his exploration than with his anxiety. The therapist is also interested to watch the parent's affect during interaction with her child on the top and bottom half of the circle, and to see where she encourages miscues, such as directing the child's attention away from her to the toys as she reenters after a separation, leaving no room for him to express sadness, anger, or a need for comfort.

Immediately following the filming, the parent is filmed responding to the Circle of Security Interview (COSI; Cooper, Hoffman, Marvin, & Powell, 1999) beginning with five questions about the experience of parent and child in the SSP (e.g., "What do you think he needed while you stood behind the mirror watching him?"). Twenty questions about the parent's perception of the child and their relationship have been adapted from the Parent Development Interview (Aber, Slade, Berger, Bresgi, & Kaplan, 1985)—for example, "What gives you the most pain and difficulty about being his parent?" Finally, there are six questions about the parent's relationships with her own caregivers during childhood (adapted from the Adult Attachment Interview; George, Kaplan, & Main, 1996). These include a request for five words that describe the parent's relationship with her own primary caregiver, followed by a request for episodic memories related to the words she has chosen. The COSI is examined for indications of the mother's representations of the child and herself as caregiver, as well as her own early attachment experiences, her reflective capacity, and her core sensitivity. The therapist is interested in her struggles, but also in identifying her strengths.

Following from what is learned in the course of the SSP and COSI, the parent–child interaction can be examined to discern where on the Circle the parent is able to meet the child's needs, and where she is not. The therapist seeks to identify a moment that exemplifies the *linchpin* struggle between mother and child—that is, the key defensive strategy represented both in the parent–child interaction and in each partner's internal working model. Learning goals are formulated for each parent: What do we want *this* parent to know about *this* child? What do we want *this* parent to understand about the way in which her caregiving practices support or constrain their relationship? How can we present these questions to her in a way that will open her to reflection upon her innermost thoughts and beliefs about herself as a person, and as a mother?

Children do not attend the group program, which involves three series of tape reviews, tailored to the specific dyadic strengths and struggles for each parent and child, and the parent's primary defensive strategy. Vignettes from the SSP are chosen to illustrate particular aspects of the relationship. Some show the parent struggling to meet her child's need, and others reveal underutilized strengths. The other parents are encouraged to reflect on what they observe, to learn from each other's tape reviews, and to support one another.

The linchpin moment is usually shown to parents in their second tape review. The third tape review focuses on improvements in the relationship but also indicates areas needing further attention and work. Some parents finish the program with a securely attached child. For others, the COS protocol begins a process of reflection, and a readiness for self-examination that will lead to more psychotherapy. Participants often maintain some therapeutic links following the program.

CLINICAL ILLUSTRATION

Clinical material helps to demonstrate a therapeutic style. We begin with some background information, and then examine 5 minutes of therapy in which a mother from the program looks at the linchpin moment during her second tape review. Her child had a disorganized attachment (D-Forced C)[1] at the start of the program, and finished with a secure classification. We will provide some discussion throughout the case illustration, in italics.

Marie was a married woman with two children: Rose, age 2 months, and Samuel, 3 years. Previously, she was a junior executive for a mining firm. Her husband had a more senior position in the same firm, working long hours. When at home, he spent a lot of time with the children, and helped her with household chores. She described him as emotionally supportive, but unable to take away the overwhelming anxiety she had been feeling since Rose was born. Marie had suffered from postnatal depression following Samuel's birth, 3 years earlier. She had believed that good mothers were able to establish routines for their babies' sleep and play, but Samuel resisted her efforts, remaining clingy and difficult throughout his first year. Eventually, her doctor had diagnosed her as depressed and helped her to recognize that she had been quite anxious—she had not seen herself as an anxious person growing up. She believed her depression had resolved once she had managed to organize Samuel's sleep using a "controlled crying" settling technique. She described their relationship prior to Rose's birth as full of lovely moments. However, although she described him as a sensitive child with special, admirable, abilities, she struggled to establish her authority with him and was concerned that he was covertly aggressive toward Rose, so that she could not leave them alone together. [*Comment:* Even though it is a good sign for a child to be special to a parent, in this context, where Marie has focused her parenting efforts on developing a routine, and has not recognized her own anxiety, a description of a child as "special" alerts us to the possibility that the mother is esteem-sensitive—a "special" or "gifted" child can serve the function of conferring some measure of reflected glory on the parent. It also implies a distorted idealized perception of the child as somehow being greater than he actually is—potentially in less need of care and protection (see George & Solomon, Chapter 6, this volume.]

During her recent pregnancy, Marie attended an antenatal education program emphasizing the role of the parent–infant relationship in child development. Following the delivery, she vigilantly watched her interaction with Rose for any sign that she was not meeting Rose's needs. She became overwhelmed with a sense of failure and anxiety if Rose did not seem to want eye contact or was unsettled. Recalling that Samuel had also been an unsettled infant, she began to feel panic, thinking that she may have been an instrument in his distress, and fearing that she may have caused him irreparable damage. At times of conflict between them, she often deferred to him, but was sometimes enraged. [*Comment:* parents struggling to keep their Hands on the Circle (i.e., to maintain a bigger, stronger, wiser, and kind stance) often vacillate between being weak and mean—the child responds to the parent's weakness with difficult behavior, the parent becomes angry and mean, and then collapses with guilt and anguish, finally taking a role-reversed conciliatory approach to the child.]

Prior to joining the COS program, Marie indicated she had a close relationship with her mother. Her father had died during her adolescence. Marie's feelings about this loss did not appear to have been resolved. She spoke of two other current sources of grief: her 4-year-old niece had been recently diagnosed with leukemia and her mother had developed a chronic debilitating illness, requiring a lot of practical and emotional support from Marie. Marie expressed a great deal of sadness that her mother was not able to enjoy her grandchildren, nor offer her much help and support. [*Comment:* At this point, there are already several indicators of attachment and caregiving disorganization. Marie's fear of Samuel's aggression (Main & Solomon, 1990), her helplessness (George & Solomon, 2008; Lyons-Ruth & Jacobvitz, 2008), and her angry loss of control (George & Solomon, 2008; Lyons-Ruth & Jacobvitz, 2008; Main & Solomon, 1990). Similarly, her grief for her father's death, her mother's illness, and her niece is unresolved (Main & Hesse, 1990) and the latter two stressors potentially undermine her confidence in her capacity to adequately protect her own children (Bowlby, 1988; George & Solomon, 1996).]

In the COSI, Marie revealed more about her representations of herself, of Samuel, and of herself as his caregiver. Asked to describe her relationship with her mother as a little child, she used the word "loving." In a separate question, she also had memories of sitting on her mother's knee when needing comfort. She was quite unable to recall an episodic memory that showed her mother as loving, or to recall whether her mother's comfort terminated her distress. However, she spoke eloquently of her mother's pressure on her to achieve. She told how she and her mother had engaged in a struggle over learning her multiplication tables—her mother had tried to "push [the knowledge] down her throat"—and mentioned another time when she had felt her mother tried to exert emotional "control" over her. She recalled her mother had pressured her to make others happy, such as her father when he became depressed during her childhood. More recently her mother had been telling her to smile, as it would make her feel better. To Marie, this advice felt similar to many other times in the past when her mother pushed her to change her demeanor, without having been sensitive to her feelings. [*Comment:* at the time, the interviewer had the impression that Marie had some anger about these incidents, but noted that it was expressed in a "watered-down" way.] When asked about her thoughts and feelings in moments where she might have felt anger, or faced Samuel's anger, Marie was unable to think of a response. [*Comment:* these stories gave a coherent representation of self as valuable if meeting external expectations and of self in service to another, more important, person's need. There is a suggestion of maternal coercion and hostility. In comparison, the self-representation of being loved seemed rather empty. In COS terms, she revealed a childhood in which her exploration was significantly valued over her needs for emotional connection or comfort. Her mother appears to have pressured her to perform and achieve, and yet Marie repeatedly took care to present her relationship with her mother only in a positive light. She defended herself from awareness of angry feelings about some of her own attachment experiences, in order to preserve an idealized representation of her mother and their relationship. Again, this defensive stance is consistent with esteem-sensitivity.]

Marie thought Samuel did not show any need for her when she left him in the first separation of the SSP. She was unable to discuss his distress in the second separation, becoming quite disjointed. She was also incoherent and uncertain in talking about how he usually shows her his need for comfort, appearing confused about whether seeking affection was the same thing as seeking comfort. She consistently struggled to find her thoughts when asked about his perspective on their interaction. She gave several instances of punitive behavior toward her—resisting, provoking, hitting, and throwing—and none of soothing. However, she did not report this with any sense of his being an adversary. Rather, she saw him as justified in being angry. In some cases, usually when his behavior was dangerous, she revealed that she effectively took a stand with him when he behaved aggressively. In every instance, she remained positively oriented toward him, and was unqualified in her love for him, and her wish to do better by him. [*Comment:* Marie represented Samuel as a child capable of determining for himself how his needs should be met. There are indications of role-reversal, and aggressive behavior toward her, suggestive of punitive–controlling disorganized attachment. In COS terms, Marie's Shark Music plays when Samuel is on the bottom half of the Circle and when he needs to feel her Hands on the Circle (to see that he is little and to sort out his needs, rather than leave him to do it for himself). Although she is able to delight in him (a strength), she frequently fails to organize his feelings or to provide comfort. She *is* able to and to take charge sometimes, when he needs protection. This can be seen as an underutilized strength in that she does not need to create the capacity to "take charge"—she already has it. But she feels fear (hears Shark Music) when Samuel has a need for her to exert some expectations regarding his behavior, or to regulate his feelings, so as much as possible she avoids seeing or responding to these particular needs.]

Marie's conscious representations of self as caregiver were of being loving, but helpless to make Samuel feel secure because of her constant anxiety. She poignantly described how she'd felt confident before Rose's birth, but now she was overcome with anxiety. She wept, saying that she saw his difficult behavior as a reflection of his distress at her failure to be happy around him: "I know he's stressing out from *my* distress." The fact that she was distressed and anxious seemed in itself to disorganize her. [*Comment:* Feeling anxiety evokes shame in Marie. She seems to have had no internal working model of having anxiety regulated by being in relationship—indeed, she had reached adulthood with no capacity to recognize herself as anxious. Managing anxiety takes practice, and in normal circumstances parents recognize and scaffold anxiety-provoking situations, so that over time children internalize a way of negotiating similar situations when alone. The only means Marie had of feeling better was to see that her child was functioning well, as this provided an external benchmark that she was achieving an appropriate standard of parenting, and restored her self-esteem. She had little sense of her own capacity to help Samuel organize his feelings or of her own real value to her children, as someone capable of looking after them, someone "Bigger, Stronger, Wiser, and Kind." In the COSI we caught a glimpse of the segregated representations lurking within her internal working model of caregiving: first, if Marie showed resistance to her mother's wishes, or a need for comfort and protection, it caused pain/displeasure to others, and brought shame upon herself; second, if Marie placed expectations on Samuel, or tried to modify (regulate) the expression of his feelings, she worried that he would grow up as she had, feeling undervalued and overcontrolled.]

Countertransference responses during the COSI can shed interesting light on the parent's primary defensive strategy. The interviewer noted consistent pressure to show acknowledgment and mirroring throughout the hour. There were many times when Marie looked for agreement that Samuel was special, or that aside from this current period of anxiety, their relationship was wonderful—a pressure on the interviewer to be of one mind with her idealized view. The overall picture was of esteem-sensitivity, but not of the obviously grandiose kind. Marie seemed to fit better with Masterson's description of the developmental course of closet narcissistic personality. "The individual with a Closet Narcissistic Disorder must continuously avoid the mother's hostility, envy and attack by mirroring the mother and denying his or her own grandiose wishes. Narcissistic supplies are then derived from basking in the glow of the idealized other's glory" (Masterson & Lieberman, 2004, p. 43).

Marie had experienced insufficient emotional responsiveness as a child, but needed to keep a representation of herself as loved, and therefore lovable. She maintained an idealized view of her relationship with her mother to avoid the feelings associated with her mother's criticism and dissatisfaction with her. Similarly, she tried to keep her relationships with her children on a happy and constantly harmonious plane to protect both them and herself from the harsh feelings that might be unleashed if either acknowledged dissatisfaction with the other.

Having had so little experience of comfort, comforting did not come naturally—she watched her children's responses to be sure her comfort was good enough, and her confidence rose and fell with Samuel's emotional tone. Her focus on her own internal experience and his outward behavior blinded her from seeing Samuel as a separate person, with his own thoughts and feelings about their interaction. In effect, Samuel functioned as emotional regulator to his mother, a reverse in the caregiving role seen in many disorganized parent–child dyads (Main & Cassidy, 1988). When Samuel needed Marie to be bigger, stronger, wiser, and kind for mutual regulation, she provided comforting behaviors, such as holding and patting, but not comforting affect. She was physically, but not mentally or emotionally present (in COS terms, "Gone"), which was frightening for Samuel. At these moments he would seek his father if available, or become aggressive with Marie. George and Solomon (2008) contend that the parent's caregiving capacity develops in tandem with the child's attachment system. Marie's experiences of caregiving were limited by her reliance on supporting Samuel's exploration and delighting in him (which were more comfortable for her) at the expense of staying bigger, stronger, wiser, and kind when his feelings became too big for him to manage alone. Marie was teaching Samuel not to rely upon her, which was at odds with his developmental needs. Controlling behaviors can be understood as a strategy to hold an inconsistently reliable parent in place. They keep child and parent engaged in interaction—children seem to find this preferable to being alone, even when a parent is frightening.

In the SSP, Samuel appeared to be a precocious, but subdued little boy. Despite his attempts to dominate his mother when she was in the room, he was distraught during the second separation. The linchpin moment occurred when Marie returned. Samuel was standing near the stranger, sobbing. He looked toward Marie as she reentered with her arms outstretched. She picked him up and took him to a chair. She uttered reassuring words, patting him, and wiping his tears, but her face showed her agonized uncertainty, and her touch had a frantic quality. Overall, her comfort seemed to be ineffective in helping him to settle his feelings. Within 30 seconds, she took him to the floor, and began to encourage him to look at the toys, defensively trying to get him onto the top half of the Circle, even though he was directly cueing her that he was on the bottom. He stopped sobbing, and then said he wanted his father, got up and walked away to the door. In this instance, he did not seem to be actively punishing her, rather just seeking the comfort of his father because hers was not enough.

Here was a clear demonstration of the dyadic struggle that promoted attachment disorganization—when Samuel was distressed, Marie became distressed too, and needed him calm so she could feel successful and organize her own feelings. Until he showed he was settled, she could not provide a bigger, stronger, wiser, and kind presence. Thus, Samuel was left psychologically to manage on his own, and he chose to look for his father for the help he needed. We will look at how this moment was presented to Marie in a group therapy setting. Marie's first tape review focused on showing her how she can sometimes take charge of their interaction to help Samuel organize his feelings (such as when she behaved warmly and confidently at the second separation) and that he is little, and finds it really helpful when she does this for him.

In this second tape review, Marie sat beside the therapist, and the five other mothers attending the program sat alongside. They watched the early part of the reunion, when Samuel was sobbing, and Marie was holding him on her lap. Asked if she could describe what was happening, Marie said confidently that she was comforting Samuel. We will go through the conversation between Marie and the therapist as it unfolded:

MARIE: I was comforting him, bringing him in, trying to make him feel safe— not that I felt safe. [*Comment:* Marie describes her behavior as comforting. This is how she would like to be seen. She does not leave much space for further comments on the observed interaction. However, she does acknowledge her own feelings in that moment. The therapist understands that Marie is sensitive to being seen as failing Samuel, but also that she is signaling some openness to talking about her difficult feelings in the moment they have been watching.]

THERAPIST: How well do you think it's going at present?

MARIE: Not extremely well, because I was anxious for him—that's my Shark Music—*I* don't feel safe on my own either—I feel more comfortable when other people are around. [*Comment:* Marie's Shark Music plays when she has to organize Samuel's feelings by providing a bigger, stronger, wiser, and kind presence. She has not had a true insight into her Shark Music at this point. She is making a guess that his distress is just about being left alone. She can resonate with his feelings about being alone without getting lost in the affects associated with her own unmet childhood attachment needs. The therapist replays the tape, stopping at the point where Marie put out her arms and gathered Samuel up.]

THERAPIST: How do you think it's going there?

MARIE: Well.

THERAPIST: Me too ... You just did absolutely what's required. There's something nice about the way you're doing it. (*Mimics Marie's gesture of embracing.*) ... You can see that it feels right to him too. [*Comment:* it is important for Marie to see that she really does have the capacity to meet Samuel's need—to have her true strengths acknowledged, especially as the later parts of the interaction are not so successful, and may bring out her defenses. The therapist replays the tape to where Marie has brought Samuel onto a chair, and holds him on her lap. He is still very upset. She invites Marie to reflect on her own experience in this moment.] What do you feel this is like for you?

MARIE: Very upsetting, because he's really distressed. I feel really upset for him, and upset for me ...

THERAPIST: And what do you think you are thinking [in the vignette]?

MARIE: I was thinking I need to help him to calm down, and trying to work out how to do that—what to do, and how to make him feel safe again. [*Comment:* Marie's recognition that Samuel needs her to help him calm down, and her accompanying sense of helplessness, is made explicit. The therapist now wants to alert Marie to the idea that she already has the skills to work out how to help Samuel, without confronting her.]

THERAPIST: How do we work out what's needed to calm someone down? (*Marie looks uncertain, so the therapist scaffolds.*) To a certain extent, the decision you make about what strategy to use depends on how upset the person is.

MARIE: (*Responds, nodding.*) If someone's really, really distressed, you might stay with them for a while ... [*Comment:* Marie is thinking about *being with* her child, rather than pushing the painful feeling away. This is self-activation.] ... and then try ... umm ... and then think about other things? To *distract* them from that real distress state, so they ... then help them think about other things, so they can feel better ... (*Her voice stumbles.*) ... so that they can relax a bit more. But it ... but I don't know, I *did* do that ... [*Comment:* Now Marie clearly outlines her current internal working model of managing distress. As she defines it in words, she recognizes that her approach is at odds with what she has been learning about children's needs in the COS model—that a need for comfort must be met with comfort, not distraction. For an esteem-sensitive person, recognizing that she has made a mistake carries with it the expectation that others might be critical. After Marie is vulnerable, she begins to defend herself by asserting that she did it right. This is a small but crucial moment. Marie has activated her true self, and allowed insight that potentially exposes herself as "wrong," or "in error," and thus unworthy of love—a very vulnerable place for her. Every time Marie expresses an authentic thought or feeling, memories of the painful affects associated with doing so during childhood threaten to break through, and she reverts to defending against feeling or knowing about them. In this instance, Marie has defended by making out that she *did* help him, and that she is *not* in error. The therapist takes her back to the point where her model was consistent with her child's need.]

THERAPIST: What did you say you had to do? (*Asks this question gently but firmly, while looking into Marie's face.*)

MARIE: Just to be with them ... to let them know that you're there, and it's okay. To spend that time, to be *with* that person. [*Comment:* Marie has returned to activating her full and true perception of what Samuel needs, rather than turning away from it.]

THERAPIST: Yes. That's the crucial thing, until they're a bit calmer. (*Plays the tape to when Marie moves with Samuel, who is still crying, to the toys on the floor.*) So what's happening here?

MARIE: I guess I was just realizing that he was still very worked up, so I was staying with him, but I was also trying to find a way to help him calm down. Because he was still very, very distressed, and maybe I should have just stayed with him. [*Comment:* She has recognized (self-activation) she may not have done the best thing for Samuel by distracting him, and now, once again, fears exposure and disapproval. She grins, claps her hands, and continues to speak, gesturing with her hands held together.] But I ... [*Comment:* She has resumed her defensive position.]

THERAPIST: Well, on the Circle, what are you doing here?

MARIE: I'm being in charge, I'm ... It's at the bottom; I'm trying to be in charge.... Mmm ... [*Comment:* Marie says she is trying to "*be*" in charge—she doesn't feel in charge, and she hopes that by *doing* comforting things (performing comforting actions) he will settle. She is watching him to see the effect of her actions, rather than taking charge to organize his feelings—thus, she is waiting for him to lead the way, a form of role-reversal.]

THERAPIST: So, what are you doing? (*Looks intently at Marie, serious but kind.*)

MARIE: I'm comforting him. And ...

THERAPIST: On the floor, now. (*Clarifies.*) You're going to comfort him on the floor?

MARIE: Oh! ... Yeah!

THERAPIST: So that's probably exploring, rather than comforting, isn't it? [*Comment:* The therapist risks a gentle confrontation. She smiles encouragingly at Marie, who is brave, and stays calm enough to stay with her vulnerability—she continues to hold onto her insight, as the therapist supports her.]

THERAPIST: Yeah.... There's a message there.

MARIE: Yeah.... [*Comment:* Marie sounds subdued—the stress of staying open and vulnerable is telling on her.]

THERAPIST: (*gently*) What's the message?

MARIE: Well, I ... the only thing I'm thinking there is that maybe I should have been ... [*Comment:* The therapist recognizes that Marie is becoming defensive by focusing on perfect performance. She interrupts in a friendly tone.]

THERAPIST: No, let's not talk about what you *should* have done—what's happening? This is what we're interested in—what's *happening* here? (*Looks at Marie.*)

MARIE: Well, I'm not comfortable with what's ...

THERAPIST: Good! Good! *You're* not comfortable.

MARIE: *That's* my Shark Music! (*Is excited at her insight.*) So I'm not comfortable with that real high emotional state, and I don't know how to manage that. [*Comment:* This is the key moment in the Shark Music tape review, where Marie is recognizing that by her actions with Samuel when he is distressed, she fails to actually provide the comfort he needs. The therapist keeps her gaze on mother's face, encouraging her to continue with her insight.] So, I'm trying to avoid it by getting down and ...

THERAPIST: That's right. (*Gives warm smile.*)

MARIE: Yeah, but I might have been able to sit there a bit longer. [*Comment:* Marie is holding onto the good feeling that came with her insight, and it allows her to remain vulnerable and open. The therapist takes this opportunity, while Marie is open and brave, to show more clearly her struggle to be with Samuel at these moments.]

THERAPIST: I just want you to see something ... (*Replays Marie's early efforts to comfort Samuel, giving a running commentary of Marie's actions.*) Patting his bottom ... giving some rocking ... looking at him ...

MARIE: He's getting worse.

THERAPIST: And what are you doing?

MARIE: What am I doing? [*Comment:* Marie begins to sound confused, which suggests she may be defending by blocking awareness. Once again, the therapist conveys compassion and interest in Marie's responses to Samuel to contain her anxiety in the moment.]

THERAPIST: *He's* winding up, and what are *you* doing?

MARIE: I'm winding up too.

THERAPIST: Good. (*looking at Marie*) So, you sort of know how he's feeling.... In your mind, you're monitoring how he's feeling, instead of holding yourself steady. (*Marie is nodding.*) And it's sort of like the *other* person's feelings are what you've got to respond to ... [*Comment:* The therapist pauses here, to see if this taps into deeper affect.]

MARIE: But I should be able to separate, somehow ... [*Comment:* The use of the word *should* alerts the therapist—Marie has once again become defensive, diverting back to focus on performance, and momentarily relinquishing the openness to vulnerability that allowed her to become more insightful to Samuel's needs.]

THERAPIST: Not what it *should* be! (*Marie laughs.*) because the minute you say "should," there's the potential for failure, and the minute you fail, then you're ashamed. Then you're disorganized, and then you're no help to him or yourself ...

MARIE: Yeah.

THERAPIST: (*smiling at Marie*) Okay, so we try to keep "should" out of this ... [*Comment:* The therapist has made a deep connection with Marie, and is aware that Marie's issues may evoke feelings in other mothers in the group. She addresses all the mothers.] ... and just think about what we're struggling to achieve for our children—where it gets hard, and how we can refine what we do, because there's no doubt about it, all of you do lovely things for your children. *All* of you get it right. Sometimes, you get it wrong. When you get it wrong, it's distressing, and it undoes you. So that's what we're trying to do. We're trying to strengthen you up, (*looking at Marie*) for those times when your own Shark Music comes in, and you start to ... get a bit undone. Okay? [*Comment:* Although these remarks are made to the whole group, and are relevant to all of them, they are an attempt to directly address Marie's self-criticism by normalizing the process. In order to stay emotionally regulated and thus available to perform the same function for her children, she needs to be able to tolerate the idea that she doesn't always get things right. This concept also ties into the notion of rupture and repair that is emphasized throughout the program.] So, what we're seeing here, is that he's winding up and up and up, and you can sort of see in the way you are touching his face that you're winding up and up and up ... and that's going to have a consequence ...

MARIE: Uh huh! (*Is engaged, and following*)

THERAPIST: So, we'll see what that is! (*Replays, as Marie leans forward, smiling. She watches the video.*) What's happening there? (*Samuel is settling a little.*)

MARIE: He's exhausted by it. He's totally exhausted by it. This feeling, and … [*Comment:* Marie hasn't recognized that Samuel is taking comfort from her up to this point.]

THERAPIST: He's seems overwrought, but he isn't limp and hanging his head. He's got his head up, and he's actually looking at you. (*The group enters with an indistinct chorus, as all are looking for an opportunity to support Marie.*) He looked at you for a moment—it was hard to catch it, but he looked for a moment, and then, … he's just going to get upset again.

MARIE: (*very engaged*) Yeah.

THERAPIST: But the opportunity's there.

MARIE: Yeah. If I was able to be … If *I* was calm, and he'd looked at me and seen that I was calm …

THERAPIST: (*Looks at Marie and smiles.*)

Marie has attained an important insight, *and* she is openly acknowledging her struggle, which is normally very difficult for her without feeling like a failure, accompanied by devastating shame. The therapist's genuine delight in this moment is a new sort of experience for her—she has exposed her real self, rather than the false self that requires an idealized response from the world, and she has been delighted in, despite having made some mistakes along the way.

This, and similar experiences within the program, made it possible for Marie to shift her internal working model of self as either perfect, or valueless and empty, to incorporate a new perception of herself as capable of giving and accepting genuine repair. Her internal working model of Samuel changed to one that was more realistic—she could see him as a little boy, who needed strength and wisdom, which she could supply. Her internal working model of "self as caregiver" began to shift towards bigger, stronger, wiser, and kind, allowing compassion for herself when she struggled. At the end of the group program, Marie said that she had observed substantial changes in Samuel's behavior, with fewer tantrums, less anger expressed toward herself and his baby sister, and more warmth between them. She felt the most useful thing she had learned was that her children were little, and she was big—"Maybe it was said before, but it had to be at the right time.… It was just wonderful to hear that, and for it to click." Her growth could be seen in the postintervention SSP when, at the second separation, she was able to reassure Samuel when he ran after her, bringing him back into the room, and saying "It'll be all right. Mummy wouldn't tell you if it wasn't."

Of note, during the program, Marie did not shift very much from her idealized views of her parents. The work focused around the relationship with Samuel, because this was where she experienced activating distress—the original caregiving relationship was kept off-limits. However, she returned to individual therapy 2 years later, when Samuel began school. At this time, she experienced a return of overwhelming anxiety—if Samuel did not make friends, other children might (in her mind) despise him, and other parents despise her for creating a child who was socially unacceptable. It made sense that her esteem-sensitivity would make Samuel's formal transition into the social world difficult for her. In this further therapy, she was able to talk more freely about the pressures she felt when growing up, and was able to examine feelings related to her upbringing, and it effects, including her current defensive process.

CONCLUSION

Preliminary results in other sites (Zanetti, 2007, 2008) have demonstrated that the COS protocol is effective in changing the attachment status of middle-class dyads from disorganized to secure, as well as in the high-risk group who formed the first cohort (Hoffman et al., 2006). The COS protocol has been modified slightly for use prenatally and with young infants, using the still-face procedure, rather than the Strange Situation. The infant protocol was utilized in "Tamar's Children," a jail-diversion program that proved highly effective in ameliorating attachment relationships, even in an extremely high-risk population (Cassidy et al., 2010).

In a recent interview, Peter Fonagy remarked that treatments can be more effective, briefer, more to the point if titrated to what is wrong with the patient, and focused on the *mechanism underlying* what is wrong (Jurist, 2009). The COS model provides a roadmap for parents who are experiencing struggles in their relationship with a particular child. In this respect, it offers an *organizing* framework to help the parent to see the child's need more clearly and to understand how she should respond in order to promote her child's healthy development.

The COS framework is organizing in a number of senses: first, by outlining the biologically based needs and behaviors within the attachment and exploration systems; second, by explicitly outlining the caregiving responses and behaviors required to support children's capacity for intimacy as well as assisting them toward autonomy; and third, by presenting this material to a parent in such a way that she can receive it without psychological defense. Finally, in all the modalities in which it has currently been developed (Hoffman et al., 2006; Cooper, Hoffman, & Powell, 2009), the COS model recognizes the parent's intrinsic motivation to be an effective, responsive caregiver, and to provide adequate care and protection for her child. This supportive and accepting stance is reflected in many aspects of the delivery of the program (see Powell et al., 2009; Cooper et al., 2005) and represents the holding environment (Winnicott, 1978b) or secure base (Bowlby, 1988) which enables parents to think about their current internal working models of caregiving and to reorganize them to promote secure attachment relationships with their children. It is very hard to give what you have not been given. When the parent experiences having her feelings organized in the bigger, stronger, wiser, and kind presence of the therapist, it helps her to know how to give the same sort of response to her child, and a sense of security in the relationship is established.

NOTE

1. Classification was made by two scorers, blind to pre- or postintervention status, and with good interrater reliability, using the Cassidy–Marvin system. "D-forced C" means that the child had a disorganized attachment (D), and an underlying insecure–resistant (C) pattern of interaction with his mother.

REFERENCES

Aber, J., Slade, A., Berger, B., Bresgi, I., & Kaplan, M. (1985). *The Parent Development Interview.* Unpublished manuscript, Barnard College, Columbia University, New York.

Ainsworth, M. B. (1972). Attachment and dependency: A comparison. In J. Gewirtz (Ed.), *Attachment and dependency* (pp. 97–137). Washington, DC: Winston.

Ainsworth, M. B. (1978). *Patterns of attachment: Assessed in the Strange Situation and at home.* Hillsdale, NJ: Erlbaum.

Ainsworth, M. B., Blehar, M. C., Waters, E., & Wall, S. (1978). *Patterns of attachment: A psychological study of the Strange Situation.* Hillsdale, NJ: Erlbaum.

Bowlby, J. (1969). *Attachment and loss: Vol. 1. Attachment.* London: Hogarth Press.

Bowlby, J. (1980). *Attachment and loss: Vol. 3. Loss: Sadness and depression.* New York: Basic Books.

Bowlby, J. (1988). *A secure base: Parent–child attachment and healthy human development.* London: Basic Books.

Bowlby, J. (1998). *Attachment and loss: Vol. 2. Separation: Anxiety and anger.* London: Pimlico. (Original work published 1973)

Cassidy, J., & Marvin, R. W. (2000). *A system for classifying individual differences in the attachment behavior of 2½ to 4½ year old children.* Unpublished coding manual, University of Virginia.

Cassidy, J., Ziv, Y., Stupica, B., Sherman, L. J., Butler, H., Karfgin, A., et al. (2010). Enhancing attachment security in the infants of women in a jail-diversion program. In J. Cassidy, J. Poehlmann, & P. R. Shaver (Eds.), *Incarcerated indi-*

viduals and their children viewed from the perspective of attachment theory. *Attachment and Human Development, 12*(4), 333–353.

Cooper, G., Hoffman, K., Marvin, R., & Powell, B. (1999). *The Circle of Security Interview.* Unpublished materials, Marycliff Institute, Spokane, WA.

Cooper, G., Hoffman, K., & Powell, B. (2009). *Circle of Security parenting: A relationship based DVD parenting program.* Spokane, WA: Marycliff Institute.

Cooper, G., Hoffman, K., Powell, B., & Marvin, R. (2005). The Circle of Security intervention. In L.J. Berlin, Y. Ziv, L.M. Amaya-Jackson, & M.T. Greenberg (Eds.), *Enhancing early attachments: Theory, research, intervention and policy* (pp. 127–151). New York: Guilford Press.

Cyr, C., Euser, E., Bakermans-Kranenburg, M., & van IJzendoorn, M. (2010). Attachment security and disorganization in maltreating and high-risk families: A series of meta-analyses. *Development and Psychopathology, 22,* 87–108.

George, C., Kaplan, N., & Main, M. (1985). *Adult Attachment Interview.* Unpublished manuscript, University of California at Berkeley.

George, C., & Solomon, J. (1996). Representational models of relationships: Links between caregiving and attachment. *Infant Mental Health Journal, 17,* 198–216.

George, C., & Solomon, J. (2008). The caregiving system: A behavioural systems approach to parenting. In J. Cassidy & P.R. Shaver (Eds.), *Handbook of attachment: Theory, research, and clinical applications* (2nd ed., pp. 833–856). New York: Guilford Press.

Hoffman, K., Marvin, R., Cooper, G., & Powell, B. (2006). Changing toddlers' and preschoolers' attachment classifications: The Circle of Security intervention. *Journal of Clinical and Consulting Psychology, 74,* 1017–1026.

Jurist, E. (2010). Elliot Jurist interviews Peter Fonagy. *Psychoanalytic Psychology, 27,* 2–7.

Lyons-Ruth, K., & Jacobvitz, D. (2008). Attachment disorganization. In J. Cassidy & P.R. Shaver (Eds.), *Handbook of attachment: Theory, research, and clinical applications* (2nd ed., pp. 666–697). New York: Guilford Press.

Lyons-Ruth, K., Bronfman, E., & Atwood, G. (1999). A relational diathesis model of hostile–helpless states of mind: Expressions in mother–infant interaction. In J. Solomon & C. George (Eds.), *Attachment disorganization* (pp. 33–70). New York: Guilford Press.

Main, M., & Cassidy, J. (1988). Categories of response to reunion with the parent at age 6: Predictable from infant attachment classifications and stable over a 1-month period. *Developmental Psychology, 24,* 1–12.

Main, M., & Hesse, E. (1990). Parents' unresolved traumatic experiences are related to infant disorganized attachment status: Is frightened and/or frightening parental behaviour the linking mechanism? In M. Greenberg, D. Cicchetti, & E. M. Cummings (Eds.), *Attachment in the preschool years* (pp. 161–182). Chicago: University of Chicago Press.

Main, M., & Solomon, J. (1990). Procedures for identifying infants as disorganized/ disoriented during the Ainsworth Strange Situation. In T. Greenberg, D. Cicchetti, & E. M. Cummings, *Attachment in the preschool years: Theory, research, and intervention* (pp. 121–160). Chicago: University of Chicago Press.

Marvin, R., Cooper, G., Hoffman, K., & Powell, B. (2002). The Circle of Security

Project: Attachment-based intervention with caregiver–preschool child dyads. *Attachment and Human Development, 1,* 107.

Masterson, J. (1976). *Psychotherapy of the borderline adult.* New York: Brunner/ Mazel.

Masterson, J. (1988). *The search for the real self: Unmasking the personality disorders of our age.* New York: Free Press.

Masterson, J., & Klein, R. (1995). *Disorders of the self: New therapeutic horizons: The Masterson approach.* New York: Brunner/Mazel.

Masterson, J., & Lieberman, A. (2004). *A therapist's guide to the personality disorders: The Masterson approach. A handbook and workbook.* Phoenix, AZ: Zeig, Tucker, & Thiesen.

Powell, B., Cooper, G., Hoffman, K., & Marvin, R. (2007). The Circle of Security Project: A case study. In D. Oppenheim & D. Goldsmith (Eds.), *Clinical application of attachment theory: Bridging the gap between theory, research, and practice* (pp. 172–202). New York: Guilford Press.

Powell, B., Cooper, G., Hoffman, K., & Marvin, R. (2009). The Circle of Security. In Charles H. Zeanah (Ed.), *Handbook of infant mental health* (3rd ed., pp. 450–467). New York: Guilford Press.

Solomon, J., & George, C. (1996). Defining the caregiving system: Toward a theory of caregiving. *Infant Mental Health Journal, 17,* 183–197.

Solomon, J., & George, C. (1999). The place of disorganization in attachment theory: Linking classic observations with contemporary findings. In J. Solomon & C. George (Eds.), *Attachment disorganization* (pp. 3–32). New York: Guilford Press.

Sroufe, L. A. (1997). Psychopathology as an outcome of development. *Development and Psychopathology, 9,* 251–268.

Sroufe, L.A., Egeland, B., Carlson, E., & Collins, W.A. (2005). *The development of the person.* New York: Guilford Press.

Sroufe, L. A., & Waters, E. (1977). Attachment as an organizational construct. *Child Development, 48,* 1184–1199.

van IJzendoorn, M., Schuengel, C., & Bakermans-Kranenburg, M. (1999). Disorganized attachment in early childhood: Meta-analysis of precursors, concomitants, and sequelae. *Development and Psychopathology, 11,* 225–249.

Winnicott, D. (1978a). The theory of the parent–infant relationship. In *The maturational processes and the facilitating environment: Studies in the theory of emotional development* (pp. 37–55). London: Hogarth Press. (Original work published 1960)

Winnicott, D. (1978b). Psychiatric disorder in terms of infantile maturational processes. In *The maturational processes and the facilitating environment: Studies in the theory of emotional development* (pp. 230–241). London: Hogarth Press. (Original work published 1963)

Zanetti, C. (2007, July). *Efficacy of the Circle of Security protocol in a middle class cohort: Preliminary findings.* Poster presented at the International Attachment Conference, Braga, Portugal.

Zanetti, C. (2008, July). *Bringing an attachment perspective to working with women with postnatal depression using Circle of Security concepts.* Workshop presented at the World Association for Infant Mental Health, 11th Congress, Yokohama, Japan.

Chapter 13

Attachment Disorganization in Borderline Personality Disorder and Anxiety Disorder

ANNA BUCHHEIM and CAROL GEORGE

This chapter presents the results and clinical implications of our research on attachment disorganization in patients with borderline personality disorder (BPD) and anxiety disorders. The symptoms associated with these disorders take the form of enduring traits, the origins of which are not easily remembered without distortion. The DSM conceives of these disorders quite differently. BPD, an Axis II disorder, is conceived in terms of symptoms of emotional and relationship instability rooted in the individual's developmental history. Anxiety disorders, Axis I disorders, include a fairly traditional list of clinical syndromes and presenting symptomology, with little or no consideration of developmental contributions. We bring these disorders together in this chapter because research has shown that experiences with attachment figures in early childhood are central to their etiology. The elusiveness of some symptoms may baffle and misdirect clinicians' search for the source of maladaptive perceptions and responses in these patients when the developmental contributions are not fully understood.

Attachment insecurity in childhood is a well-established developmental risk factor. The association between attachment and specific mental disorders has been a prominent focus in the clinical application of attachment (Cassidy & Shaver, 2008; Dozier, Stovall-McClough, & Albus, 2008; Sroufe, Egeland, Carlson, & Collins, 2005; Riggs et al., 2007). Research has established a strong correspondence between unresolved attachment and psychiatric symptoms and diagnoses in clinical and community samples

343

(Dozier et al., 2008; Fonagy et al., 1996; Riggs et al., 2007; van IJzendoorn & Bakermans-Kranenburg, 1996; Warren, Huston, Egeland, & Sroufe, 1997).

Unresolved attachment is conceived as a representational form of disorganized attachment in adolescents and adults and is typically described in terms of attachment state of mind (George, West, & Pettem, 1999). "State of mind" refers to the elements and process that integrate and permit conscious access to memories, thoughts, and feelings about attachment. Empirical investigations of unresolved attachment are based on Main and Goldwyn's operational definition of lack of resolution (i.e., unresolved) using the Adult Attachment Interview (AAI, George, Kaplan, & Main, 1984/1985/1996; Main & Goldwyn, 1984/1998). The AAI is a semistructured interview about childhood attachment experiences. Unresolved state of mind on the AAI is evidenced by discourse dysregulation defined by Main and Goldwyn as lapses in discourse and metacognitive capacities when describing deceased loved ones or abusive experience during the interview. Dysregulation at the representational level is analogous to the disorganized and disoriented attachment behaviors observed in infants in the Strange Situation (e.g., freezing behavior in infants—see Main & Solomon, 1990—as comparable to long silences in adults during the AAI—see Main & Goldwyn, 1984/1998).

The association between unresolved attachment with psychiatric symptoms is consistent with Bowlby's original predictions regarding psychiatric instability as related to pathological mourning (Bowlby, 1980). We draw the reader's attention to the resemblance between Main's definition of unresolved attachment on the AAI and Bowlby's (1980) description of a form of pathological mourning he termed "chronic mourning." Bowlby viewed normal mourning as the prolonged yearning and searching for the lost attachment figure that is naturally accompanied by a heightened state of activation of the attachment system and behavioral and ideational disorganization. He postulated, however, that chronic mourning was pathological because the individual remained in the yearning and searching state and was unable (consciously and unconsciously) to reorganize and reintegrate his or her mental representation of the attachment figure as inaccessible (i.e., deceased). The chronic mourner continues to hope for a reunion that cannot be realized and activation of the attachment system can result in seemingly irrational distress, including disorientation, anxiety, angry aggressive outbursts, depersonalization, delusions, and suicidal ideation.

Attachment researchers have shown that understanding attachment disorganization and psychiatric risk in adults must be extended beyond the concept of unresolved loss (Lyons-Ruth, Yellen, Melnick, & Atwood, 2003; Hennighausen, Bureau, David, Holmes, & Lyons-Ruth, Chapter 8, this volume; Solomon & George, 2006, Chapter 2, this volume; Spieker, Nelson, DeKlyen, Jolley, & Mennet, Chapter 4, this volume). Bowlby (1973) conceptually posited difficult separations or threats of separations from the attachment figure, not loss per se, as the foundation of pathology. He emphasized the debilitating conflict that resulted when a parent blocked a child's ability to seek the parent for protection. Loss was conceived to be only one of many kinds of examples of potentially debilitating separations that included threats to send the child away, threats of parental departure, suicide, or abuse. Faced with threatened abandonment by or harm from the attachment figure, the child is helpless and vulnerable and desperately seeks proximity and protection from the attachment figure (Solomon & George, 1996). Bowlby further theorized that extreme conditions elicited a fundamental biologically based attachment conflict between seeking the attachment figure and withdrawing if the attachment figure was the source of the child's fear. It was this experience that he posited as the foundation of pathological forms of anxiety, worry, and anger. Main and Solomon (1990) placed this mechanism conceptually at the core of attachment disorganization.

Expanding on this model, Solomon and George (2006; Chapter 2, this volume) suggested that separation, complicated loss, abuse, and parental rage that block a child's access to the attachment figure or protection from others might be best conceived as assaults to attachment. These experiences threaten the essence of attachment; they undermine the protective capacity of the caregiving–attachment relationship; and, ultimately, they threaten self-integrity.

We still know very little about how unresolved attachment and attachment assaults relate to psychiatric problems. The goal of this chapter is to begin to delve more deeply into these associations for the patient groups in our research: those with BPD and those with anxiety disorders. The sections that follow provide an overview of attachment theory and research regarding these disorders. We then describe how we have used the Adult Attachment Projective Picture System (AAP; George & West, 2001, in press) to unravel what may be diagnosis-specific nuances of unresolved attachment in these two groups. We present the findings from our most recent studies and two clinical cases that exemplify using the AAP in this clinical context.

ATTACHMENT STUDIES OF BPD AND ANXIETY DISORDERS

Before we summarize the attachment research related to these disorders, the reader needs to understand that the attachment literature is bifurcated into two different approaches and that these approaches have developed their own sets of assessment measures (George & West, 1999; Waters, Crowell, Elliott, Corcoran, & Treboux, 2002). The approach of this chapter and this volume is developmental, which is an extension of the Bowlby–Ainsworth model of development and risk beginning in infancy. The developmental approach defines attachment in terms of patterns of behaviors and their associated mental and affective regulation processes that differentiate among secure and insecure attachment groups, termed "attachment status." Attachment status in adults represents individual differences in the representational processes that regulate attachment state of mind, and is most frequently assessed using the AAI. As designated by the term *status*, stability is governed by lawful continuity or changes in attachment experience (Waters & Hamilton, 2000). The other approach conceives of attachment as a personality trait, termed "attachment style." *Attachment style* is defined as social-cognitive schemas of experiences and feelings in romantic relationships (i.e., dating couples, marriage), originating from social-personality research that applied the Ainsworth infant attachment prototypes to the study of adult loneliness (Feeney, 2008). Attachment style is assessed using self-report questionnaires (Crowell, Fraley, & Shaver, 2008) and the empirical association of measurement based on these two approaches is poor. Developmental and social-personality attachment researchers now agree that these two approaches and their associated measures tap different and not necessarily overlapping aspects of attachment relationships (Crowell et al., 2008; Riggs et al., 2007). Researchers have approached studying the attachment correlates and contributions to psychopathology from both approaches. We review studies from both approaches in this section in order to provide a comprehensive view of the intersection between the development of *unconscious* processes built from *past* experiences and the social-cognitive evaluation of *conscious* cognitions and appraisals of *current* romantic attachment figures.

Borderline Personality Disorder

BPD is a serious mental disorder defined by a characteristic pervasive pattern of extreme emotional fluctuations, together with instability in affect regulation, impulse control, interpersonal relationships, and self-image (American Psychiatric Association, 2000). Childhood maltreatment is one of the most important developmental factors documented in the etiology of BPD (Riggs et al., 2007; Zanarini, 2000). Zanarini found that 91% of the 358 patients with BPD in this study reported abuse and 92% reported neglect before age 18. The patients with BPD in this study were significantly more likely than the 109 patients with other personality disorders to report having been emotionally and physically abused by a parent figure and sexually abused by a nonparent figure. Patients with BPD were more likely than other patients to report parents' emotional withdrawal, inconsistent treatment, denial of thoughts and feelings, role inversion (i.e., parentification), and failure to provide protection (Lyons-Ruth, Melnick, Patrick, & Hobson, 2007; Zanarini, 2000).

The main diagnostic criteria for BPD are a constellation of interpersonal problems (American Psychiatric Association, 2000). One element of this constellation is the profound *fear of abandonment*, typically shown by desperate efforts to avoid being left alone (e.g., calling people on the phone repeatedly, physically clinging). A second is *intolerance of aloneness*. Gunderson (1996) suggested that intolerance of aloneness might be a deficit that is associated with the borderline patient's typical clinging and attention seeking or also, paradoxically, seemingly detached forms of attachment. A third is *tumultuous close relationships* (e.g., frequent arguments, repeated breakups, relying on maladaptive strategies that anger and frighten others). A fourth is *affective dysregulation*, evidenced by the inability to modulate emotional responses, including extreme anger and hostility, impulsivity and self-damaging behavior, and dissociative symptomology (e.g., Bohus, Schmahl, & Lieb, 2004; Lyons-Ruth et al., 2007; Scott, Levy, & Pincus, 2009). Affective dysregulation is thought to result from a combination of emotional vulnerability factors, including extreme swings between idealization and devaluation and hypersensitivity to emotional stimuli.

Every developmental attachment study and approximately half of the attachment style studies report a strong association between BPD and indices of unresolved, fearful, preoccupied, or angry/hostile attachment (Aaronson, Bender, Skodol, & Gunderson, 2006; Fossati et al., 2005; Critchfield, Levy, Clarkin, & Kernberg, 2009; Agrawal, Gunderson, Holmes, & Lyons-Ruth, 2004; Levy et al., 2006; Levy, Meehan, & Weber, 2005; Lyons-Ruth et al., 2007; Minzenberg, Poole, & Vinogradov, 2006; Morse et al., 2009). Fonagy et al. (2006) emphasized abuse as the core state of mind associated with BPD, combined with underlying traumatic angry preoccupation. The association between BPD and unresolved and preoccupied attachment was recently demonstrated in a meta-analysis of developmental studies using the AAI to assess adult attachment in clinical and nonclinical samples (Bakermans-Kranenburg & van IJzendoorn, 2009).

These studies suggest that BPD is associated with past and present traumatic preoccupation with relationships and frightening abuse. Disorganized in their attachment, patients with BPD appear to be caught in a vicious cycle. Current situations and attachment figures (including adult romantic partners) likely activate past memories of abuse and aloneness and attempts to organize current attachment relationships would therefore be derailed by chronic mourning of loss, abuse (i.e., unresolved state of mind), and a complex spectrum of assaults to attachment. We would expect, then, that the borderline state of mind demonstrates chronic yearning and searching for attachments in order to prevent isolation and aloneness, yet simultaneously demonstrates the failure to remedy these feelings by establishing new relationships.

Anxiety Disorders

Anxiety disorders are among the most common mental disorders. Lifetime prevalence rates range from 14.4 to 28.7%. Anxiety disorders fill people's lives with overwhelming fear due to debilitating anxiety and worry. The clinical range of anxiety disorders includes panic disorder, social phobia (or social anxiety disorder), specific phobias, agoraphobia, and generalized anxiety disorder. Patients with *panic disorder*, for example, have feelings of terror that strike suddenly and repeatedly with no warning. They cannot predict when an attack will occur and many develop intense anxiety between episodes, worrying when and where the next one will strike.

The etiology of most anxiety disorders is not well understood. Anxiety disorders are thought to involve a heterogeneous combination of early life experiences (e.g., parent–child interaction, separation, abuse, or rape), psychological traits (e.g., temperament, behavioral inhibition), and/or genetic factors (Elizabeth et al., 2006; Matthew, Coplan, & Gorman, 2001; Peleikis, Mykletun, & Dahl, 2004; Peter, Brackner, Hand, & Rufer, 2005). In terms of symptoms, all of the anxiety disorders, with the exception of a specific phobia, involve debilitating fears that are not necessarily directed to a specific event or object. These fears include high levels of latent anxiety, which some understand as extreme responses to feelings of uncontrollability and helplessness triggered by fantasized or real-life events (Barlow, Chorpita, & Turovsky, 1996; Busch, Milrod, & Singer, 1999).

Bowlby (1973) viewed anxiety as rooted in separation and ambivalence. He emphasized two parallel attachment contributions. One was actual separation threat, which he proposed was especially debilitating in a family climate of fear, rage, or alcoholism that Solomon and George (Chapter 2, this volume) conceive as parental rage patterns. The other was parent's denial of the importance or reality of the separation threats. The contradictory juxtaposition of competing attachment experience and affect has been shown in some studies that have been linked empirically to ambivalent attachment (George & Solomon, 2008; Solomon, George, & De Jong, 1995) and was conceived by Bowlby to contribute to chronic mourning (Bowlby, 1980). The link between ambivalent attachment and anxiety symptoms in children has also been demonstrated in longitudinal studies of infant attachment (Bar-Haim, Dan, Eshel, & Sagi-Schwartz, 2007; Bosquet & Egeland, 2006; Dallaire & Weinraub, 2005; Shamir-Essakow, Ungerer, & Rapee, 2005; Warren et al., 1997).

There is little developmental attachment research on adult anxiety disorders. Most studies report an overrepresentation of unresolved attachment, especially unresolved loss (Buchheim & Benecke, 2007; Buchheim, George, Liebl, Moser, & Benecke, 2007; Fonagy et al., 1996; Manassis & Bradley, 1994; Riggs et al., 2007; Rosenstein & Horowitz, 1996). The prevalence of unresolved attachment was not supported, however, in one study of volunteer outpatients with anxiety disorder participating in cognitive-behavioral treatment. This study reported a predominance of secure and dismissing attachment (van Emmichoven, van IJzendoorn, De Ruiter, & Brosschot, 2003). It is possible in our view that these patients' ability to describe their childhood experiences without becoming dysregulated may be directly linked to cognitive-behavioral treatment, since the goal of this treatment approach is to change the structure of how patients think (and presumably talk about) their experience.

Attachment style studies describe patients with anxiety as having personality traits consistent with Bowlby's (1973) view of anxiety, including ambivalence, anger, fear, depression, maternal rejection/neglect, enmeshed role-reversal, and adult separation anxiety (Bifulco et al., 2006; Cassidy, Lichtenstein-Phelps, Sibrava, Thomas, & Borkovec, 2009; Eng, Heimberg, Hart, Schneier, & Liebowitz, 2001; Lee & Hankin, 2009; Manicavasagar, Silove, Marnane, & Wagner, 2009; Strodl & Noller, 2003). One study found a significantly higher incidence of preoccupied attachment associated with high anxiety ratings in patients diagnosed with panic disorder than in nonpatient controls (Marazziti et al., 2007). Another study, however, reported a high proportion of secure attachment (Eng et al., 2001), a surprising finding given that the participants were hospitalized. This finding may also be attributed to the intersection of the self-report assessment methodology of attachment style and a cognitive-behavioral treatment approach.

Overall, these two bodies of research suggest that patients with anxiety are likely to have attachment and personality qualities associated with unresolved and preoccupied attachment.

THE AAP

The AAP (George & West, 2001; in press), a relatively new measure of adult attachment status, has been central to our clinical research. A complete description of the measure and coding system is beyond the scope of this chapter. Here we provide an overview of the AAP with special emphasis on the representational elements and processes associated with unresolved attachment and traumatic assaults to the attachment system.

The AAP is a set of eight picture stimuli. The stimuli are line drawings of a neutral scene and seven attachment scenes (e.g., illness, separation, solitude, death, and threat). The stimuli are administered in a standard order: *Neutral*—two children playing ball; *Child at Window*—a child looks out a window; *Departure*—an adult man and woman stand facing each other with suitcases positioned nearby; *Bench*—a youth sits alone on a bench;

Bed—a child and a woman sit facing each other at opposite ends of the child's bed; *Ambulance*—a woman and a child watch someone being put on an ambulance stretcher; *Cemetery*—a man stands by a grave site headstone; and *Child in Corner*—a child stands askance in a corner with hand and arm extended outward. The interviewee is asked to describe the events that comprise a "story" for each picture, following a modified apperceptive projective administration technique.

The AAP classification system designates the four main adult attachment groups identified using the AAI classification system (secure, dismissing, preoccupied, unresolved).[1] Classifications are based on the analysis of verbatim transcripts of the narratives of the seven attachment stimuli responses. One of the main features of the AAP coding system is the evaluation of attachment-based defensive processes. The AAP defines the defenses associated with unresolved attachment following Bowlby's (1980) conceptualization of defensive exclusion in pathological mourning. He viewed defense as the regulating mechanism that maintained a steady representational state, the goal of which is representational, behavioral, and physiological homeostasis (Bowlby, 1973; see also Spangler, Chapter 5, this volume). Pathological mourning, including the unresolved state of mind that we view as linked especially to chronic mourning, is associated with a particular form of defensive exclusion that Bowlby (1980) termed the "segregated system" (see also George & West, in press). Homeostasis is extremely difficult to maintain in the face of threats to attachment. Bowlby proposed that such memories and their associated affects must literally be segregated, or blocked from conscious processing, in order to prevent debilitating emotional dysregulation.

In essence, then, Bowlby reformulated the psychoanalytic concept of repression into an attachment concept that is consistent with attachment theory's adaptive function (protection) and goal (to maintain proximity and access to attachment figures). Segregated systems defenses provide the individual with a rigid protection mechanism that works to prevent becoming overwhelmed and flooded by severe attachment distress, anger, sadness, and fear. However, because of the defensive rigidity, emotional cues or events could trigger dysregulation and threaten the integrity of relationships and self. Research has established that the segregated system is the core of defensive processing associated with disorganized attachment in children (Solomon et al., 1995) and is linked with the helpless abdication of parental caregiving that is associated with attachment disorganization in the child (George & Solomon, 1996, 2008; Solomon & George, Chapter 2, this volume). Assessing evidence of segregated systems using the AAP has been central to our clinical research.

The AAP operationally defines segregated systems in terms of a designated set of specific story response elements that are empirically and theoretically established indicators of attachment disorganization (termed "markers"—George & West, 2001, in press; drawing in part from Solomon et al., 1995). These include features of the response narrative that evidence danger, failed protection, helplessness, being out of control, isolation, spectral ideation, or response constriction. The AAP is judged "resolved" (i.e., reintegrated and contained as designated by the secure, dismissing, preoccupied classifications) or unresolved by evaluating if segregated systems markers are contained and reorganized in the narrative response. Resolution can take several forms, including descriptions of a character's ability to think about attachment distress (the "internalized secure base"; see George & West, 2001, in press), descriptions of the character as taking constructive action, and depictions of others providing care. The failure to reorganize (i.e., unresolved) is designated by uncontained dysregulation or constriction. Evidence of uncontained markers includes themes in which characters remain unprotected, descriptions of dysregulating distress are not diminished or transformed, or descriptions of frightening autobiographical experiences. Constricted responses are evidenced by the inability to engage in the narrative task in response to a picture stimulus, which is conceived as the individual totally shutting down attachment so as to block overwhelming feelings of being out of control and dangerously unprotected (following Solomon et al., 1995).

Classifying a transcript as resolved or unresolved is the first step in using the AAP. In our work, we have been interested in the patterns of dysregulation that appear in the transcript above and beyond the classification category, in order to determine especially if there are different patterns in patient and nonpatient responses. The second author noted during the blind classification coding of several hundred AAPs in a range of different samples that some segregated systems markers were common and others were unusual. As a result, this author developed a supplementary set of AAP coding instructions that differentiated between what was considered "normative" (SS_{Norm}) and "traumatic" (SS_{Tr}) markers. Normative markers seemed to be related to the stimulus "pull," for example, a death in *Ambulance* or the isolation associated with the breakup of teenage romance in *Bench*. Traumatic dysregulation markers (SS_{Tr}) were particularly frightening or bizarre responses to the AAP stimulus. These included themes of abuse, entrapment, abandonment, murder, suicide, or incarceration, or eerie descriptions of characters or events (e.g., girl floats over the bench). Some responses included descriptions of personal trauma (e.g., loss or abuse experiences), indicating merging with the depicted character and becoming flooded by personal memories. Table 13.1 provides examples that contrast SS_{Norm} and SS_{Tr} story responses.

TABLE 13.1. Transcript Examples of "Resolved" and "Unresolved" AAP Bench Story

Resolved AAP story	Unresolved AAP story
Normative dysregulation (control participant)	Normative dysregulation (control participant)
"A women is *afraid*, feels bad, had a fight with a friend, sits on a bench to be alone and by herself. She is sitting and crying. Her friend was very disappointed that she has not told him the truth for several times, so he broke up with her. Now *she feels abandoned* and is *afraid* of the future. She thinks about the fight and realizes that she has to say sorry. But she is *afraid* that her friend would not talk to her, like her mother often did when she was young. She is *afraid*. She is sitting there for a long time, thinking about the problem. After a while she gets up and is trying to get in contact with the friend to talk about everything."	"She is very sad, wants to *hide herself under the bench*; she is very *frightened*, feels *abandoned* by everybody. Life can be so cruel. Her friend does not love her anymore, because she is overweight. Her mother *broke up* contact with her because she is not interested in her life anymore. She is *frightened* about the future and she doubts that she ever will meet someone who finds her attractive. I have no idea how this could end. I think she sits there forever, I really don't know."

	Traumatic dysregulation (patient with BPD)
	"She feels **homeless**, it seems that she is **incarcerated in jail**, wants to **escape** from this **isolation, she thinks about suicide.** It is also possible that she is in a **mental institution**, because **she has already tried to commit suicide** and now she has to be **alone in an empty room. Nobody helps her, and she has no relatives or friends.** I have no idea. (Long pause) I think **she only dreams of running away.**"

Note. "Normative dysregulation markers" are in *italics*; "traumatic dysregulation markers" are **bold**.

TRAUMATIC DYSREGULATION IN BPD AND ANXIETY DISORDERS IN THE AAP

We now describe a study that examined attachment status and traumatic dysregulation (using SS_{Tr}) in a combined patient and control sample drawn from several studies (Buchheim, George, Kächele, Erk, & Walter, 2006; Buchheim, Erk, et al., 2006; Buchheim & Benecke, 2007; Buchheim, George, Liebl, Moser, & Benecke, 2007; Buchheim et al., 2008). This sample included 34 patients with BPD, 20 patients with anxiety disorders, and 21 healthy controls. All of the patient participants in these studies were German women recruited from psychiatric hospitals and psychotherapeutic settings. Control participants were recruited by advertisement in local newspapers and fliers posted for hospital employees. The participants with BPD included 13 inpatients and 21 outpatients. All patients with BPD met the criteria for a severe borderline disorder according to DSM-IV criteria. All of the patient participants with anxiety disorders were hospitalized inpatients (12 with panic disorder, two with agoraphobia, two with social phobia, four with generalized anxiety disorder). Exclusion criteria for all participants included serious medical or neurological illness, including comorbid psychotic disorders. Diagnoses and comorbidity were assessed by a trained psychiatrist and psychologist using the Structured Clinical Interview I and II for DSM-IV (First et al., 1995). The mean age for patients with BPD was 26.96 years (SD = 6.70, range = 18–39 years), 33.35 years (SD = 10.08, range = 28–60 years) for patients with anxiety disorder, and 27.81 years (SD = 6.82, range = 21–43 years) for controls.

Participants were administered the AAP using the procedure described earlier. All patients with anxiety disorders, 21 outpatients with BPD, and five controls were administered the AAP in a clinical setting. Thirteen inpatients with BPD and 17 controls were administered the AAP using our fMRI procedure, which has been shown to be a valid procedure (see Buchheim et al., 2008; Buchheim, Erk, et al., 2006). All AAPs were classified independently by the authors. The second author was blind to all information about the participants. The classification reliability calculated for four attachment groups was 97% (kappa = .95, p < .000). The SS_{Tr} markers coding system was developed and applied for the first time in this study and only coded by CG.

AAP Validity in a German Population

The first step was to determine if the AAP was a valid assessment in our German-speaking sample. The AAI is an established developmental assessment for adult attachment and has been used in a large range of cross-cultural studies in normative and clinical populations (Hesse, 2008). We examined AAP validity in the German-speaking population by administering the AAI to all 75 participants on an average of 6 weeks following the AAP administration. The AAIs were classified by two AAI judges (AB and a second judge who had no information about this study). Both AAI judges were trained and achieved reliability in AAI training institutes.[2] The AAPs were coded by the authors; the second author was blind to all information about the participants. The first author coded AAPs from the original German language transcript. The second author coded AAPs from an English translation transcript. Interjudge reliability calculated for four attachment groups was 98% (kappa =.97, p < .000). AAP/AAI concordance was 84% for four classification groups (kappa = .71, p < .000), 91% for secure versus insecure (kappa = .70, p < .000), and 88% for unresolved vs. resolved (kappa = .75, p < .000). These results provide evidence that the AAP is a valid attachment assessment to use in the German language.

Attachment Classification Distributions in Patients with BPD and Patients with Anxiety Disorders

The next step was to examine the attachment classification distributions for each of participant groups. These distributions are shown in Tables 13.2 and 13.3. There were significant differences in the four-group classification distributions (secure, dismissing, preoccupied, and unresolved) for all three participant groups (borderline, anxiety, control; Fisher's exact test, p < .001). Controls showed significantly more secure and dismissing attachments compared to both clinical groups. The patient groups with BPD and anxiety disorders showed significantly more unresolved attachment than the controls. The distribution of unresolved attachment for the psychiatric patients is consistent with the clinical attachment studies in the field. The relative proportion of unresolved classifications in our patient versus control groups is larger than that reported by van IJzendoorn and Bakermans-Kranenburg (1996). These investigators reported 40% of the clinic participants as unresolved, as compared with 80% of our patients; 19% of their control participants were unresolved, as compared with 38% of our controls. Their study was a meta-analysis of studies that included a broader range of psychiatric disorders than ours. Therefore, their analysis was more likely to capture a distribution of psychiatric problems associated with other insecure classification groups, for example, the broader attachment classification spectrum associated with depression (West & George, 2002). We do not know why there were so many unresolved individuals in our control group. One explanation may be recruitment. Our methods of recruiting in the hospital

TABLE 13.2. Distribution of Four-Group Classification in Patients with BPD versus Patients with Anxiety Disorders versus Controls

AAP classification	BPD	Anxiety	Controls	Total
Secure	2	3	7***	9
Dismissing	2	1	6***	8
Preoccupied	5***	0	0	5
Unresolved	25	16~	8	33
Total	34	20	21	55

Note. Generalized Fisher's exact test: ***p < .001; ~ designates trend-level significance. Table cells: One-sided Fisher's exact test (direction: observed > expected).

TABLE 13.3. Distribution of Four-Group Classification: Pairwise Two-Group Comparisons

AAP classification	BPD	Controls	Anxiety	Controls	BPD	Anxiety
Secure	2	7*	3	7	2	3
Dismissing	2	6*	1	6~	2	1
Preoccupied	5~	0	0	0	5~	0
Unresolved	25*	8	16**	8	25	16
Total	34	21	20	21	34	20
Generalized Fisher's exact test	.001***		.022*		.280 n.s.	

Note. Table cells: One-sided Fisher's exact test (direction: observed > expected).
*$p < .05$; **$p < .01$; ***$p < .001$; ~ designates trend-level significance.

may have attracted an overrepresentative proportion of hospital staff who wished to talk about their lives in a "psychology" study.

There were no significant differences in classification distributions for patients with BPD and the patients with anxiety disorders (see Table 13.3). Only the patients with BPD in our study showed preoccupied attachment. This finding is consistent with other reports of attachment in BPD as associated preoccupied attachment, likely to be in the angry and traumatic spectrum (E2 and E3) (Dozier et al., 2008, Fonagy et al., 1996). However, the proportion of preoccupied classifications in our study did not differentiate between the patient groups. The majority of each patient group was unresolved: 75% of the patients with BPD and 80% of the patients with anxiety disorders. This finding indicates that a strong association between clinical status and disorganized/unresolved states of mind and is consistent with the results of other clinical studies (Dozier et al., 2008; Fonagy et al., 1996), although one study failed to find a significant difference for patients with anxiety symptoms related to unresolved attachment (Riggs et al., 2007).

Traumatic Attachment Dysregulation in Patients with BPD and Patients with Anxiety Disorders

Our finding regarding unresolved attachment, however, does not provide specific information about the *severity* and *quality* of the representational manifestation of attachment disorganization in the patient or control participants. The next step was to determine if we could identify specific representational disorganization patterns, irrespective of attachment classification group status, that might be associated with these two disorders. For this goal, we applied the new traumatic dysregulation coding scheme and examined three hypotheses.

First, we predicted that there would be no differences among groups in the overall indications of attachment disorganization (i.e., all segregated systems markers in the transcript). Given the proportion of unresolved individuals in the control sample, we could examine this hypothesis with a sufficient representation of unresolved individuals. Second, we predicted a greater degree of traumatic dysregulation in the patient groups as compared with the control group in response to the alone stimuli but not for dyadic stimuli. Fears of being alone are at the core of both BPD and anxiety disorders. We reasoned that dyadic stimuli might help regulate the patients because these stimuli portray some kind of potential attachment relationship or at least an interaction with another person. Third, we expected to see differences in the traumatic dysregulation in the two patient groups. We predicted that traumatic dysregulation would be associated with abuse and loss for patients with BPD and predominantly only with loss for patients with anxiety disorders, as evaluated using ratings from AAI scales for lack of resolution of loss and physical abuse.

We tested the first hypothesis by comparing the frequency of segregated systems markers ($SS_{Norm} + SS_{Tr}$) in the AAP transcripts for all groups. There were no differences among groups in total segregated systems markers (Kruskal–Wallis H-test, $p = .388$).

We tested the second hypothesis by comparing the frequencies of SS_{Tr} markers for the alone and dyadic stimuli for all groups. The results are shown in Table 13.4. As predicted, patients with BPD showed a significantly greater frequency of SS_{Tr} markers in response to alone pictures than controls. The *Window, Bench,* and *Corner* alone scenes activated significant levels of dysregulation for patients with BPD. The effect was strongest in response to *Window* and *Corner*, scenes that can be easily interpreted to depict confinement. This response pattern did not reach significance for *Cemetery*. Unexpectedly, patients with BPD also demonstrated a significantly greater frequency of SS_{Tr} markers than controls in response to the dyadic stimulus *Ambulance*.

The alone stimuli also elicited a greater frequency of more SS_{Tr} markers for patients with anxiety disorders than controls. As with the BPD patients, this pattern was evident especially in *Window, Bench,* and *Corner*. Patients with anxiety disorders did not differ from controls in their response to the dyadic pictures.

The SS_{Tr} analyses also demonstrated a pattern that we did not expect. The alone pictures elicited traumatic *personal experiences* in the patients with anxiety disorders, but not the patients with BPD (see Table 13.4). This means that patients with anxiety disorders were prone to becoming distracted and described their own traumatic life events; their attention shifted away from the task of responding to the hypothetical character and their stories temporarily or permanently focused on themselves. This attentional shift was especially prevalent in response to the alone stimuli.

TABLE 13.4. Three-Group Comparison of Traumatic Dysregulation Markers in the AAP: Pairwise Two-Group Comparisons, Two-Tailed Tests

Frequency of traumatic marker in the AAP	BPD (n = 34)		Anxiety (n = 21)		Controls (n = 21)		Exact U-test					
							BPD × control		Anxiety × control		BPD × anxiety	
	M	SD	M	SD	M	SD	Z	p	Z	p	Z	p
Total in all "alone" pictures	6.15	5.72	7.35	6.82	0.19	0.60	3.43	.001	2.97	.003	−0.333	.74
Window	1.12	2.17	1.10	1.58	0.43	1.36	3.00	.003	1.99	.05	0.330	.74
Bench	1.79	2.19	2.60	2.87	0.67	1.28	2.36	.02	2.92	.003	−0.993	.32
Cemetery	1.06	1.65	1.05	1.79	0.38	0.81	1.67	.10	1.28	.12	0.190	.85
Corner	2.18	2.15	2.60	3.99	0.67	1.62	2.94	.003	1.95	.05	0.262	.80
Total in all "dyadic" pictures	1.24	2.05	0.60	1.14	0.52	1.08	1.74	.08	0.715	.48	1.09	.28
Departure	0.15	0.44	0.20	0.696	0.10	0.43	0.817	.41	0.635	.52	0.148	.89
Bed	0.26	0.93	0.00	0.00	0.24	0.89	0.256	.80	−1.39	.16	1.57	.12
Ambulance	0.82	0.16	0.40	0.598	0.19	0.60	2.20	.03	1.71	.09	0.513	.61
Personal Experience "alone" pictures	0.15	0.61	1.20	2.35	0.00	0.00	1.12	.27	2.41	.02	0.208	.04
Personal Experience "dyadic" pictures	0.12	0.48	0.05	0.224	0.00	0.00	1.12	.27	1.02	.31	0.180	.86

We tested the third hypothesis by examining SS_{Tr} frequency patterns in relation to loss and abuse. There were two ways to approach this hypothesis. One approach was to examine the AAP stimuli responses to *Cemetery* and *Corner* responses. There were no differences between patient groups in response to these two stimuli. When we examined the transcripts, we found that themes of loss or abuse were elicited throughout the AAP across a range of stimuli, including *Bed, Bench,* and *Ambulance* in a way that appeared to be consistent with individuals' own personal histories.

The other approach was to compare the AAI loss and abuse scale ratings. We found differences between the two clinical groups in the intensity of dysregulation due to these experiences observed during the interview. The AAI unresolved loss ratings were significantly higher in patients with anxiety disorders; the AAI unresolved physical abuse ratings were significantly higher in patients with BPD (see Table 13.5).

We then correlated the SS_{Tr} frequencies separately for the alone and dyadic pictures with the unresolved loss and abuse ratings (see Table 13.6). Significant correlations were again only found for the AAP alone stimuli. We noted too that in this analysis, the correlation patterns were significant for the *Cemetery* stimulus. There were significant correlations for AAI U_{loss} and $U_{physical\ abuse}$ ratings in the group with BPD but only for AAI U_{loss} ratings in the group with anxiety disorders.

These results take on particular meaning in the context of our studies of neural attachment activation patterns. Using fMRI procedure, Buchheim and her colleagues (2008) demonstrated significantly higher neural activation patterns associated with pain and fear in response to the alone AAP stimuli in patients with BPD compared to healthy controls. The fMRI scans of 13 unresolved patients demonstrated significantly greater activation in the anterior medial cingulate cortex (aMCC) than both resolved and unresolved controls. The aMCC is innervated by the midline and intralaminar thalamic nuclei belonging to the medial pain system (Vogt, Finch, & Olson, 1992), and also receives direct input from the amygdala (Vogt & Pandya, 1987). Thus, the aMCC is linked to aspects of pain, especially fear avoidance. The ACC activation in the Buchheim et al. study was located in this subregion. This finding may represent dysregulation or imbalance in the

TABLE 13.5. Two-Group Comparison of AAI Unresolved State of Mind

Scores in the AAI	BPD (*n* = 30)		Anxiety (*n* = 20)		Exact U-test	
	M	*SD*	*M*	*SD*	*Z*	*p*
Unresolved loss	3.10	2.22	4.55	2.35	−2.05	.040*
Unresolved abuse	4.64	2.96	2.45	2.46	2.73	.006**

*p < .05; **p < .01.

TABLE 13.6. Correlations between AAP Traumatic Dysregulating Markers and AAI Lack of Resolution of Loss and Abuse Ratings in Patients with BPD and Patients with Anxiety

Frequency of AAP traumatic dysregulation markers	AAI loss rating ($n = 30 + 20$)		AAI abuse rating ($n = 33 + 20$)	
	BPD ($n = 30$)	Anxiety ($n = 20$)	BPD ($n = 33$)	Anxiety ($n = 20$)
All "alone" stories	.36*	.33~	.54***	.02
Window	.05	.39*	.25~	−.24
Bench	.06	.11	.40**	−.25
Cemetery	.48**	.43*	.48**	.15
Corner	.19	.29~	.14	.18
All "dyadic" stories	−.12	−.05	.08	−.29
Departure	−.27~	−.26	.06	−.21
Bed	.24	—	.25~	—
Ambulance	−.23	.09	.09	−.23

Note. Nonparametric Spearman correlations.

*$p < .05$; **$p < .01$; ***$p < .001$; ~ designates trend-level significance.

ACC's integrative function in pain and emotion processing and may be a neural signature of the emotional pain associated with fear of aloneness described as one core clinical criteria of patients with BPD. Furthermore, abandonment concerns and intolerance of aloneness are reported to be the most persistent and painful experienced symptoms in patients with BPD after 6 years of prospective follow-up (Zanarini, Frankenburg, Hennen, & Silk, 2003).

CLINICAL CASE EXAMPLES

We now present case examples of the AAP material from a patient with BPD and a patient with an anxiety disorder. The discussion first presents background information based on descriptions from the patient's AAI. The AAP and our analysis of traumatic dysregulation and other attachment dimensions are then discussed. The reader will note that we have grouped the alone and dyadic responses together in order to highlight discussion of the different patterns evoked by these stimuli and, as described earlier in the introduction to the AAP, that this not the order in which the stimuli are administered.

BPD Case: Clara

Clara is a 21-year-old student. She was a hospitalized patient with BPD at the time of this study. She and her brother grew up in a rural community.

Clara was sexually abused by her father for about 6 years when she was a young girl. Her mother shut her down, rejecting Clara's efforts to tell her about the abuse. Despite the abuse, she felt close to her father because she experienced him as strong in contrast to her weak mother.

When asked to think about the influence of her childhood experiences on her present personality, Clara described strong pathological behavioral consequences. She described her emotional instability, relationship problems, and insecurity concerning her sexual identity. She feels that being a woman means being weak and unprotected. As an adult, Clara described how she feels betrayed by her father; she views him as not loving her but rather as a man who was obsessed with uncontrollable sexual motives.

Clara's beloved uncle died about a year prior to the onset of her father's abuse. She recalls her uncle as the only adult to whom she was close as a child and she believed that she would not have been abused by her father if her uncle had lived.

Clara was judged unresolved on the AAI and the AAP. Her AAP transcript is provided below; traumatic dysregulation markers (SS_{Tr}) are indicated in the narrative by **bold** font.

Alone Responses

STIMULUS 2: WINDOW

"Oh there is a girl standing by the window looking outside and wishing to *be away*. It happened ... the girl is **half naked.** Perhaps she **doesn't feel safe** at all. Actually she wants to go someplace else. She is looking outside, maybe, maybe looking at the other houses, perhaps where her teacher lives, or she ... anyhow wants to go away, is **without protection** in a large room. **Everybody can uh, somehow touch her.** She looks very **unprotected.** The long hair, they, they make her to be somehow, she looks very much **at someone's mercy.** She is wearing a skirt. Very feminine, very small, very **much at their mercy** actually, **terrible.** Well she is looking outside because naturally she wants to go away and she is hoping for a better life. She probably is with her family a big room at her parents' house or ... but she is **defenseless, utterly defenseless.** Yes, she wants to get away from her parents, especially from her father perhaps. Her home is **the most horrible place.** That's why the child looks like an orphan. **The child knows that she has to watch out for herself.** The girl wants to get away. If she is wise then she wants to get away."

Window elicits immediate and strong traumatic dysregulation, and Clara never reorganizes or contains the dysregulation elicited by this stimulus. The narrative describes terror and helplessness. The girl's home is horrible and dangerous and the girl is defenseless and at the mercy of her father's sexual abuse. Clara's feelings of utter abandonment in this situation are evidenced in her reference to the girl as an "orphan." Although the child knows that she must watch out for herself, there is no evidence that the girl can act on this knowledge and take any self-protective action. In the language of the AAP coding system, she has no personal agency (a representational strength associated with self-protection) and she has no one to protect her.

STIMULUS 4: BENCH

"An adult woman is sitting there alone on a bench, crying. She has too much pity for herself. Uh, she should have taken charge of her life more often, should not cry so much; be more tough. She looks very feminine somehow, that is quite weak. **Someone could do anything with her, really do everything with her,** if somebody is so **unrestrained** that **it's almost his fault,** isn't it? Well she is **unprotected.** She will **kick the bucket** if she keeps carrying on this way. She is on her way. **Everything can be done with her.** Is feeling? I actually don't want to know how she is feeling. Well, being **at the mercy of, weak, little most of all.** Perhaps she doesn't realize any longer how much **at the mercy of others she is** and uh. The ending? If she is in good graces she is eventually going home or she is searching or **will be dragged off by some guy** or something else. **She is going up in smoke,** this woman. She is going downhill. Yes, **nothing more to be said about it.**"

This adult woman, like the girl in *Window*, is helpless and defenseless. Clara appears to want to block awareness of these feelings at one point, stating that she does not want to know what this woman is feeling. She had the opportunity at this point to stop telling a story, but she instead continues to develop a narrative that perseverates on the helplessness theme. Clara introduces the possibility of the woman going home at the end, which would have been an indicator of personal agency and resolution in the AAP. But she undermines the woman's agency and returns to the theme of powerlessness and defeat. The woman leaves the bench taking the road to her demise. Clara again also cannot envision seeking or receiving care from others. The reader will also note the disgusted and deprecating tone Clara uses when describing the woman's utter helplessness.

STIMULUS 7: CEMETERY

"Here is a man in front of a tombstone. A tombstone. Yes. I'm thinking of my uncle. He remembers somebody who perhaps would have been well meaning but died a little too soon. Perhaps this man returned to his hometown and is going to his uncle's grave. Uh, he is **no longer welcome in his native place, he cannot show up any place.** But he is going to the grave because it was his ..., he had an attachment to the one who died. He feels a little **homeless** standing in front of the grave. Uh, a little **homeless** because only the grave belongs to him and otherwise **his home is gone, all lost, everything destroyed, all gone.** And that's the feeling the man might have just now, yes he, he will think, he will realize that he does not belong and he will soon move on from there and his new life and his present life, which very different from then. He is going to leave. A tombstone always is such a, such a sort of pain, symbol for the home which has been lost."

The loss portrayed in this stimulus activates more traumatic dysregulation. Clara states clearly how this picture makes her think of her own deceased uncle and could easily at that point merge with the depicted character. She maintains a boundary between him and her, even though we clearly see her speaking about her loss through his feelings. The man is described as abandoned and homeless, returning to his home town to visit his beloved uncle's grave. His uncle's death symbolized a profound loss of home and we once again see the theme of orphan in Clara's representation of self. Resigned and alone, Clara acknowledges through the man's eyes that somehow a new life must be made, but she again fails to describe a life that includes relationships or help.

STIMULUS 8: CORNER

"Well there is a boy, um, a boy maybe 7 or 8 years old. It would be better if he were wearing a leather jacket. He is a little sloppily dressed, uh, somehow he looks a little unmanly. A boring guy. Boring, he is not able to fight, he ... little lax, yes he looks like my brother actually, a little soft, well somehow a little soft. He came to this place, because he is somehow a little boring, he has nothing to do, doesn't know what to do with himself. And is very, has a lot of feelings and so, yes has a lot of feelings. Yes indeed he has a lot of feelings. Uh ... actually he is indigent and small, but nevertheless a boy. Later when he grows up he will be more attractive. He is going to be big and strong. Actually it's a good thing to be a boy but he should be looking a little bit stronger. A little more robust, a little cooler with pocket knife or something."

There is no evidence of attachment dysregulation in Clara's response to *Corner*. We might have expected a narrative of threat and abuse, similar to the *Window* response. What unfolds, however, is Clara's response to abuse that was echoed in her AAI. She deprecates weakness and admires the strength associated with adult men. The narrative describes a soft and boring boy who will be transformed to become a big, strong, attractive, and dangerous (pocket knife) man. Clara can envision the transformation that she desires. However, the people and events associated with this transformation are elusive and undefined. As with *Bench*, Clara's response contains elements of disgust at weakness, described by her evaluation of the boy as unmanly, soft, boring, and indigent.

Dyadic Responses

STIMULUS 3: DEPARTURE

"This picture shows a man and a woman standing at the railway station and, uh, they want to leave. Perhaps it's a vacation. They came by car. Maybe somebody brought them there. And now they are standing by the track and are waiting for the train to arrive. Yes, the two of them seem to like each other well enough. But perhaps there they are bored. They have to go someplace, perhaps on vacation. You know, if it's delightful to go on vacation, probably not. Vacation is another of those things one has to do. A rule of life. I believe the woman probably looks at it as an obligation. She has to go on vacation, that's the way it is. It's time and everybody does, but I don't think she is very pleased about it. The man probably does not know what is going on inside her, he. I think he is feeling better than the woman, for sure. He too is bigger and more powerful and the like. Probably the train arrives, they take their suitcases, get on board, the man looks for a seat, the woman follows and the train leaves."

There is no evidence of dysregulation in Clara's response to *Departure*. The narrative describes a typical event. However, they are a disconnected couple and do not share any feelings of mutuality or togetherness. The images of masculine and feminine sex roles are powerful in this response. The woman is unhappy, unimportant, and essentially invisible. By contrast, the man has a better emotional state, which is associated with being big and powerful. The man is in the lead and the woman is passively compliant.

STIMULUS 5: BED

"There is a sick child lying in bed and there is a mother sitting, uh, giving the child soup. The child is glad to get the warm soup. Well the child is sick, stayed at home from school. The mother, she is quite nice, well this day she is quite nice because she is taking care of the child, bringing him hot soup. The child is reaching for the soup. Yes. The mother is relatively far away from the child, but that's actually always the case. But at least she is concerned, is bringing soup and uh.... That's by itself good for the child, the feeling that somebody is giving to him something that is **necessary for life, so he can survive**; because the child right now cannot help himself and—well he is getting food, that's at least something. Naturally the mother will be getting a little less reliable as soon as the child is feeling a little better. And the child will then again be very much on his own. The child can go to school again. He will once again be very lonely. Somehow such an illness suggests at least a little closeness."

This is the only stimulus in the AAP set that activates a story about an attachment figure providing care. Even then, Clara slowly removes the caregiver from the narrative with the mother never really knowing about the boy's pathetic and helpless desperation (necessary for life, so he can survive). The boy is described as understanding very clearly that his mother will soon withdraw and return to her usual unreliable state as he gets better. The boy is ultimately alone.

STIMULUS 5: AMBULANCE

"I was just thinking whether the child is looking at a picture or is looking out of the window. Well, probably he is looking out of the window. Uh, you can see an ambulance with a **corpse**, that's to say someone who will soon **die**. Yeah, like my uncle somehow at that time, um well, uh somebody is being taken away and **he never comes back**. Maybe an uncle, or an aunt. The child thinks, yes the child somehow realizes that this is something serious. The older woman doesn't have to say anything, the child gets it all on his own and uh ... the ambulance men are **covering him**, he perhaps is already even already **dead**. **Won't come back**, he was a nice guy. The child was fond of his uncle. Yeah, **it's in such a moment when nobody speaks. Nobody speaks but everybody knows what is the matter. The end. Following that one has to cut it off and put away. One has to go away.** This reminds me very much of my uncle, I was young at the time."

Clara's first response to this stimulus is to try to distance herself from reality by suggesting that the child may be looking instead at a picture instead of a real event. Once she accepts that the boy is witnessing his uncle's death, she reminds us of her own uncle's death. The narrative becomes dysregulated when Clara mentally shifts the story back to the boy. The child is looking at his uncle's corpse with the sorrow of the knowledge that his attachment figure will never return. The older woman, a potential but unidentified alternative attachment figure, is essentially invisible; she might as well be made of stone. She provides neither comfort nor explanation. Nobody speaks, and the boy faces the death alone. Once again, even though Clara can visibly see a potential attachment figure in the stimulus, she cannot describe care or help. The boy remains alone in the presence of others.

Clara's AAP protocol clearly reveals the continued traumatic elements of her life's story. How does the AAP add to our understanding of Clara's unresolved attachment? The AAP narratives provide a unique perspective on Clara's interpretation of her life events, and of how she evaluates self and other in potential attachment–caregiving relationships. The traumatic dysregulation patterns in Clara's transcript are consistent overall with the group BPD pattern we observed in this study. She describes experiences of unresolved abuse and loss, and moreover reveals how this unresolved state of mind is related to a complex set of attachment assaults. Her stories evidence tremendous abandonment fears and intolerance of aloneness, even in the presence of others.

This pattern was confirmed by our neuroimaging study using the AAP-fMRI-paradigm (Buchheim et al., 2008). As described earlier, patients with BPD showed significantly more activation in regions associated with pain and fear in response to the alone AAP pictures compared to healthy controls. For Clara, representations of the desperately alone self not only emerged in her responses to the alone stimuli (*Window, Bench, Cemetery*) but were also created in response to stimuli that portray potential attachment figures (*Bed, Ambulance*). Even more than some of the patients with BPD in our fMRI study Clara's unifying representation of self is as helpless, frightened, isolated, and desperate. Attachment figures are viewed as threatening or absent. She continues to mourn the death of the single person that she believed could save her. And although she desires to find safety, she is not able to conceive of how this end result would occur or of any personal agency that might assist her. She is incapable of productive action and not connected to other people.

It is striking that Clara becomes dysregulated in response to the very first attachment stimulus. Buchheim et al.'s fMRI study on neural correlates of attachment representation in a normative sample (Buchheim, George, et al. 2006; Buchheim, Erk, et al., 2006) showed that neural activity in the amygdala and hippocampus was activated increasingly *over the course* of the AAP task. These activations became stronger in participants with an unresolved attachment status when the attachment system was increasingly activated induced by the order of the AAP pictures. Participants were challenged to tell a story to the pictures in the fMRI scanner. Emotional involvement and memory processes were stronger in the last part of the AAP-set rather than in the beginning of the task. We interpreted this as a neural signature of the activation of the attachment system (Buchheim, George, et al., 2006; Buchheim, Erk, et al., 2006). In normative samples, the typical *Window* responses describe a girl getting up in the morning, going to bed, getting ready to go to school or preparing to go out to play with friends. Clara's response demonstrates her hypersensitivity and susceptibility to interpreting seemingly unthreatening events in which one is alone as threatening from the very beginning of the AAP assessment; her attachment system was immediately triggered by what is clearly the clinically relevant stimulus of being alone in a room.

The *Corner* story is uniquely Clara's story. *Corner* activated her fantasy self of becoming strong and dangerous. As with the other alone response, she cannot envision the processes or the people that might help her achieve this goal. And although not formally coded in the AAP classification system, we can see that Clara's representation of self in the *Corner* response demonstrates an identification with the aggressive attachment figure, a central feature of BPD as described by Lyons-Ruth and her colleagues (2007).

Clara's overpowering sense of aloneness is also evident in her responses to the dyadic stimuli. Clearly, Clara feels alone even when she is in the company of potential attachment figures. The stories portray disconnected relationships and vulnerable characters (i.e., the self) are unnoticed or invisible (woman in *Departure*, children in *Bed* and *Ambulance*). *Bed* also demonstrates Clara's yearning for an attachment relationship and her desire to "seize" onto a relationship that hints at care (as the boy in *Bed* seizes his soup). Her response demonstrates the conflict between yearning and searching for attachment and mistrust using images that support Gunderson's (1996) description of paradoxically clinging and detached BPD behavior.

Clara's response to the dyadic pictures is consistent with a dyadic stimuli response pattern found for patients with BPD using the AAP fMRI paradigm (Buchheim et al., 2008). The patients with BPD showed significantly more activation of the right superior temporal sulcus (STS) than controls in response to the dyadic AAP pictures. The right STS is thought to be associated with theory-of-mind capacities (Gallagher & Frith, 2003). Theory-of-mind studies confirm that, when asked to remember and describe attachment experiences, patients with BPD show low reflective function, which can be identified either in the lack of mentalizing capacity or in a exaggerated *hyperanalytical* way to think and talk about relationships (Fonagy, Gergely, Jurist, & Target, 2003). They often demonstrate a misleading hypersensitivity for the mental state of the other during interaction in order to manipulate and control potentially threatening relationships. A history of traumatic experience requires individuals to be hyperattentive to their surroundings and, more generally, unresolved attachment has been linked to fear-based hypervigilance in relationships (Solomon & George, 1999, 2000). The STS activation pattern in response to the dyadic AAP pictures by patients with BPD indicates fear-based hyperarousal in relationships and interactive contexts; these individuals are compelled to pay attention to social interactive cues (Buchheim et al., 2008). Clara's AAP demonstrates hyperarousal surrounding interactions that might ultimately leave her abandoned and alone.

Finally, in addition to uncontained dysregulation patterns, several of Clara's responses indicated her annoyance and disgust with the character's state of being. The tone of the *Departure* narrative was loathing for the vacation ritual and the woman's passivity and invisibility. She was disgusted by the woman's self-pity and feminine weakness in *Bench*. She was repulsed by the boy's unmanliness in *Corner*. The disgust patterns in Clara's narratives are consistent with the results from another of our studies in which we examined the AAP as related to affective facial activity patterns using the Emotional Facial Action Coding System (EMFACS; Friesen & Ekman, 1984). This study found a predominance of disgust responses, especially for unresolved patients with BPD over the course of the AAP task (Buchheim et al., 2007). This recent finding may objectify a clinically relevant aspect of emotional regulation in BPD: when these patients are confronted with attachment-relevant material that reminds them of their traumatic experiences (e.g., sexual abuse, physical abuse), they project severe negative emotions in their narratives while reacting on a behavioral level with disgust in their face.

Anxiety Disorder Case: Monica

Monica was 38 years old and hospitalized with severe panic disorder at the time of our study. She grew up with her three older brothers in a rural community. Her parents had blue-collar jobs and worked full time.

Monica experienced many different kinds of attachment assaults and parental rage patterns, including parental alcoholism and sexual assault by her father, that had severe consequences of her life choices and her self-confidence. Her grandmother was the only other person who sometimes cared for her and her brothers. Monica loved her grandparents and spent most of her vacation time and holidays with them. She recalled that they were the only ones who visited her in the hospital when she broke her arm as a young child. They wanted to adopt Monica, but her parents refused. Her brother was her closest attachment figure. She described him as being "father-like" to her and she recalled that she wanted to marry him when she was a little girl.

Monica said she adored her father, yet she felt deserted by his empty promises, unavailability, and cruelty. She remembered vividly how he never allowed her to play outside, so she would often stand looking out of her window. Once when she asked him to go outside, he threw her out of the house and locked the door. Locked out, he forced her to wait until nightfall before he would unlock the door and let her in. She said that she never asked to play outside again and, from that point forward in her life, she was frightened to go outdoors.

Monica described her relationship with her mother as absent. She remembered her mother as being very jealous of her because she was her father's favorite. Her mother was so enraged that she would physically punish Monica until she had bruises.

The conflicting images of father and mother were particularly poignant in Monica's description from adolescence of a time when she and her father were walking together. She remembered that her father was drunk and accosted her. She got away from him and ran home, but her mother punished her without ever knowing about what had happened. His attack was a family secret for 10 years.

Monica said that she married to escape home when her mother's drinking became intolerable. Her husband, however, turned out to be violent and threatening. She later divorced him and married a different man.

Monica's life was filled with loss, following a pattern that Solomon and George (Chapter 2, this volume) term "complicated bereavement." Her grandmother died when she was 19. Monica said that she reacted to her grandmother's loss with tremendous anxiety and insecurity, as if the mourning was endless and her loss left a "big hole" in Monica's life. Her mother died of alcoholism shortly after Monica had left home to marry for the first time. Her closest boy friend died suddenly while they were on vacation together—he collapsed and died without warning. Monica explained that she viewed this loss as catalyst for her panic attacks because she felt so guilty about her friend's death. Since that time, Monica had developed several full-blown forms of anxiety problems, including panic, claustrophobia, and agoraphobia.

There were other losses around this time of her life as well. She lost the baby she was carrying from her second marriage, and her father, having become severely depressed and ill, also died. She said she had tried to talk to him about accosting her, and he told her that he was very ashamed before he died. Three days after her father died, Monica's oldest brother (her attachment figure) told her that he had terminal cancer. Monica said that she almost went crazy. She visited her brother every day when he was hospitalized. Ultimately, she explained that she still felt responsible for his death and believes that she could have prevented his death if she had stayed with him longer in the hospital.

Monica was judged unresolved on the AAI and the AAP. Her AAP transcript is presented below. Traumatic dysregulation markers are marked in the narrative in bold font; interview prompts are indicated in square brackets.

Alone Responses

STIMULUS 2: WINDOW

"Oh no. So I see myself standing at a window. A girl that is not allowed to go outside and would want, outside wants and wants to play like the others. But it is not allowed. Instead must do homework. And the girl has no other choice except to stand in front of the window and to dream about playing with others. That makes me very sad. I always also wanted as a child to play and I was not allowed. And once I told my father about it and he said, 'You want to play? Inside when it is dark.' And I did not know my way around in the village because I never was allowed to go outside and was afraid outside. And then my brother came and said, 'What are you doing here outside? What do you want here? And I said, 'Father said I should play. I do not know where I should go.' He then took me with him up to the church and simply ran away. And I was tremendously afraid that I could not find my way home. And there a woman who helped me to find my way home and I rang the bell and wanted back inside because I was afraid. And my father slammed the door in my face and said, 'You stay outside until it is dark. You wanted to play and now you can play.' I never again asked to go out to play. Yes, I still stand in front of the window today. What happens next? It is still not finished for me. I still stand in front of the window. I cannot, cannot find any end to it in the moment. No. Because it is exactly where I actually stand now. I could now outside and, and am afraid to go outside. As I said, I am still standing, still in front of the window and dreaming what it is like to be outside. And I do not find the courage to go outside. Out of fear. I would like to go outside and do something. It would be good for me to go for a walk or maybe go swimming."

Monica immediately put herself into the picture and was immersed with dread—"Oh no," she said. Her narrative shifted to the hypothetical character portrayed in the stimulus, describing a girl who is not allowed to play

outside and dreams of playing outside with friends. She must stay inside and
do her homework. Monica cannot maintain the distinction between the fic-
tional character and the self, and mentally shifts back to her own childhood
experience. She was overcome by her father's cruelty, which was an extreme
response to a child simply asking to play outside. Her request elicited rage
and threat of abandonment (stay outside until dark). She became lost, and
was found but abandoned yet again by her brother (he runs away). After
a stranger's assistance to find her home, her arrival to potential safety was
demolished by her father's rage and continued abandonment (locked outside of the house).

STIMULUS 4: BENCH

> "Yes. There I see a woman who seems **very desperate.** Protecting herself
> by embracing herself and she cries, **because there is no one else who
> can comfort her. She appears totally lost.** Her posture shows that **she
> feels lost.** I think there was a quarrel before that. A quarrel with a per-
> son who is very, yes, important to her and she does not know any way
> out, what she should say. Maybe she tried to clear up something or to
> push through something and did not succeed. A nice ending would be
> if now someone would really come and comfort her and give her cour-
> age. But mostly that doesn't happen. Instead she will collect herself and
> say, "Life goes on and I must now get through it." And she continues
> like that until now. Doubts herself and hopes that next time it will be
> better."

Monica's *Bench* response demonstrates the traumatic desperation
and abandonment that is elicited by anger in a relationship. The narrative
described a woman who had a quarrel and sits alone with no one to comfort
her. She hopes for a stranger to provide the care and comfort she needs, but
she knows that this is unlikely. The woman tries to reorganize (collects herself), but she has no resources. As with the girl in *Window*, the woman lives
in a dream world of hope for change that is unlikely when the self does not
have the personal agency to seek out an effective solution or another person
who can provide help or comfort.

STIMULUS 7: CEMETERY

> "Yes, there is someone standing at a grave. **I don't want to talk about
> that. My brother has died, I really don't want to respond to that** [long
> pause]. Okay, then I will take the picture away? Hm."

Monica's response to *Cemetery* is constricted. She is overwhelmed by
her grief of her brother's death. She cannot engage with the stimulus.

STIMULUS 8: CORNER

"There a child is standing in the corner. And has his hands in front of him to protect himself. His head is turned away so that he does not see what can happen. The child has done something ... from father, mother yes I think so father, mother, child, no idea. The child must have done something that **has totally enraged someone.** Hm. The child was caught lying. And the mother talks about that to the child and **goes quite aggressively toward the child so that the child has no choice any more except to go to a corner.** The mother comes closer and the child moves into the corner and is already anticipating the punishment which he is going to get. **The child is feeling totally helpless, is afraid** does not know any more what he should do and hopes then actually that it is over as fast as possible. And when it is over he just goes to his room **or into another corner** and is sad and cries until he can calm himself. And then maybe goes outside to friends to tell them about it. Maybe. Hmhm. Yes. Okay."

The traumatic dysregulation in *Corner* is revealed by parental rage and the child's helplessness. The narrative described a boy caught lying by one of his parents (Monica becomes confused as to which one). The parent is enraged and the boy is forced into the corner, and can only try to protect himself with a hand gesture. Unlike the utter helplessness of the other responses, Monica demonstrates signs of self-protection (hands in a protective position), agency (going to his room and seeking others), and connectedness to peer relationships for support (friends). These elements of her narrative suggests that Monica may have stood up for herself against her mother's rage in a way that she was not able to do against her father's abuse.

Dyadic Responses

STIMULUS 3: DEPARTURE

"Vacation. [Laughs.] Yes I see there a man and a woman with suitcase. What disturbs me about the picture is that both have their hands in their pockets. It is for me somehow as if something is unclear. I think, one of the two will probably have said we will go there and there and the other does not feel like it. I assume that the man decided and knows exactly that she goes along although she really does not feel like it. And also she does not say anything more about it. What are they feeling or thinking? Yes. Yes. They can also be angry about the fact that he again decides where to go. And he cannot understand it at all. He is rather totally surprised or also bored because he knows it. I think the two will drive away. For him it will be as always and she will sit aside well behaved and pretend as if it were fun. They are standing so strangely toward each other that it is as if they have nothing to say to each other. [Laughs.] I do not know. So I, I think so really uh they have nothing to tell each other. That looks to me so old-fashioned like such an old married couple. Where everything is already established, hanging in some tracks and no one is happy with it. Yes. [Anything else?] No."

There are no signs of traumatic dysregulation in this response. However, there continued to be underlying themes found in other responses of relationship anger and confusion. The narrative described a man and woman going on vacation. The woman did not feel like going to this place, and she is angry that it is the man who has made this decision and that he is so oblivious to her state. He is confused, surprised, but did not seem interested in seeing her point of view. As a couple, they are disconnected, bored, and unhappy and the woman acquiesces—Monica's prototype of a long-standing romantic attachment relationship.

STIMULUS 5: BED

"There I see a mother with a child. The child stretches his arms out to the mother and the mother also makes a movement to take the child. The child is ill, is ill and seeks comfort. And mother takes the time to sit next to the child and to comfort, to converse. A nice picture. And if a mother handles such an ill child like that then the child will get well faster. And he will soon be back up and play. What are they feeling or thinking? The child wants the mother to hug him. And she also already makes this gesture so.... The child can only be glad for the hug because he wants it and mother, she is glad too that the child wants to be hugged. So they are sitting actually rather apart there because of the flu. I, I have always relished when my children have embraced me. I think that it is here the same. Because so much comes back. Therefore, I also said, it is a nice picture. It is the give-and-take in harmony for me. Which is good for the child and also for the mother. So it should be, yes. And what happens next? That the child then is gets well again. As a mother I then also knew that I had done the right thing when the child gets well again. Yes. Yes? Hmhm."

There are no signs of traumatic dysregulation in this response. The narrative describes a sensitive and responsive relationship in which a mother comforts and cares for a sick child. Monica commented about her own experiences as a mother, emphasizing the mutual joys and benefits to child and mother in a harmonious embrace.

STIMULUS 5: AMBULANCE

"I just want to look, is that a child or should that be an adult? [Laughs.] [It is your story.] Yes? Looks already bigger. So there is a grandmother and that must be a teenager, because of his height. So, hmm I now assume that the teenager is ill so ill that the ambulance has to come. Uh so that the ambulance has to come and his grandmother comforts him, stands at the window and already expects the help of the ambulance, so actually is watching over everything. Uh to comfort the teenager and when help is coming? The teenager looks rather, yes, for me the way he is sitting there, **frightened**, he has **his hand in front of his mouth** and is thinking 'What is happening now?' Nice I find that he is not alone. 'You will come to the hospital, the grandmother will take care of that she can drive after them or she is allowed to drive along,' so as all grandmothers are and she will take care of the child. The grandmother is holding the boy somewhere tight or is holding him, that one cannot see everything, no, the arms are both free. She has, however, contact with the child. I think she tries to comfort, but is **helpless because she cannot help him the way she wants to** and the teenager is probably **afraid** about what then there is now going to happen. One does become **panicked** when one sees the ambulance when one is so injured or so ill that the ambulance must come. But he is fully dressed so he surely is injured. At first he will be totally insecure until he knows what is going to happen with him. The story will end like this that he is being taken care of medically and maybe also the grandmother, that the grandmother informs the mother and then she comes and the two women will care for him until he is healthy again. [Laughs.] Yes. Not that easy. Yes that's it. It is not so easy to get out there, to invent a story."

The *Ambulance* stimulus elicits traumatic fear and helplessness. The narrative described a boy who is frightened by the prospect of going away in the ambulance to the hospital. His grandmother comforts him, although the narrative acknowledges her own feelings of helplessness as a caregiver. Monica associates the *Ambulance* scene with potential panic that is prevented because the boy is with attachment figures. He gets good medical attention and the both the grandmother and mother are with him in the hospital.

How does the AAP add to our understanding of Monica's unresolved attachment? The traumatic dysregulation patterns in this case follow the overall pattern that we identified for patients with anxiety disorders in our study. Every alone stimulus elicited traumatic dysregulation and Monica is clearly unresolved regarding loss. She became dysregulated by her personal

memories related to two of the alone stimuli. The themes of separation anxiety are consistent with a constellation of views reviewed earlier, including
Bowlby's (1973).

Following Solomon and George's (2006; Chapter 2, this volume)
model of complicated grief and assaults to attachment, Monica's life is a
horror story of loss and attachment threats. Her parents were alcoholics,
her father sexually accosted her, her mother beat her, both parents would
become unpredictably enraged, she married an abusive man, and she lost
five attachment figures and her baby. What aspects, if any, of her threatening experiences might be the most overwhelming for her and contributing
to her anxiety disorder? Monica's AAP responses suggest that debilitating separation anxiety and unresolved loss are her most influential attachment experiences. Her characters were portrayed as "holding their own"
against parental rage (e.g., *Corner*). This is not to say that the other threats
of attachment are unimportant. Following Solomon and George's model,
Monica's anxiety problem were likely the product of the constellation of
attachment-based fears. Drawing from the attachment style research, we
might expect Monica's anger and fear states to become enduring personality
traits. The question that emerges then is whether her anger is an enduring
personality trait, or if it is a by-product of attachment fear and frustration
(as proposed by Bowlby, 1973).

One of the major features of anxiety in Bowlby's model was the development of and conscious access to parallel contradictory representations of
the self and attachment figures. Monica's AAP demonstrates these contradictions. The alone stories represent extreme attachment disorganization.
The alone self is helpless, frightened, and abandoned, rarely receiving care
or contact with others or taking initiative to protect the self. Attachment
figures were portrayed as hostile and threatening abandonment. Separation
is terrifying. Monica's dyadic stories involving children epitomized security.
These children and their attachment figures were engaged in flexibly integrated goal-corrected partnerships. Monica represented the dyadic child-self
as worthy of care. Attachment figures were portrayed as present, sensitive,
responsive, and following through with care.

The origins of these opposing representations are not exactly clear. Monica had a caring grandmother who tried to adopt her as a child. We believe
that this is likely to be the source of her description of the grandmother
figure in *Ambulance*. The descriptions of her own mother and her portrayal
of mother in the alone pictures, however, do not match the described mothers in these dyadic stories. West and Sheldon-Keller (1994) propose that
individuals must mourn the loss of the "wished for" attachment figure, irrespective of their real loss. Clearly, the mothers in Monica's child dyadic
stimuli responses portray this defensive process. She clearly states how hard
she is working in *Ambulance* to "invent" this situation (i.e., the fantasy). So

embedded in these opposing models of attachment, it appears that the AAP has also uncovered another form of unresolved mourning. This interpretation is also supported by Monica's report in response to *Bed* about her own experience in providing care for her children. Instead of describing the joys of providing care for her children, Monica inverts the situation and describes the joys of receiving their care. This type of role inversion is consistent with Bowlby's view of chronic mourning and forms of compulsive caregiving in which the mourning individual provides care for others in order to receive care him- or herself (Bowlby, 1980).

CONCLUSIONS

This chapter describes a new approach to understanding unresolved attachment in BPD and the anxiety disorders by delving deeply into the AAP assessment narrative to examine traumatic content. This narrative material was rich for interpretation when combined with knowledge of life events (e.g., as told in the AAI) and new models of attachment disorganization that have sought to define more broadly than the AAI unresolved loss or abuse scales Bowlby's (1980) original perspective on pathological mourning in terms of helplessness, rage patterns and complicated grief (Solomon & George, Chapter 2, this volume). We succeeded in uncovering important group differences in the traumatic underlying patterns of unresolved attachment related to these disorders. In order to do this, we used the AAP, a validated projective measure of attachment that assesses attachment using a standardized set of attachment-activating stimuli. Our study also added to AAP research that has demonstrated the validity of its use in German-speaking populations and with clinical groups.

Consistent with the overall consensus of previous research with the BPD and anxiety disorder patient populations, we found that the two patient groups were overrepresented by unresolved attachment, as compared with the nonpatient controls. The amount of traumatic dysregulation demonstrated in response to the AAP alone stimuli was significantly greater for the patient groups than for the controls. The traumatic dysregulation patterns observed in the two patient groups supported our hypotheses regarding the role of aloneness in these two disorders. This study also successfully took the first steps in the field of attachment to document patterns of traumatic dysregulation patterns that may differentiate unresolved attachment in nonclinical groups and also between these two disorders. There were some similarities between these patients, including fears of being alone and the importance of loss of attachment figures in their lives. But there were important differences between the patient groups. The patients with BPD tended to demonstrate the strongest dysregulation in response to fears of being alone combined with isolation, which are related to severe abuse combined with loss of protective attachment figures. The fear and certainty of being alone was so pervasive in our borderline case study that this individual transformed every dyadic picture stimulus into a situation of being or becoming alone.

The patients with anxiety disorders were also dysregulated by the alone stimuli, but less so than the patients with BPD. Our findings importantly demonstrated how patients with anxiety disorders seem to build opposing contradictory models of attachment, and how sometimes these models produced sudden shifts in attention that put the self and fear in the center of focus. This finding is consistent with Bowlby's view of the roots of anxiety (Bowlby, 1973) and this seemed to occur when attachment was activated, even when this was inappropriate (e.g., the AAP task).

Our first steps in this research approach are, of course, tempered by small samples and need to be replicated by others. We also do not know if these patterns are uniquely associated with patients with BPD and with anxiety disorders or if the patterns we described might also be found in other clinical groups.

Our research demonstrated that the AAP provides a rich picture of attachment representation and other clinical material. We only presented material in this chapter that was related to disorganization by trauma and threats of attachment, with corollary discussions that tied the differential responses to the AAP alone and dyadic stimuli to neurobiological and emotion expression studies. The AAP analysis differentiating normative and traumatic segregated systems narrative markers provided us with a more detailed level of understanding of representational markers regarding organization and threats to attachment than exists in the literature to date. The AAP results confirmed that patients with BPD manifested more "traumatic" as compared to "normative" attachment dysregulation, the form of dysregulation that predominated in nonpatient unresolved controls. This unique dimension has been fruitful in several of our studies, including our fMRI analysis (Buchheim et al., 2008) and EMFACS facial activity analysis (Buchheim et al., 2007) of patients with BPD. In both studies, the AAP served as an excellent assessment in paradigms developed to assess the neural and emotional correlates of attachment disorganization.

NOTES

1. George and West have found in their studies using the AAP that the CC (i.e., Cannot Classify classification group) in the AAI is found to be judged unresolved on the AAP. The overlap in this classification fits the notion that CC is a particular attachment state of mind in which lapses of discourse and the disorganization of thinking is associated with severe attachment threats, such as sexual abuse.
2. Anna Buchheim as first AAI judge and Fabienne Becker-Stoll as second AAI judge

are both certified AAI raters, trained by Mary Main and Eric Hesse at the AAI Institute in Berkeley, California.

REFERENCES

Aaronson, C. J., Bender, D. S., Skodol, A. E., & Gunderson, J. G. (2006). Comparison of attachment styles in borderline personality disorder and obsessive–compulsive personality disorder. *Psychiatric Quarterly, 77,* 69–80.

Agrawal, H. R., Gunderson, J., Holmes, B. M., & Lyons-Ruth, K. (2004). Attachment studies with borderline patients: A review. *Harvard Review of Psychiatry, 12,* 94–104.

American Psychiatric Association. (2000). *Diagnostic and statistical manual of mental disorders* (4th ed.). Washington, DC: Author.

Bar-Haim, Y., Dan, O., Eshel, Y., & Sagi-Schwartz, A. (2007). Predicting children's anxiety from early attachment relationships. *Journal of Anxiety Disorders, 21,* 1061–1068.

Bakermans-Kranenburg, M. J., & van IJzendoorn, M. H. (2009). The first 10,000 Adult Attachment Interviews: Distribution of adult attachment in clinical and non-clinical groups. *Attachment and Human Development, 11,* 223–263.

Barlow, D. H., Chorpita, B. F., & Turovsky, J. (1996). Fear, panic, anxiety, and disorders of emotion. *Nebraska Symposium on Motivation, 43,* 251–328.

Bifulco, A., Kwon, J., Jacobs, C., Moran, P., Bunn, A., & Beer, N. (2006). Adult attachment style as mediator between childhood neglect/abuse and adult depression and anxiety. *Social Psychiatry and Psychiatric Epidemiology, 41,* 796–805.

Bohus, M., Schmahl, C., & Lieb, K. (2004). New developments in the neurobiology of borderline personality disorder. *Current Psychiatry Reports, 6,* 43–50.

Bosquet, M., & Egeland, B. (2006). The development and maintenance of anxiety symptoms from infancy through adolescence in a longitudinal sample. *Development and Psychopathology, 18,* 517–550.

Bowlby, J. (1969). *Attachment and loss: Vol. 1. Attachment.* New York: Basic Books.

Bowlby, J. (1973). *Attachment and loss: Vol. 2. Separation.* New York: Basic Books.

Bowlby, J. (1980). *Attachment and loss: Vol. 3. Loss.* New York: Basic Books.

Buchheim, A., & Benecke, C. (2007). Mimisch-affektives Verhalten bei Patientinnen mit Angststörungen während des Adult Attachment Interviews: Eine Pilotstudie [Affective facial behavior of patients with anxiety disorders during the Adult Attachment Interview: A pilot study]. *Psychotherapeutic and Psychological Medicine, 57,* 343–347.

Buchheim, A., Erk, S., George, C., Kächele, H., Martius, P., Pokorny, D., et al. (2008). Neural correlates of attachment dysregulation in borderline personality disorder using functional magnetic resonance imaging. *Psychiatry Research: Neuroimaging, 163,* 223–235.

Buchheim, A., Erk, S., George, C., Kächele, H., Ruschow, M., Spitzer, M., et al.

(2006). Measuring attachment in an fMRI environment: A pilot study. *Psychopathology, 39,* 144–152.

Buchheim, A., George, C., Kächele, H., Erk, S., & Walter, H. (2006). Measuring adult attachment representation in an fMRI environment: Concepts and assessment. *Psychopathology, 39,* 136–143.

Buchheim, A., George, C., Liebl, V., Moser, A., & Benecke, C. (2007). Mimische Affektivität von Patientinnen mit einer Borderline-Persönlichkeitsstörung während des Adult Attachment Projective [Affective facial behavior of borderline patients during the Adult Attachment Projective]. *Zeitschrift forPsychosomatic Medicine and Psychotherapy, 53,* 339–354.

Buchheim, A., Ziegenhain, U., Peter, A., von Wietersheim, H., Vicari, A., Kolb, A., et al. (2007). Unverarbeitete Verlusterfahrungen bei Müttern mit einer Angststörung und ihre Kinder: Eine transgenerationale Pilotstudie [Unresolved experiences of loss and anxiety disorders: A transgenerational pilot study with mothers and their children]. *Nervenheilkunde, 26,* 1130–1135.

Busch, F. N., Milrod, B. L., & Singer, M. B. (1999). Theory and technique in psychodynamic treatment of panic disorder. *Journal of Psychotherapy Practice and Research, 8,* 234–242.

Cassidy, J., Lichtenstein-Phelps, J., Sibrava, N. J., Thomas C. L. Jr., & Borkovec, T. D. (2009). Generalized anxiety disorder: Connections to self-reported attachment. *Behavior Therapy, 40,* 23–38.

Cassidy, J., & Shaver, P. R. (Eds.). (2008). *Handbook of attachment: Theory, research, and clinical applications* (2nd ed.). New York: Guilford Press.

Critchfield, K. L., Levy, K. N., Clarkin, J. E., & Kernberg, O. F. (2009). The relational context of aggression in borderline personality disorder: Using attachment style to predict forms of hostility. *Journal of Clinical Psychology, 64,* 67–82.

Crowell, J., Fraley, R. C., & Shaver, P. R. (2008). Measurement of individual differences in adolescent and adult attachment. In J. Cassidy & P. R. Shaver (Eds.), *Handbook of attachment: Theory, research, and clinical applications* (2nd ed., pp. 599–634). New York: Guilford Press.

Dallaire, D. H., & Weinraub, M. (2005). Predicting children's separation anxiety at age 6: The contributions of infant–mother attachment security, maternal sensitivity, and maternal separation anxiety. *Attachment and Human Development, 7,* 393–408.

Dozier, M., Stovall-McClough, K. C., & Albus, K. E. (2008). Attachment and psychopathology in adulthood. In J. Cassidy & P. R. Shaver (Eds.), *Handbook of attachment: Theory, research, and clinical applications* (2nd ed., pp. 718–744). New York: Guilford Press.

Elizabeth, J., King, N., Ollendick, T. H., Gullone, E., Tonge, B., Watson, S., et al. (2006). Social anxiety disorder in children and youth: A research update on aetiological factors. *Counselling Psychology Quarterly, 19,* 151–163.

Eng, W., Heimberg, R. G., Hart, T. A., Schneier, F. R., & Liebowitz, M. R. (2001). Attachment in individuals with social anxiety disorder: The relationship among adult attachment styles, social anxiety, and depression. *Emotion, 1,* 365–380.

Feeney, J. A. (2008). Adult romantic attachment: Developments in the study of couple relationships. In J. Cassidy & P. R. Shaver (Eds.), *Handbook of attachment:*

Theory, research, and clinical applications (2nd ed., pp. 456–481). New York: Guilford Press.

Fonagy, P., Gergely, G., Jurist, E. L., & Target, M. (2003). *Affect regulation, mentalization, and the development of the self.* New York: Other Press.

Fonagy, P., Leigh, T., Steele, M., Steele, H., Kennedy, R., & Mattoon, G. (1996). The relation of attachment status, psychiatric classification, and response to psychotherapy. *Journal of Counseling and Clinical Psychology, 64,* 22–31.

Fossati, A., Feeney, J. A., Carretta, I., Grazioli, F., Milesi, R., Leonardi, B., et al. (2005). Modeling the relationships between adult attachment patterns and borderline personality disorder: The role of impulsivity and aggressiveness *Journal of Social and Clinical Psychology, 24,* 520–537.

First, M. B., Spitzer, R. L., Gibbon, M., Willians, J. B. W., Davies, M., Howes, M. J., et al. (1995). The Structured Clinical Interview for DSM-III-R Personality Disorders (SCID-II): Part II. Multi-site test–retest reliability study. *Journal of Personality, 9,* 92–104.

Friesen, W. V., & Ekman, P. (1984). *EMFACS-7. Emotional Facial Action Coding System,* Unpublished manual, University of California.

Gallagher, H. L., & Frith, C. D. (2003). Functional imaging of "theory of mind." *Trends in Cognitive Science, 7,* 77–83.

George, C., Kaplan, N., & Main, M. (1984/1985/1996). *The Adult Attachment Interview.* Unpublished manuscript, University of California at Berkeley.

George, C., & Solomon, J. (1996). Representational models of relationships: Links between caregiving and attachment. *Infant Mental Health Journal, 17,* 198–216.

George, C., & Solomon, J. (2008). The caregiving system: A behavioral systems approach to parenting. In J. Cassidy & P. R. Shaver (Eds.), *Handbook of attachment: Theory, research, and clinical applications* (2nd ed., pp. 833–856). New York: Guilford Press.

George, C., & West, M. (1999). Developmental vs. social personality models of adult attachment and mental ill health. *British Journal of Medical Psychology, 72,* 285–303.

George, C., & West, M. (2001). The development and preliminary validation of a new measure of adult attachment: The Adult Attachment Projective. *Attachment and Human Development, 3,* 30–61.

George, C., & West, M. (in press). *The Adult Attachment Projective Picture System.* New York: Guilford Press.

George, C., West, M., & Pettem, O. (1999). The Adult Attachment Projective: Disorganization of adult attachment at the level of representation. In J. Solomom & C. George (Eds.), *Attachment disorganization* (pp. 462–507). New York: Guilford Press.

Gunderson, J. G. (1996). The borderline patient's intolerance of aloneness: Insecure attachments and therapist availability. *American Journal of Psychiatry, 153,* 752–758.

Hesse, E. (2008). The Adult Attachment Interview: Protocol, methods of analysis, and empirical studies. In J. Cassidy & P. R. Shaver (Eds.), *Handbook of attachment: Theory, research, and clinical applications* (2nd ed., pp. 552–598). New York: Guilford Press.

Lee, A., & Hankin, B. L. (2009). Insecure attachment, dysfunctional attitudes, and low self esteem predicting prospective symptoms of depression and anxiety during adolescence. *Journal of Clinical Child and Adolescent Psychology, 38,* 219–231.

Levy, K. N., Meehan, K. B., Kelly, K. M., Reynoso, J. S., Weber, M., Clarkin, J. F., et al. (2006). Change in attachment patterns and reflective function in a randomized control trial of transference-focused psychotherapy for borderline personality disorder. *Journal of Consulting and Clinical Psychology, 74,* 1027–1040.

Levy, K. N., Meehan, K. B., & Weber, M. (2005). Attachment and borderline personality disorder: Implications for psychotherapy. *Psychopathology, 38,* 64–74.

Lyons-Ruth, K., Melnick, S., Patrick, M., & Hobson, R. P. (2007). A controlled study of hostile–helpless states of mind among borderline and dysthymic women. *Attachment and Human Development, 9,* 1–16.

Lyons-Ruth, K., Yellin, C., Melnick, S., & Atwood, G. (2003). Childhood experiences of trauma and loss have different relations to maternal unresolved and hostile–helpless states of mind on the AAI. *Attachment and Human Development, 5,* 330–352.

Main, M., & Goldwyn, R. (1984/1998). *Adult Attachment Interview scoring and classification system.* Unpublished manuscript, University of California at Berkeley.

Main, M., & Solomon, J. (1990). Procedures for identifying infants as disorganized/disoriented during the Ainsworth Strange Situation. In M. T. Greenberg, D. Cicchetti, & E. M. Cummings (Eds.), *Attachment in the preschool years* (pp. 121–160). Chicago: University of Chicago Press.

Manassis, K., & Bradley, S. (1994). Attachment in mothers with anxiety disorders and their children. *Journal of the American Academy of Child and Adolescent Psychiatry, 33,* 1106–1113.

Manicavasagar, V., Silove, D., Marnane, C., & Wagner, R. (2009). Adult attachment styles in panic disorder with and without comorbid adult separation anxiety disorder. *Australian and New Zealand Journal of Psychiatry, 43,* 167–172.

Marazziti, D., Dell'Osso, B., Dell'Osso, M. C., Consoli, G., Del Debbio, A., Mungai, F., et al. (2007). Romantic attachment in patients with mood and anxiety disorders. *CNS Spectrums, 12,* 751–756.

Matthew, S. J., Coplan, J. B., & Gorman, J. M. (2001). Neurobiological mechanisms of social anxiety disorder. *American Journal of Psychiatry, 158,* 1558–1567.

Minzenberg, M. J., Poole, J. H., & Vinogradov, S. (2006). Adult social attachment disturbance is related to childhood maltreatment and current symptoms in borderline personality disorder. *Journal of Nervous and Mental Disease, 194,* 341–348.

Morse, J. O., Hill, J., Pilkonis, P. A., Yaggi, K., Brovden, N., Stepp, S., et al. (2009). Anger, preoccupied attachment, and domain disorganization in borderline personality disorder. *Journal of Personality Disorders, 23,* 240–257.

Peleikis, D. E., Mykletun, A., & Dahl, A. A. (2004). The relative influence of childhood sexual abuse and other family background risk factors on adult adversities in female outpatients treated for anxiety disorders and depression. *Child Abuse and Neglect, 28,* 61–77.

Peter, H., Brackner, E., Hand, I., & Rufer, M. (2005). Childhood separation anxiety and separation events in women with agoraphobia with or without panic disorder. *Canadian Journal of Psychiatry, 50,* 941–944.

Riggs, S. A., Paulson, A., Tunnell, E., Sahl, G., Atkison, H., & Ross, C. A. (2007). Attachment, personality, and psychopathology among adult inpatients: Self-reported romantic attachment style versus Adult Attachment Interview states of mind. *Development and Psychopathology, 19,* 263–291.

Rosenstein, D. S., & Horowitz, H. A. (1996). Adolescent attachment and psychopathology. *Journal of Consulting and Clinical Psychology, 64,* 244–253.

Shamir-Essakow, G., Ungerer, J. A., & Rapee, R. M. (2005). Attachment, behavioral inhibition, and anxiety in preschool children. *Journal of Abnormal Child Psychology, 33,* 131–143.

Scott, L. N., Levy, K. N., & Pincus, A. L. (2009). Adult attachment, personality traits, and borderline personality features in young adults. *Journal of Personality Disorders, 23,* 258–280.

Solomon, J., & George, C. (1999). The place of disorganization in attachment theory: Linking classic observations with contemporary findings. In J. Solomon & C. George (Eds.), *Attachment disorganization* (pp. 3–32). New York: Guilford Press.

Solomon, J., & George, C. (2000). Toward a theory of caregiving. In J. Osofsky & H. Fitzgerald (Eds.), *World Association for Infant Mental Health handbook of infant mental health* (pp. 323–368). New York: Wiley.

Solomon, J., & George, C. (2006). Intergenerational transmission of dysregulated maternal caregiving: Mothers describe their upbringing and childrearing. In O. Mayseless (Ed.), *Parenting representations: Theory, research, and clinical implications* (pp. 265–295). New York: Cambridge University Press.

Solomon, J., George, C., & De Jong, A. (1995). Children classified as controlling at age six: Evidence of disorganized representational strategies and aggression at home and at school. *Development and Psychopathology, 7,* 447–463.

Sroufe, L. A., Egeland, B., Carlson, E. A., & Collins, A. W. (2005). *The development of the person.* New York: Guilford Press.

Strodl, E., & Noller, P. (2003). The relationship of adult attachment dimensions to depression and agoraphobia. *Personal Relationships, 10,* 171–186.

van Emmichoven, I. A. Z., van IJzendoorn, M. H., De Ruiter, C., & Brosschot, J. F. (2003). Selective processing of threatening information: Effects of attachment representation and anxiety disorder on attention and memory. *Development and Psychopathology, 15,* 219–237.

van IJzendoorn, M. H., & Bakermans-Kranenburg, M. J. (1996). Attachment representations in mothers, fathers, adolescents, and clinical groups: A meta-analytic search for normative data. *Journal of Consulting and Clinical Psychology, 64,* 8–21.

Vogt, B. A., Finch, D. M., & Olson, C. R. (1992). Functional heterogeneity in cingulate cortex: The anterior executive and posterior evaluative regions. *Cerebral Cortex, 2,* 435–443.

Vogt, B.A., & Pandya, D. N. (1987). Cingulate cortex of the rhesus monkey: II. Cortical afferents. *Journal of Comparative Neurology, 262,* 271–289.

Warren, S. L., Huston, L., Egeland, B., & Sroufe, L. A. (1997). Child and adolescent anxiety disorders and early attachment. *Journal of the American Academy of Child and Adolescent Psychiatry, 36,* 637–644.

Waters, E., Crowell, J., Elliott, M., Corcoran, D., & Treboux, D. (2002). Bowlby's secure base theory and the social/personality psychology of attachment styles: Work(s) in progress. *Attachment and Human Development, 4,* 230–242.

Waters, E., & Hamilton, C. E. (2000). The stability of attachment security from infancy to adolescence and early adulthood: General introduction. *Child Development, 71,* 678–683.

West, M., & George, C. (2002). Attachment and dysthymia: The contributions of preoccupied attachment and agency of self to depression in women. *Attachment and Human Development, 4,* 278–293.

West, M., & Sheldon-Keller, A. E. (1994). *Patterns of relating: An adult attachment perspective.* New York: Guilford Press.

Zanarini, M.C. (2000). Childhood experiences associated with the development of borderline personality disorder. *Psychiatric Clinics of North America, 23,* 89–101.

Zanarini, M. C., Frankenburg, F. R., Hennen, J., & Silk, K. R. (2003). The longitudinal course of borderline psychopathology: 6–year prospective followup of the phenomenology of borderline personality disorder. *American Journal of Psychiatry, 160,* 827–832.

Chapter 14

Attachment Disorganization and the Clinical Dialogue
Theme and Variations

GIOVANNI LIOTTI

Both clinical reflections and empirical studies support the hypothesis that early attachment disorganization is causally linked to a group of adult disorders consequent to attachment-related childhood traumas (Buchheim & George, Chapter 13, this volume; Dozier, Stovall-McClough, & Albus, 2008; Fonagy, 2002; Fonagy, Target, Gergely, Allen & Bateman, 2003; Hesse, Main, Abrams, & Rifkin, 2003; Liotti, 1992, 1999, 2004, 2006; Lyons-Ruth, Melnick, Patrick, & Hobson, 2007; Schore, 2009). This group of disorders, including most cases of dissociative disorders and a substantial subgroup of borderline personality disorders, is characterized by three interrelated and partially overlapping key features: (1) dissociation, splitting, or other forms of nonintegrated self-representations; (2) metacognitive deficits hampering the ability to reflect on mental states (mentalization deficits); and (3) serious disturbances in the regulation of emotions. The basic hypothesis is that early attachment disorganization fosters dissociative responses to later traumatic events, and that the cumulating effect of dissociative experiences throughout the developmental years leads to different types of complex and chronic adult disorders (Liotti, 2004). Specific risk factors, besides disorganized attachment, should account for the differential characteristics of these disorders (e.g., the characteristics of traumas that may intervene in depersonalization disorder, and their difference from those intervening in dissociative identity disorder, as discussed by Simeon, 2009).

The role of early attachment disorganization in the genesis of complex and chronic trauma-related disturbances has induced clinicians to propose

383

attachment-based strategies for better dealing with some typical difficulties in psychotherapy with patients suffering from these disorders. Three main aspects of attachment disorganization have been considered as the focus of these strategies: (1) the multiplicity of nonintegrated representations of self and others (Liotti, 1995, 1999, 2007); (2) metacognitive or mentalization deficits (i.e., the hindrance to the ability to reflect on one's own and other people's mental states; Bateman & Fonagy, 2004; Fonagy, 2002; Fonagy et al., 2003); and (3) relational dilemmas implied in disorganization of attachment (Blizard, 2001, 2008; Gold, 2000; Holmes, 2004; Howell, 2005; Van der Hart, Nijenhuis, & Steele, 2006). Each of the above attachment-based therapeutic strategies emphasizes a different aspect of attachment disorganization; disorganization of attachment is a single theme in developmental psychopathology, but it allows for many variations when it is considered as a focus for therapeutic interventions with adult patients.

This chapter's clinical illustrations are lessons drawn from the author's personal experience (his own "variations on the theme") of treatment and case supervision based on the concept of attachment disorganization. Other variations on the theme, like the ones cited above (Bateman & Fonagy, 2004; Blizard, 2001, 2008; Gold, 2000; Holmes, 2004; Howell, 2005), are admirable for their clinical wisdom and practical usefulness, and are often the source of inspiration for the author's clinical work, but the length and the purpose of this chapter does not allow for their detailed description. Before dwelling on a few variations concerning its clinical application, an overview of the basic aspects of attachment disorganization may assist the reader in capturing the unity of the underlying theme. The aim of this chapter is such that the overview will focus on the developmental pathways that may proceed from early attachment disorganization to adult psychopathology. It must be emphasized, however, that by no mean all, or even the majority, of infants who have been disorganized in their attachments develop clinically significant disturbances (Liotti, 1992; Main & Morgan, 1996). What is asserted in this chapter is only that attachment disorganization is a risk factor for the development of trauma-related disorders implying fragmentation of the self, and that psychotherapists may better understand the interpersonal difficulties of these patients if they have a working knowledge of attachment disorganization.

ANTECEDENTS, BASIC FEATURES, AND CONSEQUENCES OF EARLY ATTACHMENT DISORGANIZATION

The Intergenerational Effects of Traumas and Losses

Empirical research has evidenced that attachment disorganization in the infant is the relational consequence of one or a combination of the following: (1) unresolved attachment-related traumas or losses in the caregiver (Hesse & Main, 2000); (2) a caregiver's state of mind characterized by non-integrated, hostile, and helpless representations of self and others (Lyons-Ruth, Yellin, Melnick, & Atwood, 2005; Lyons-Ruth et al., 2007); and (3) caregiver's self-description of childhood experiences where he or she felt threatened and helpless in the face of his or her attachment figure's behavior (Solomon & George, 2006; Chapter 2, this volume). Like any other type of experience in the domain of attachment–caregiving interactions, attachment disorganization is part of a wider reality—both intergenerational (Solomon & George, 2006; Chapter 2, this volume) and intersubjective (Lyons-Ruth, 1999, 2003)—where the caregiver's state of mind, characterized by lack of resolution of traumatic experiences and/or by hostility and helplessness, meets with the infant's state of mind, characterized by the need to be soothed, helped, and protected from dangers.

The Disorganized Infant's Motivational Dynamics: Defense and Attachment

Being exposed to frequent interactions with a helplessly frightened, hostile and frightening, or confused caregiver, infants are caught in a relational trap, created by the dynamics of two inborn motivational systems, the attachment system and the defense (fight–flight) system. The attachment and the defense systems normally operate in harmony (i.e., flight from the source of fear to find refuge in proximity to the attachment figure). They, however, clash in such a type of infant–caregiver interaction where the caregiver is at the same time the source and the solution of the infant's fear ("fright without solution": Main & Hesse, 1990, p. 163). The consequence of the simultaneous activation of the defense and the attachment systems is the "failure to terminate" attachment interactions, due to the fact that fear is in itself a powerful activator of the attachment system (Solomon & George, 1999). Solomon and George (1996) linked this "failure to terminate" hypothesis to an abdicating attitude of the caregiver: the mothers of disorganized babies seem to be unwilling to repair or incapable of repairing the errors in their attitude that are frightening to their children.

The interaction between a frightened–frightening, helpless, or abdicating caregiver and a disorganized infant experiencing fright without solution is an extreme example of emotional misattunement, that is, of threatened failure in the intrinsic intersubjectivity of human experience (Stern, 1985, 2004). Instead of preserving secure intersubjectivity, the infant's experience is alike to feeling utterly alienated from one's own primary relatedness, that is, to feeling alone while being in the perceptual (as opposed to the communicational and affectional) presence of another person. This experience may be understood as a type of early relational trauma that exerts an adverse influence on the development of the stress-coping system in the infant's brain (Schore, 2009). Such an adverse influence is mediated by the internal working model (IWM) of attachment. The IWM, it should be emphasized, is a cognitive structure that (1) is constructed on the basis of *implicit* memories of attachment experiences (Amini et al., 1996), (2) influences meaning and expectations concerning requests for help and comfort, and (3) is expressed in the form of enactments (Lyons-Ruth, 1999).

The Dramatic Multiplicity of the Disorganized IWM

The IWM of early disorganized attachment is conceived, on theoretical grounds, as multiple, nonintegrated, and conveying dramatic expectations (Hesse et al., 2003; Liotti, 1995, 1999, 2004; Main, 1991; Main & Hesse, 1990). This conceptualization of the IWM of disorganized attachment in infancy, although it cannot be directly assessed in present-time research, is in keeping with observations on the state of mind of school-age children and adults who have likely been disorganized infants (see Hesse et al., 2003, for a review). Adults who report histories of traumatic attachments, and whose children have developed disorganized attachments toward them, typically show multiple, nonintegrated (dissociated) dramatic representations of self and attachment figures, shifting from hostility to helplessness and to compulsive caregiving (Lyons-Ruth et al., 2005, 2007). Liotti (1995, 1999, 2006) suggested that this multiple, dramatic, and dissociated representation of self and attachment figures is captured, in a clinically useful way, by the metaphor of the "drama triangle," in which both self and significant others are represented, simultaneously or in quick sequence, according to the reciprocally incompatible roles of the helpless victim, the powerful-benevolent rescuer, and the equally powerful but malevolent persecutor (for the original description of the drama triangle, see Karpman, 1968). Data collected by Solomon, George, and De Jong (1995) support this view, showing that at age 6 children who had been disorganized in their infant attachment display helplessness, caregiving, and aggression in a doll play task.

Besides being intrinsically multiple, incoherent, and very likely compartmentalized in its content (Liotti, 1992, 2004; Main, 1991; Main & Morgan, 1996)—so that the construction of a single representation of self and the caregiver is hindered—the IWM of disorganized attachment may be selectively and defensively excluded (i.e., segregated; Bowlby, 1980) from conscious scrutiny. The reader should be alerted to the fact that clinical applications of the notion of disorganized attachment focusing on segregated systems may lead to "variations on the theme" that are slightly different from those expressed in this chapter.

Attachment Disorganization, Dissociative Processes, and Mentalization

One of the consequences of early disorganized attachment is a proneness toward dissociative experiences and toward developing clinically relevant dissociative symptoms throughout development. The link between dissociation and disorganized attachment has been evidenced by longitudinal research extending from infancy to adolescence (Carlson, 1998; Ogawa, Sroufe, Weinfield, Carlson, & Egeland, 1997) and by other controlled studies in nonclinical populations (Hesse & van IJzendoorn, 1999). These research findings are in keeping with the results of other controlled studies exploring the relationship between variables indicative of disorganized attachment and dissociative or borderline disorders in adolescents and adults (Liotti, Pasquini & Italian Group for the Study of Dissociation, 2000; Pasquini et al., 2002; West, Adam, Spreng, & Rose, 2001). Taken cumulatively, all these studies suggest that dissociation is a feature of disorganized attachment, independent from later traumas. Many research findings (reviewed by Levy, 2005) suggest that attachment disorganization, in itself, is a rather nonspecific risk factor in the development of many types of emotional disorders. This is in keeping with theories that regard dissociation as a widespread feature of many types of mental disorders (see, e.g., Bromberg, 2009). Even if attachment disorganization seems to be a risk factor in the development of many types of mental disorders, it can be argued that *when it is co-opted in reactions to later traumas*, it leaves the ground open for the development of adult disorders mainly in the dissociative and borderline spectrum—that is, disorders characterized by a fragmented experience of the self (Howell, 2005; Lieberman, 2004; Liotti, 1992, 2004, 2006; Ogawa et al., 1997). This assertion does not imply that all cases of borderline personality disorders (BPD) and dissociative disorders are caused by attachment disorganization followed by later traumas (indeed, traumas may play a secondary role, or even no role, in the genesis of a subgroup of BPD cases; see Paris, 1995). It only means that *if later and severe traumatic experiences impinge upon the IWM of disorganized attachment*, then one likely consequence is a disorder in the borderline or in the dissociative spectrum (cf. Bradley, Jeney, & Westen, 2005).

The link between mental disorders implying dissociation and disorganized attachment has been explained on the ground that (1) infant disorganized attachment is in itself a dissociative process (Liotti, 1992, 2004, 2006; Main & Morgan, 1996), and (2) it makes dissociative experiences more likely when one is facing traumas. Traumas involve the activation of the attachment motivational system (i.e., of wishes to be soothed and helped). When this activation switches on over the operations of a disorganized

IWM that is intrinsically disassociated and yields catastrophic expectations linked to the experience of fright without solution, both peritraumatic and posttraumatic dissociative experiences become likely. In contrast, the IWM of early secure attachment, providing expectations to be soothed and helped by competent caregivers, very likely reduces the likelihood of peritraumatic dissociation, and therefore acts as a protective factor in the face of later traumas, against the development of chronic and complex types of trauma-related disorders (Liotti, 1999, 2004, 2006).

Besides facilitating pathological dissociation, early disorganized attachment hampers the proper development or fruition, from childhood to adult age, of metacognitive or mentalizing capacities (Fonagy et al., 2003). Emotional dysregulation (i.e., abnormally intense and durable emotional reactions in the face of stressors) may be a further untoward consequence of early attachment disorganization (see Buchheim & George, Chapter 13, this volume; Hesse et al., 2003; Lyons-Ruth & Jacobvitz, 2008; Schore, 2009). Mentalization deficits and emotional dysregulation are among the basic features of disorders characterized by the fragmentation of self-experience.

The Controlling Strategies

The hypothesis that the developmental sequels of early disorganized attachment may include proneness toward dissociative reactions, metacognitive deficits, and emotional dysregulation does not imply that children who have been disorganized infants constantly show, during their development, disassociated, utterly incoherent, and dysregulated mental states (and behavior) in their interactions with other people. On the contrary, before they reach school age, the great majority of children who have been disorganized in their infant attachments develop an organized behavioral and attentional strategy toward their caregivers. They achieve such an organization by exerting active control on the parent's attention and behavior either through caregiving or through domineering-punitive strategies (Hesse et al., 2003; Lyons-Ruth & Jacobvitz, 2008). These observations may be explained as follows (cf. Liotti, 2004).

When a disorganized IWM dominates them since infancy, the activities of the attachment system tend to be defensively inhibited throughout development, in order to protect both the child and his or her relationship with parents from the unbearably chaotic experience of disorganization. The relative inhibition of the attachment motivational system is achieved through co-opting another, equally inborn interpersonal motivational system during the daily interactions with the caregiver. Another system tends to intervene instead of the attachment system to regulate the interactions between child and parent, so that behavior and intersubjective experience can achieve at least a degree of organization. Attachment is not the only motivational system with an inborn basis that regulates interpersonal behavior. Other motivational systems were described by Bowlby (1979) and have also been described by Lichtenberg (1989) and by Gilbert (1989). While the attachment system regulates mainly careseeking interactions, the sexual system, the adversative or ranking system, the caregiving system, and the cooperative system regulate, respectively, the sexual, the antagonistic, the nurturant, and the cooperative aspects of human interactions. At least two of these systems seem to be summoned in the developmental sequels of early disorganized attachment: the caregiving system (George & Solomon, 2008) and the adversative system (Lichtenberg, 1989), that bears many similarities to Gilbert's (1989) ranking system (Gilbert calls "ranking system" the aspect of Lichtenberg's adversative system that intervenes in regulating competitive, antagonistic interactions whose aim is to define the rank of dominance and submission). The activation of the caregiving system in the service of a defensive inhibition of the attachment system yields controlling–caregiving strategies in the child. The activation of the ranking system lies at the root of controlling–punitive strategies (for the dynamic interplay between attachment and ranking motivations in distorted family communications, see Sloman, Atkinson, Milligan, & Liotti, 2002).

The defensive activation of another motivational system in response to an IWM of disorganized attachment should not necessarily be construed as a purely intrapsychic process. Rather, a few empirical observations suggest that the choice of the motivational system that defensively substitutes for the disorganized attachment system is influenced by the caregivers' attitudes. Parents who show frightened–frightening behaviors toward their children may also be more likely than other parents to display unusual arrays of submissive, care-seeking, or violently domineering behaviors together with caregiving (Hesse et al., 2003). Solomon and George (2006; Chapter 2, this volume) provided evidence of correlations between mothers' descriptions of their upbringing, their own child-rearing behaviors, and the type of controlling strategy shown by their child. George and Solomon (C. George, personal communication, November 21, 2007) are collecting data showing that controlling–punitive children are often in relationship with confrontational, punitive mothers, while controlling–caregiving children more often interact with fragile, "disappearing" mothers who seem in constant need of being nurtured back into the real world.

Dissociation as Collapse of the Controlling Strategies

The competitively aggressive or the caregiving interactions substituting for the activation of the attachment system limit the disassociating influence of the disorganized IWM on the child's current thought, emotion, and behavior. They, however, do not correct or cancel the IWM of disorganized attachment from the child's mind, as becomes obvious when the child's attachment system is activated by conditions that are able to overcome its relative inhibition. For instance, 6-year-old controlling children appear well oriented and organized in their thinking, behavioral, and attentional strategies until they are shown the pictures of a version of the Separation Anxiety Test (Main, Kaplan, & Cassidy, 1985). These pictures portray situations that are able to powerfully activate a child's attachment system (e.g., parents leaving a child alone). Once the system is thus activated, the formerly organized strategies of thought and behavior collapse in the controlling children: the underlying disorganization of their mental operations is suddenly revealed by the unrealistic, catastrophic, and *utterly incoherent* narratives generated in response to the pictures (an illustration of these narratives may be found in Hesse et al., 2003). Solomon et al. (1995) provided similar data, and emphasized the failure to terminate attachment themes that accompanies the catastrophic, chaotic, and disintegrated content of the doll-play stories narrated by controlling/disorganized children (the characters in the stories are left in a state of fright and despair because, e.g., the house blows up, the child dies, or a wicked witch kidnaps the child).

The collapse of the seemingly coherence-yielding strategy of controlling/disorganized children in the face of a powerful activation of the attachment system illustrates an important process in the pathogenesis of trauma-related disorders based on a disorganized IWM. The relative inhibition of the attachment system through the defensive activation of other equally inborn motivational systems (the caregiving, the social-ranking, and/or perhaps the sexual system, as may occur in some sexually abusive families) allows for coherent styles of relating. These relational styles can meet social approval and be appraised as pleasant and healthy (as it often happens with controlling–caregiving children), or on the contrary they can be regarded as problematic but not necessarily indicative of a disorder (as with controlling–punitive children). Adult survivors of childhood abuse and early attachment disorganization may therefore live a life that is not regarded as abnormal/pathological, either subjectively or by standard diagnostic psychiatric criteria, until the controlling strategy is forcefully suspended under the influence of a powerful stressor that activates the attachment system. This stressor need not necessarily be an obviously traumatic event: changes in the balance of affectional bonds because of separations or the making of new bonds can also activate the attachment system beyond the limit imposed on it by the controlling strategy. It is on these occasions that unmistakable psychopathological symptoms make their appearance. Because these symptoms imply emotional dysregulation, reduced mentalizing capacity, dissociative experiences (e.g., depersonalization, dissociative amnesias, trance-like states), and dramatic nonintegrated self-representations, they may lead to a diagnosis of dissociative or borderline disorder.

A particularly clear extraclinical example of how dissociated self-representations (previously unnoticed both by the person and by his or her relatives and doctors) can appear *in the context of an intense and durable activation of the attachment system* is provided by the Adult Attachment Interview (AAI) leading to the coding "Cannot Classify" (CC; Hesse, 1996). Sometimes, the response of the interviewed person that is coded CC is formally undistinguishable from the symptoms of a patient diagnosed as suffering from a dissociative identity disorder (Steele & Steele, 2003). Research findings in keeping with the hypothesis that dissociative symptoms emerge from a strong activation of the attachment system are emerging in a recent neuroimaging study (Buchheim,George, Kächele, Erk, & Walter, 2006; Buchheim & George, Chapter 13, this volume). Only subjects with unresolved–disorganized attachment showed increasing activation of medial temporal regions, including the amygdala and the hippocampus, in the course of attachment activation caused by the pictures of the Adult Attachment Projective (AAP: George & West, 2001). This pattern was demonstrated especially at the end of the AAP task, where the pictures are drawn to portray traumatic situations. The abnormal pattern of brain activity during the AAP task may be explained by dissociative processes and emotional dysregulation consequent to the activation of a disorganized IWM.

IMPLICATIONS FOR CLINICAL PRACTICE

The above overview of research findings and theoretical reflections concerning attachment disorganization is far from exhaustive (see the other chapters in this book). Its aim is to provide clinicians with the essential notions that enable them to understand, during their dialogues with patients suffering from trauma-related complex disorders, a series of interrelated clinical phenomena whose meaning becomes clearer when they are regarded as aspects of attachment disorganization. These phenomena can be summarized as follows:

1. Dissociative symptoms (and/or other types of nonintegrated, split representations of self-with-other) either appear or are exacerbated, both in the patient's life and within the therapeutic relationship, by events and interpersonal processes that bring on intense and durable activation of the attachment motivational system, previously inhibited through controlling strategies. That is, dissociative symptoms are contingent upon the activation of attachment needs, coincident with the collapse of controlling interpersonal strategies either of the compulsive caregiving or of the ranking (punitive) type. This implies that dissociative pathology is best understood in an intersubjective perspective (Lyons-Ruth, 1999, 2003).

2. Fear ("fright without solution") plays a key role, albeit often a concealed or utterly unconscious one, during difficult phases of the therapeutic relationship. Multiple simultaneous transferential responses (the drama triangle) are to be expected when fright without solution underpins the patient's construal of the therapeutic relationship. On the other hand, countertransferential fear—that is by no means unlikely given the proneness of these patients toward acting aggressively (Bradley & Westen, 2005)—can retraumatize the patient by re-creating the relational atmosphere of attachment disorganization (i.e., interaction with a frightened and therefore frightening attachment figure).

3. The IWM of disorganized attachment is likely to be segregated from consciousness, and operates only at the implicit level. This means that the therapists face, during the clinical dialogues, patients' interpersonal behaviors that are to be seen as enactments of elements of the disorganized IWM (Howell, 2005; Lyons-Ruth, 1999).

4. Since the patients' enactments are closely related to hindered mentalization (also contingent upon disorganized attachment), interventions that imply self-reflective abilities may not be understood properly by the patient in the beginning phases of the treatment. On the other side, empathic (or compassionate and solicitous) therapists' responses may open the road to intense activation of the patients' attachment system within the therapeutic relationship, and therefore to a worsening of symptoms and increasing relational difficulties in the clinical dialogue. This is because the attachment system is activated in any suffering person by appraisals of supportive availability in another interacting individual perceived as "stronger and/or wiser" than the self (Bowlby, 1979, p. 129), such as solicitous therapists are likely perceived by patients. In other words, two features are likely to activate the attachment system: fear and pain on the one side, and on the other side the perceived availability of empathy and support from another, well-known person. In the context of a strong and durable activation of the patients' attachment system within the therapeutic dialogue, the concurrent activation of a disorganized IWM, besides facilitating the surfacing of dramatic representations of self-with-other (the drama triangle), hinders the integrative, organizing functions of consciousness (metacognition is a key aspect of these functions). Research data supporting this hypothesis have been collected by Prunetti et al. (2008): at the beginning of their psychotherapy, patients with borderline personality disorder (BPD) tend to respond with reduced coherence of discourse to the therapist's empathic and emotionally supportive remarks, while their response to more neutral therapist's remarks are formally more coherent (if the therapy is successful, this paradoxical response subsides in later phases of the treatment).

5. Difficult-to-solve relational dilemmas are therefore the rule during

clinical dialogues with patients coming from histories of early disorganized attachment and later traumas. Therapists should strive, in the therapeutic relationship with these deeply suffering patients, for a difficult dialectical balance between sympathetic emotional closeness and a more egalitarian cooperative attitude of exploration and co-construction of new meaning structures. The knowledge of attachment disorganization is instrumental in achieving this balance, both in individual psychotherapy and in parallel integrated interventions where the treatment is conducted by different clinicians operating in separate settings (e.g., individual and group settings, as in dialectical behavior therapy [DBT] and in mentalization-based psychotherapy of BPD: Bateman & Fonagy, 2004; Linehan, 1993: cf. also Liotti, Cortina, & Farina, 2008).

A series of clinical vignettes will illustrate how the knowledge of the aspects of attachment disorganization summarized above may become of practical value during clinical work.

DISSOCIATION CONTINGENT UPON THE ACTIVATION OF THE ATTACHMENT SYSTEM

It is often held that dissociative symptoms, when they appear during the adult life of survivors of childhood abuse, should be explained as the reactivation of traumatic memories that had previously been defensively forgotten. A better explanation may be that life events (not necessarily traumatic ones) lead to a collapse of the controlling strategies that have until then kept at bay the full activation of the attachment system and of the disorganized IWM (Liotti, 2004, 2006). This explanation has its roots in Bowlby's idea that life events, not necessarily overtly traumatic, may reactivate a formerly segregated cognitive–emotional system, based on traumatic attachment experiences, and that such a reactivation may lead to feelings and behaviors that are utterly extraneous to the patient's usual sense of self (Bowlby, 1980).

Diana, a 32-year-old physician, had remembered throughout her life that her father had sexually abused her when she was a school-age child. Diana knew that her mother failed to protect her because she suffered from recurrent major depression since well before Diana was born. Depression is a possible maternal antecedent of attachment disorganization in the children (Radke-Yarrow, Cummings, Kuczynski, & Chapman, 1985; DeMulder & Radke-Yarrow, 1991; Teti, Gelfand, Messinger, & Isabella, 1995). We may therefore assume that Diana had been disorganized in her early attachments. Memories of Diana's childhood suggest that she developed a controlling–caregiving strategy in the relationship with her fragile mother.

The controlling–caregiving strategy may have later motivated her choice of profession.

Diana had reacted to the incest by making an adamant decision to protect her younger sister from her father's abusive behavior. For almost 20 years, she had been convinced of having been totally successful in this task. By devoting herself to preventing and alleviating other people's illnesses, she had also been able to attribute meaning to her own sufferings. As an adult, Diana never manifested either subjectively felt or observable dissociative symptoms. She did suffer from recurrent depressive episodes that, since when she was a medical student, she treated through self-prescriptions of antidepressant drugs (the tendency to avoid asking for other people's help when she felt depressed is a sign of an at least relative inhibition of the attachment system).

Diana was 32 years old when her sister, then 26, told her that she too had been sexually abused by their father. Immediately thereafter, Diana started having problems with memory, concentration, and sleep (she had terrifying nightmares). She also experienced episodes of derealization and depersonalization: she had the uncanny feeling of impending grotesque transformations both of outside reality and of her own body.

Diana's therapist, who was well aware both of the links between dissociation and disorganized attachment and of controlling strategies, focused on the interpretation of his patient's ailments as the consequence of a collapse of her controlling–caregiving strategy, which had been based on the representation of self as an almost omnipotent rescuer. The collapse followed the revelation that, contrary to what she had believed for almost 20 years, she had been unable to shelter her sister from her father's incestuous approaches. As a consequence, Diana lost confidence in her ability to take care of others, and realized that she too needed help and comfort. For the first time in her life, she asked for therapy. However, the experience of the need for help was frightening to her: it emerged in her consciousness together with fragmented, contradictory expectations of how her therapist would respond to it. For instance—as she gradually become able to reveal during the clinical dialogues—while regarding the therapist as available to provide sympathetic listening to her suffering, she also imagined that he could suddenly reveal himself as a "monsters of evilness," or that he would cease to listen empathically because he could begin to feel threatened by "such a difficult patient." To the therapist, Diana's ambivalent attitudes toward her psychotherapy were hints at the shifts between the multiple, dissociated representations of self and the source of help linked to her reactivated IWM of a disorganized attachment (the drama triangle).

Besides explaining the sudden appearance of dissociative symptoms in the patient's life, as illustrated by Diana's case, the activation of attachment motivations within the clinical dialogue may also explain the exacerbation of the patients' dissociative symptoms in the context of a therapeutic relationship that seems to evolve favorably. The following clinical vignette illustrates this possibility.

Rita is a 19-year-old girl suffering from bulimia nervosa comorbid with BPD. She is an adopted child. Her biological mother, suffering from schizophrenia, threw her in a bonfire when Rita was 3-years-old: an extreme instance of frightening maternal behavior. Rita still needs periodic interventions of plastic surgery to correct the consequences of the burns.

Rita had dropped out of two previous psychotherapies after a few sessions. The third attempt seemed more acceptable to her until when, after 3 months of regular attendance, she skipped two sessions without advance notice. During the following session, the therapist tried to understand what happened during the previous week, when Rita did not come for her sessions. She (quite confusedly) reported having had a continuous "dreaming" state where she was unable "to distinguish between dreams and reality." She reported having "met" people while in this state who could not really be there, while she "forgot" having met people living at home, including her adoptive parents. This experience frightened her so much that she decided to "stay in bed all the time" until she felt "connected" again. Rita also stated that she could not remember any immediate antecedent of this "dreaming" state. Her therapist insisted on asking Rita to remember the "real people" she had just met *before* entering the dissociative state:

THERAPIST: ... [IT] it should be frightening not to remember having met a single real human being in this week, since the people you remember having met in your room could not possibly have been there ... people from your past, I suppose.

RITA: Yeah ... somebody that now lives in another country. My mates in the orphanage. The nuns. [Rita spent 3 years in an orphanage before being adopted by adoptive parents who came from a foreign country.]

THERAPIST: Who is the last human being you remember having met before this horrible period began?

RITA: (*smiling*) You.

THERAPIST: It was me. What else is coming to your mind now?

RITA: It must have been a Friday afternoon.

THERAPIST: Yeah.

RITA: I do not remember anything else.

THERAPIST: Maybe that Friday while talking we stumbled upon something that was emotionally significant to you.

RITA: We talked of my adoptive parents ... and of my having been a child.

THERAPIST: Yeah, I too remember that we talked of your adoptive parents, and of your childhood before they adopted you.

RITA: And I remember that I was in my father's car, he was driving, my mother was sitting in the front and I in the back when we headed home from here [Rita's adoptive parents used to accompany her for the sessions and to wait in their car until the session ended.] There was a conversation among them.

THERAPIST: Do you remember now what they were saying?

RITA: They were worried, ... 'cause they had seen me crying. My mother said she never saw me crying....

The therapist thought that maybe, after 3 months of empathic listening during the clinical dialogues, Rita's attachment system had become active during the last session. Her longing for care and understanding had surfaced after years of chaotic and (on her part) aggressive exchanges with her adoptive parents. She was beginning to look at him as an attachment figure. The tears in her eyes when she was leaving the last session supported this hypothesis. Her adoptive parents, who were as usual waiting for her in the car at the end of the session, had witnessed with surprise these tears. Rita's attitude toward them (as it had been described both by the patient and by her adoptive mother during the incoming interview) had been "constantly defiant"—a stable controlling–punitive strategy leaves no room for tears. Thus—the therapist thought—the inhibition of the attachment system had been obtained through the activation of the dominance–submission (ranking) system. Now, within the therapeutic relationship, Rita's defiant attitude subsided (the controlling–punitive strategy based on the ranking system collapsed), leaving room for a long-forgotten wish to be helped and soothed. The surfacing of this need meant, however, that an IWM of disorganized attachment had also become active, all of a sudden, bringing with it the propensity toward dissociation. The dissociative episode could then be understood as contingent upon the activation of a previously dormant attachment motivation.

THE DRAMA TRIANGLE

When a patient disorganized attachment system is active during a session, it is likely that his or her narratives contain self-representations that are both dramatic and multiple, as in the drama triangle mentioned above. An example is provided in the continuation of Rita's session, when the therapist inquired about how his young patient had been able "to get out of her room" at the and of her dreaming state, in order to reach his office.

THERAPIST: What might have helped you, today, in getting out of bed and deciding to come and see me?

RITA: The new cat. My mother bought a kitten this morning, and I decided to accompany her to the store. (*Smiles.*)

THERAPIST: Are you fond of the kitten already?

RITA: Indeed. A female cat. Queer, ah …

THERAPIST: What, queer, the kitten?

RITA: Queer feeling. It seems as if I am betraying the other two cats, those who are dead now, but at the same time I am already fond of this kitten. Maybe I'll be able to take care of it. She is scared.

THERAPIST: The kitten is scared?

RITA: I am so big and she is so tiny. I am scaring her. But maybe it is my room. A large, large room, and she is so tiny. She may feel lost in such a large space. Maybe this time I'll be able to take care of the cat.

THERAPIST: You said "Maybe this time I'll be able to take care of the cat." You mean that you were not with the other two cats, those that are dead?

RITA: I was not able to feed them properly. I was rude with them. And I felt at a loss when they were ill.

The therapist construed this exchange as an expression of the fragmented IWM of attachment disorganization that was tacitly governing Rita's state of mind during the clinical dialogue. She perceived herself as (1) dangerous, and, in the attitude she attributed to the kitten, hostile ("rude," "scaring": the persecutor); (2) wishing to take care of the kitten ("Maybe this time I'll be able to take care": the caregiving rescuer); and (3) utterly helpless in the face of danger and pain ("I felt at a loss when they were ill": the victim). The possibility of such a multiple self-perception was evidenced by the literature on attachment disorganization the therapist was well aware of. For instance, he knew from the Solomon et al.'s (1995) doll-play study that some controlling–disorganized children show evidence of both representational models, caregiving (the rescuer) and punitive (the persecutor). They might switch during the doll play from constricted responses associated with caregiving to chaotic dysregulated ones associated with punitive attitudes.

FRIGHT WITHOUT SOLUTION

Fear, quite understandably, dominates the patients' state of mind during and after dissociative experiences, as the reported cases of Rita and Diana illustrate. The model of attachment disorganization, however, alerts clinicians to pay particular heed to the possibility that fear, in its particularly troublesome variant of "fright without solution," underlies those dissociative and borderline patients' relational experiences that are motivated by the attachment system, even when the interpersonal exchanges are momentarily angry, sad, or seemingly joyful and serene. Latent fear, in other words, is always to be expected, on the basis of the assumption that the patient's state of mind comes to be influenced by a disorganized IWM whenever the patient's motivation during the clinical dialogue is governed by the attachment system.

Ugo, 27 years old, had asked for psychotherapy in a tragic circumstance: he had been diagnosed as suffering from primary pulmonary hypertension (PPH), a fatal disease that usually leads to death within 5 years from the diagnosis, and whose only possible cure is a heart and lungs transplant (the prospects of a successful transplant, however, are not high). Ugo had suffered from BPD since his late teens. He had considered committing suicide repeatedly before receiving the PPH diagnosis. A previous psychotherapy did not help him significantly: he quit the treatment after some months with an unchanged intention to put an end to his life. His reason for a new psychotherapy was to reconstruct his life experiences, in order to achieve a less vague and less unpleasant sense of self. "Before dying," he said, "I wish to know who I really am."

During the intake interview, Ugo stated quite clearly that he was planning to refuse the transplant (indicated when heart failure, about 2–3 years from the diagnosis in most cases of PPH, becomes imminent). He was determined to avoid both the pain of surgery and the anxieties linked to its low probability of success. He had wished, for years, to put an end to his life, and now the prospect of dying within a few years came, in part, as a relief. His therapist usually followed the prescription of the dialectic behavioral model of psychotherapy with patients with BPD who were suicidal (Linehan, 1993): namely, to begin psychotherapy only after the patients have signed a contract stating that they renounce committing suicide during the planned 2 years of treatment. However, to ask for such an explicit contract seemed illogical in the face of his idea *not* to commit suicide, but simply to let his illness run its inevitable course.

During the first months of psychotherapy Ugo came, as many patients with BPD do, to idealize his therapist: he felt deeply understood, accepted, and well guided in the exploration of his past life experiences. The therapist was inclined to regard this idealization as the outward sign of a progressive activation of his patient's attachment system within the therapeutic relationship. Having reasons for expecting that the early IWM was disorganized (Ugo reported that his mother had suffered from recurrent major depression since after her marriage), the therapist was, in the same period, looking for any sign in the clinical dialogue that could foretell either a state of latent fear within the seemingly pleasant dialogue (fright without solution) or the surfacing of fragmented interpersonal perceptions linked to the drama triangle. There was one sign that—beyond his idealizing attitude and his seemingly relaxed (sometimes even joyful) mood during the clinical dialogues—less pleasant feelings were present in Ugo's mind while he interacted with the therapist. It was the moist, cold hand the therapist felt while shaking hands at the end of each session (a customary formal substitute for saying goodbye in Italy). This could be the indication of latent anxiety during the session, but it could also be understood as a symptom of Ugo's poor circulatory and respiratory balance.

During the fourth month of psychotherapy explicit signs of discomfort suddenly appeared in the clinical dialogue. Ugo began to hint at the emerging idea that it was pointless to wait till the illness ran its fatal course. In the following sessions, he repeatedly expressed self-attacking thoughts that grew quickly in intensity to the point that he come to despise himself quite crudely. Then Ugo stated with strong, convincing determination that he had decided to kill himself soon. Every attempt the therapist made at expressing disagreement with Ugo's violent self-attacks and at trying to convince him to give up suicidal intentions was sternly rejected. Ugo, however, added to his dismissal of the therapist's arguments that his psychotherapeutic experience had been a very positive one, and that he wished to continue the dialogue until the very last days of his life: "I will come here til the very end, 'till I'll eventually kill myself."

The therapist thought that, by expressing self-disgust, Ugo might be unconsciously testing a pathogenic belief (Weiss, 1993) stemming from his IWM of disorganized attachment, namely, to be such a bad person (the "persecutor") as to be an unbearable burden to any attachment figure. By threatening suicide, Ugo might unconsciously test his belief that attachment figures would feel relieved by his disappearing from this world. The therapist imagined that such a belief could stem from Ugo's construing, as a child, the depression of his mother as caused by his misbehavior. On the basis of such an hypothesis, the therapist decided to offer a strong refutation of the pathogenic beliefs he supposed were underlying Ugo's self-despising and suicidal ideation. The therapist stated that he had tacitly accepted, at the beginning of the treatment, Ugo's expressed intention to renounce the transplant once it could had been offered to him as an extreme attempt at saving his life. Now, however, the therapist thought that such a tacit acceptance had been a mistake, and that he wanted to correct it: the therapist asked explicitly for Ugo's commitment not only to renounce committing suicide, but also to dispose himself to accept the prospect of the transplant. The reason the therapist offered to Ugo for this request was that life is more important than any relationship, however good the relationship might be, since there is no possible relationship when there is no life anymore. If, therefore, Ugo thought (as he seemed to do) that the relationship with the therapist was more important than his own life, their dialogue would be based on such a logical and affective paradox that it could not possibly be productive. In order to go on with their dialogue, this paradox should have been dismissed by accepting first to live as long as possible.

Ugo reacted to the challenge with sheer rage. When he somehow calmed down, he said that the therapist had betrayed him, and that he would quit the treatment. The therapist disagreed: he could not have possibly betrayed their shared therapeutic contract, since Ugo had not been able to refute the idea that to regard a relationship as more important than life is an unmanageable paradox. Therefore, he would have waited for Ugo on the next scheduled appointment, and would remain committed to their joint enterprise at least until Ugo could show him that it is not paradoxical to value a relationship in which one is involved more than one values his own life. Ugo came to the next session, seemingly only to state again that he was determined to quit the treatment. He also restated energetically his disappointment for having lost forever the possibility of a dialogue, which had been so free and accepting as to have constituted the best experience in his life. The therapist replied that he was convinced that their dialogue should continue, at least until Ugo could prove that a dialogue could be more important than life. Ugo was still saying "I'll not come to the next session" while he and the therapist shook hands at the end of their meeting. And then the therapist noticed that, for the first time since he had first met Ugo, his patient's hand was warm and dry. Ugo's hand witnessed that he had been, but now was no longer afraid of meeting his therapist.

Thus, the therapist thought, the possibility of resorting to a controlling–punitive strategy during the angry exchanges with his therapist could have afforded a defensive way of keeping at bay the fearful mental states linked to attachment disorganization. When Ugo seemed relatively serene in the clinical dialogue, he was instead deeply frightened because of the activation of disorganized attachment, not defensively modulated by a controlling strategy, that was reproducing the original mental state of fright without solution within the therapeutic relationship. Furthermore, Ugo might have been unconsciously harboring a pathogenic belief, linked to his disorganized IWM, that attachment figures (such as now the therapist was to him) would have somehow welcomed his disappearing from their world. By not having explicitly challenged at the beginning of the treatment Ugo's intention to avoid the transplant, the therapist had not provided any hint that could refute this pathogenic belief. Now the belief had been efficiently refuted. Ugo, while feeling disappointed at the conscious level of mental activity, was not experiencing any more, at the unconscious level, the fear of being destined to afflict, because of his equally unbearable suffering, his attachment figures—people whom he desperately needed—with an equally unbearable suffering. Ugo's warm and dry hand during the last clinical dialogue bore witness to his having found a way out of his relational dilemma linked to his disorganized attachment state.

Further evidence that the therapist's intervention had hit an important therapeutic target came with the following session, when Ugo both affirmed that he had decided to continue in the treatment and reported, for the first time, his worrying over his mother's physical illness and over her lifelong depression that was now inducing her to refuse dieting. Since his mother was obese and suffering from diabetes and hypertension, her decision not to diet was equivalent to committing a slow type of suicide, Ugo said of his mother. He then recalled how much he had been distressed by his mother's explicit threats to commit suicide when he was a child (a traumatic memory that had never surfaced before). This theme immediately allowed for important insights. It became clear then that a "transformation from passive to active" (Weiss, 1993) had taken place within the therapeutic relationship. Ugo unconsciously reproduced the central theme of his relationship to his primary attachment figure within the therapeutic relationship, which led to his enactment: he had behaved toward the therapist in a way similar to his mother's behavior toward himself when he was a child. Witnessing the difference between his reaction to his mother's threats to kill herself and the therapist's response to Ugo's suicidal threats, a radical change begun to take place in Ugo's attitudes toward life, suicide, and attachment relationships. This change was accompanied by a spontaneous insight on the origins of his previous attitudes, as predicted by the research on the therapeutic process produced by the San Francisco Psychotherapy Research Group (Weiss, 1993).

The reader may be interested in knowing that Ugo's treatment proceeded without interruptions and without further idealization or devaluation of the therapist for the following 4 years, until Ugo, who in the meantime had asked to be listed in a national waiting list for heart–lung transplants, died of heart failure before a suitable donor had been found.

RELATIONAL DILEMMAS AND PARALLEL INTERVENTIONS

Fright without solution is the likely source of typical dilemmas within the therapeutic relationship. Blizard (2001), Holmes (2004), and Van der Hart et al. (2006) have discussed these relational dilemmas using attachment theory in different but converging perspectives. While the patient oscillates between "phobia of attachment" to and abnormally clinging dependency on the therapist (Van der Hart et al., 2006), the therapist feels that every clinical choice leads to a blind alley. For instance, searching for meaning in the clinical dialogue may be the only way of increasing the patient's sense of security, but at the same time the very words used in such a quest for meaning may arouse terrifying memories of attachment trauma (Holmes, 2004).

Having two therapists engaged in the treatment, in two parallel settings, for the more severely disordered patients—as suggested by the guidelines of the American Psychiatric Association (2001) for the treatment of BPD—may assist in protecting the therapeutic program from the risk of premature interruptions caused by these relational dilemmas. Parallel interventions offer precious opportunities for corrective relational experiences that do not require in advance the use of mentalization capacities, but can foster these capacities when one therapist helps the patient in the process of elaborating the difficulties in the other therapeutic relationship (Liotti et al., 2008). The two-therapists model, however, is a double-edged weapon since it may easily become "a recipe for dangerous splitting with one professional being idealized and the other denigrated" (Bateman & Fonagy, 2004, p. 146). In order to achieve corrective relational experiences rather than to instigate dangerous splitting, the knowledge of attachment dynamics suggest that the idealized therapist (T1) understands the patients' devaluing of the other therapist (T2) as an aspect of the possible activation of the disorganized IWM. As a consequence of such an understanding, T1 strives to cooperate on equal grounds with the patient *toward the very same goal that is now hindered in the relationship with T2*, carefully avoiding taking sides, however subtly, with the patient against T2 and interpreting the reported problems in the other therapeutic relationship. The advantages of a therapeutic strategy based on the active search for cooperative exchanges between T1 and the patient when the disorganized IWM is surfacing in the therapeutic relationship with T2 are illustrated by an incident taking place in the first phase of Bianca's treatment.

Bianca, a 26-year-old patient with BPD, had tried to kill herself three times in the past 4 years. She also tried to strangle her mother with a telephone wire, and had threatened her father with a knife. She suffered from dissociative amnesias and sudden, terrific blank spells (states of mental emptiness). Because of the risk of repeating suicidal or homicidal acts, Bianca was referred to a treatment entailing partial hospitalization.

In the first assessment session Bianca reported to the referring psychiatrist a vague, confused memory: she had been induced by her paternal grandmother, when she was a school-age child, to masturbate her younger brother, then still a toddler. Bianca's mother confirmed these memories to the referring psychiatrist in a further assessment session. She reported that she refused to believe Bianca's first (and only) timid attempt at telling her that "something was happening" when she (then 6 years old) and her 3-year-old brother were left in the grandma's care. Two years later Bianca's mother dramatically discovered the reality of the sexual abuse her daughter had tried to reveal: on coming back home unexpectedly, she saw her children, both naked, caressing each other's genitals while the old woman and her lover were "showing them how to do it" and were commenting on the sexual excitement children may feel or not feel. She stopped thereafter leaving the children in the custody of her mother-in-law, but—fearing that to do so could lead to a divorce—never reported the abuse to her husband. The relationship with her husband deteriorated, notwithstanding her silence on the abuse. Bianca, during her childhood, had repeated opportunities to witness physical violence between her parents.

Relevant to a formulation of the case according to attachment theory is the information that the paternal grandmother was the main attachment figure in the first years of Bianca's life: Shortly after Bianca's birth her mother suffered a miscarriage in the fourth month of pregnancy, became depressed, and later on was bedridden in an attempt to preserve a new pregnancy from the risk of miscarriage. During this period of time, Bianca was left almost exclusively in the care of her grandmother. Since the grandmother had been diagnosed as suffering from bipolar depression, and Bianca's mother was grieving over a loss that was obviously unresolved during Bianca's infancy, one can hypothesize that Bianca's early attachments to her two primary attachment figures had been disorganized. The mother's description of Bianca's relational style toward her parents during her childhood suggested that the child had resorted to a controlling–punitive strategy in order to cope with attachment disorganization.

Bianca's treatment was based on an individual and a group setting, involving two different therapists. In the group settings, the participants' emotions were discussed according to a plan of exploration of different aspects (modules) of emotional experience. At the end of each group session, the patients were assigned homework, in order to reinforce their understanding of the module that had been the theme of the group session. During the individual sessions, each patient had the opportunity of commenting on her experience in the group: individual sessions were explicitly aimed at applying to various aspects of the patient's life the skills acquired in the group (cf. Linehan, 1993).

During the first 2 months of treatment, Bianca openly appreciated both the individual and the group sessions. Then a dialogue took place between the individual psychotherapist (T1) and Bianca, where she for the first time commented negatively on her relationship with the group therapist (T2). At the very beginning of this individual session Bianca stated, quite confusedly but with unmistakable anger, that she understood what was going on in the group sessions as an attempt at making her feel what she *could not feel*. This was an evident distortion of the meaning of the group psychopedagogic techniques, aimed merely at familiarizing all the participants with the observation and description of basic emotions, their antecedents, and their consequences. Then Bianca added: "You know, I'm getting confused in this place. I don't know who I am anymore. All I feel is one big confusion. I mean Dr. Q [T2] is going 'bang-bang-bang!' That is, I feel as if I were just a bag of rubbish that's being filled up with all sorts of things.... I will not accept this anymore. In the last group session, I think I really made Dr. Q get a bit mad at me."

T1 listened to Bianca's statement, thinking that it was a distortion of the meaning of the therapeutic dialogue possibly caused by Bianca's traumatic memories: maybe Bianca was construing T2's comments on how to observe one's own emotional experience according to the memory of the grandmother suggesting sexual feelings to children that "*could not feel*" them. This would also mean that the IWM of disorganized attachment toward the grandmother was surfacing in the therapeutic relationship with T2. Besides, T1 thought that maybe the patient was trying to keep at bay the disoriented–disorganized state of mind ("I'm getting confused") through her usual controlling–punitive strategy ("I really made Dr. Q get a bit mad at me"). On the basis of this line of reasoning, T1 decided to avoid any type of intervention that could further activate either the patient's attachment system (because it was disorganized) or her ranking system (because it was used defensively in a controlling–punitive strategy). A possible way out of the risk of further activating either the attachment or the ranking system was to concentrate on the cooperative enterprise of examining, together with Bianca, the emotional module proposed in the group setting that was the object of the patient's expressed perplexity. Before proceeding to this task, however, T1 explored how Bianca was feeling at the moment, thinking that if she reported emotions related to fear this would support the hypothesis that an IWM of disorganized attachment was surfacing in the therapeutic relationship.

THERAPIST: How are you feeling just now?

BIANCA: I'm feeling a bit nervous. This is anxiety ... because when I speak quickly ... yes, I'm feeling a bit anxious ... also in the chaos of the group I get disorientated and I find myself saying, "But here, who am I?" That is, I no longer know who I am; I find it hard to understand where my problem lies, and what the goal is that I have to attain. But you know, it's true: I don't feel these emotions; but then, it seems to be quite the opposite, and then in the end I can actually feel some emotions. So why do they tell me I can't feel them? Eh? Well, maybe I can't after all ... and when I feel them, I say, "Oh, damn, here's another emotion! ... Wham! ... Oh, God, and now what do I do?" I shut it out. I can't feel emotions ... I mean, I'm a bit panicky about all of this!

T1 thought that, "in the chaos of the group," Bianca had felt protected by T2; the activation of the attachment system toward T2 might have
caused the disorganized IWM to surface; the fear she was reporting ("This
is anxiety"; "I'm a bit panicky") was, then, an emotion related to attachment disorganization. These thoughts confirmed T1 in her decision to pursue a cooperative exchange with her patient. A success in this task could
create the basis for a corrective relational experience, showing implicitly
to the patient that shifting from attachment to a controlling–punitive interpersonal strategy is not the only way out of (1) fear without solution and
(2) disorientation–disorganization in interactions motivated by attachment
needs. This is how T1 proceeded in the dialogue:

THERAPIST: You know, Bianca, while you're speaking to me I'm thinking
    about the fact that a week ago you mentioned things that were quite
    the opposite of what you're saying today.

BIANCA: Well, yes, because I've been thinking about it.

THERAPIST: Definitely. But what I mean is, your thinking that this way of pro-
    ceeding was helping you a lot and was somehow giving you a frame-
    work you could put everything in; you spoke to me about a series of
    things ...

BIANCA: Yes, but not the emotional module ... because I've always had prob-
    lems with the emotional module.

THERAPIST: All right. Let's try to understand all of this to find out which way
    we have to go. You're saying two things in particular: on the one hand,
    "Perhaps I don't need this emotional module because I'm running the
    risk of turning something I feel spontaneously into a technical process."
    Is that right?

BIANCA: Yes, that's a possible hypothesis.

THERAPIST: That's one hypothesis. Then there's the other hypothesis—and I
    don't know whether you said it yourself or whether I've begun thinking it
    on account of what you've just said—which is almost quite the opposite;
    and that is, we're touching on a point you're having difficulty with.

BIANCA: So what do I have to do?

THERAPIST: Precisely! What do *we* have to do? We have to try to start seeing
    the light in all this confusion. Perhaps right now, you shouldn't try to
    do anything specific. What I mean is, if you go into a crisis state when
    you do one of the modules ... how can I put it ... you can just let it be
    for the moment.

The patient's question "What should *I* have to do?" is, it should be
noticed, a ranking question, that is, it entails perceiving T1 as a dominant

person who is in the position of giving directions as to what Bianca is supposed to do. T1 thought that to accept enacting the dominant role, by suggesting what Bianca could do instead of completing her homework on the emotional module, would have implied the type of interaction between a dominant and a submissive individual that is typical of controlling–punitive strategies. Therefore, in order to create a type of interpersonal exchange as far removed as possible from the influence of Bianca's disorganized attachment and controlling strategy, T1 reformulated, implicitly, the roles in the relationships by stating that she was looking at their interactions as a cooperative one ("What do *we* have to do?"). The dialogue that followed suggested that T1's intervention had been successful: suddenly, Bianca's attack about the homework and about the psychotherapy came to an end.

BIANCA: You know, I can do the homework, but I don't seem to be able to grasp the main thing ... the emotions. I don't know ... and I say, "But what the devil do these guys want with this question?" I don't know.

THERAPIST: Where is it you feel you can't make it in this module, ... in these handouts?

BIANCA: It's difficult to explain ... the only thing I know is that some feelings are fast, and that's it! And in a certain sense it's the only way I have of experiencing emotions. I can't write them down as the homework intends I do.

THERAPIST: Can you tell me about the last emotion you felt?

BIANCA: Well, ... yesterday I felt afraid. I was coming back from the cinema; I was walking alone, and there was a dog ... and a woman on a bicycle. They passed by very close to me and I got alarmed. I thought it was a man. I don't know ... and I felt my muscles becoming taut and my cheeks were burning and got red ... and my heart started beating faster.

THERAPIST: Why don't we look at one of the handouts for the emotional module ...

BIANCA: Which one?

THERAPIST: Let's take a look together. Shall we give it a try ... do you feel up to it?

BIANCA: Okay.

The remaining part of the session confirmed the drastic change in Bianca's mentalizing capacity coincident with the activation of the cooperative motivational system within the clinical dialogue. Bianca, now in an exploratory rather than a controlling–punitive mood, asked the therapist to examine with her another instance of emotional experience, involving a recent episode of painful–angry interaction with her mother. The joint exploration of this episode provided useful insights on the controlling–punitive interactions between Bianca and her mother that regularly followed interactions where Bianca expected to be helped and her mother, after having provided a beginning caregiving response, quickly shifted to a subtly or openly aggressive attitude toward her daughter. The difference in the exercise of mentalizing capacity between the second part of the session and the first one—when the patient was motivated by her attachment system and was trying to keep the disorganized state of mind at bay through the activation of the competitive-ranking system (controlling–punitive strategy)—is remarkable.

This clinical vignette exemplifies a formulation, based on attachment theory, of the typical problem that faces psychotherapists treating patients with BPD or with dissociative disorders: while their traumatic memories and their disorganized IWM distort the construing of the therapeutic dialogue, the metacognitive (or mentalizing) deficit hampers the fruition of any intervention that addresses the patient's capacity for self-reflection. Since this problem is linked to the reactivation of a disorganized IWM and of controlling strategies involving the caregiving, the ranking, and the sexual systems, the therapist may solve it by resorting to relational attitudes that foster cooperative exchanges, that is, by using the only basic motivational system that is not negatively influenced by early attachment disorganization and its developmental sequels in traumatic environments. Opportunities for cooperative patient–therapist interactions may be offered by parallel integrated treatments. When the exercise of cooperative interactions has yielded sufficient corrective relational experiences and related insights, the IWM of disorganized attachment can be consciously revised within the therapeutic dialogue.

CONCLUDING REMARKS

The clinical illustrations and comments in the above paragraphs are not meant to assert that an understanding of complex disorders based on attachment disorganization provides guidelines for treatment that lead to more favorable psychotherapy outcomes with respect to other approaches. In order to support such an assertion, controlled outcomes studies are mandatory, and these studies are, at the present moment, altogether lacking.

It is interesting, however, to remark that the mentalization-based treatment (MBT) for BPD, that has been proved effective by controlled outcome and follow-up studies (Bateman & Fonagy, 2004), involves an understanding of attachment dynamics in general, and attachment disorganization in particular, among its theoretical underpinnings. The basic strategy of DBT—whose efficacy in the treatment of BPD has also been evidenced by controlled studies and 2-year follow-up (Linehan, 1993; Linehan et al., 2006)—may be understood in terms of attachment theory (for this understanding, see Liotti, 2007, pp. 153–159). Furthermore, the outcomes of the transference-focused psychotherapy of BPD, that seems as successful as MBT and DBT in a comparative study, has been assessed with regard to changes in the patients' attachment patterns. The findings of this study (Levy et al., 2006) are compatible with the idea that attachment disorganization plays a key role in many cases of BPD. Thus, there is at least indirect evidence that a proper understanding of attachment disorganization may be of great practical importance to psychotherapists dealing with complex disorders characterized by chaotic and dramatic interpersonal styles. The clinical vignettes in this chapter provide illustrations of the manifold guidelines provided by the knowledge of attachment disorganization that may orient, in daily clinical practice, the therapist's choices during clinical dialogues. It is the author's hope that detailed single-case studies of adult psychotherapies based on attachment theory may yield more such illustrations in the not-too-distant future.

REFERENCES

American Psychiatric Association. (1994). *Diagnostic and statistical manual of mental disorders* (4th ed.). Washington, DC: Author.

American Psychiatric Association (2001). Practice guideline for the treatment of patients with borderline personality disorder. *American Journal of Psychiatry, 158*(Oct. Suppl.), 1–52.

Amini, F., Lewis, T., Lannon, R., Louie, A., Baumbacher, G., McGuinnes, T., et al. (1996). Affect, attachment, memory: Contributions toward psychobiologic integration. *Psychiatry, 59*, 213–239.

Bateman, A. W., & Fonagy, P. (2004). *Psychotherapy for borderline personality disorder: Mentalization based treatment*. Oxford, UK: Oxford University Press.

Blizard, R. A. (2001). Masochistic and sadistic ego states: Dissociative solutions to the dilemma of attachment to an abusive caregiver. *Journal of Trauma and Dissociation, 2*, 37–58.

Blizard, R. A. (2008). The role of double binds, reality testing and chronic relational trauma in the genesis and treatment of borderline personality disorder. In A. Moskowitz, I. Schaefer, & M. J. Dorahy (Eds.), *Psychosis, trauma and dissociation* (pp. 295–306). London: Wiley-Blackwell.

Bowlby, J. (1979). *The making and breaking of affectional bonds*. London: Tavistock.

Bowlby, J. (1980). *Attachment and loss: Vol. 3. Loss: Sadness and depression*. London: Hogarth Press.

Bradley, R., Jeney, J., & Westen, D. (2005). Etiology of borderline personality disorder:Disentangling the contribution of interrelated antecedents. *Journal of Mental and Nervous Disease, 193*, 24–31.

Bradley, R., & Westen, D. (2005). The psychodynamic of borderline personality disorder: A view from developmental psychopathology. *Development and Psychopathology, 17,* 927–957.

Bromberg, P. M. (2009). Multiple self-states, the relational mind, and dissociation: A psychoanalytic perspective. In P. F. Dell & J. A. O'Neill (Eds.), *Dissociation and the dissociative disorders: DSM-V and beyond* (pp. 637–661). New York: Routledge.

Buchheim, A., George, C., Kächele, H., Erk, S., & Walter, H. (2006). Measuring attachment representation in an fMRI environment: Concepts and assessment. *Psychopathology, 39,* 136–143.

Carlson, E. A. (1998). A prospective longitudinal study of disorganized/disoriented attachment. *Child Development, 69,* 1970–1979.

DeMulder, E. K., & Radke-Yarrow, M. (1991). Attachment with affectively ill and well mothers: Concurrent behavioral correlates. *Development and Psychopathology, 3,* 227–242.

Dozier, M., Stovall-McClough, K. C., & Albus, K. E. (2008). Attachment and psychopathology in adulthood. In J. Cassidy & P. R. Shaver (Eds.), *Handbook of attachment: Theory, research, and clinical applications* (2nd. ed., pp. 718–744). New York: Guilford Press.

Fonagy, P. (2002). Multiple voice versus meta-cognition: An attachment theory perspective. In V. Sinason (Ed.), *Attachment, trauma and multiplicity: Working with dissociative identity disorder* (pp. 71–85). Hove, UK: Brunner-Routledge.

Fonagy, P., Target, M., Gergely, G., Allen, J. G., & Bateman, A. W. (2003). The developmental roots of borderline personality disorder in early attachment relationships: A theory and some evidence. *Psychoanalytic Inquiry, 23,* 412–459.

George, C., & Solomon, J. (2008). The caregiving system: A behavioral systems approach to parenting. In J. Cassidy & P. R. Shaver (Eds.), *Handbook of attachment: Theory, research, and clinical applications* (2nd ed., pp. 833–856). New York: Guilford Press,

George, C., & West, M. (2001). The development and preliminary validation of a new measure of adult attachment: The Adult Attachment Projective. *Attachment and Human Development, 3,* 55–86.

Gilbert, P. (1989). *Human nature and suffering.* London: LEA.

Gold, S. N. (2000). *Not trauma alone: Therapy for child abuse survivors in family and social context.* Philadelphia: Brunner/Routledge.

Gunderson, J. C., & Sabo, A. (1993). The phenomenological and conceptual interface between borderline personality disorder and post-traumatic stress disorder. *American Journal of Psychiatry, 150,* 19–27.

Hesse, E. (1996). Discourse, memory and the Adult Attachment Interview: A note with emphasis on the emerging cannot classify category. *Infant Mental Health Journal, 17,* 4–11.

Hesse, E., & Main, M. (2000). Disorganized infant, child and adult attachment: Collapse in behavioral and attentional strategies. *Journal of the American Psychoanalytic Association, 48,* 1097–1127.

Hesse, E., Main, M., Abrams, K. Y., & Rifkin, A. (2003). Unresolved states regarding loss or abuse can have "second-generation" effects: Disorganized, role-inversion and frightening ideation in the offspring of traumatized non-maltreating parents. In D. J. Siegel & M. F. Solomon (Eds.), *Healing trauma: Attachment, mind, body and brain* (pp. 57–106). New York: Norton.

Hesse, E., & van IJzendoorn, M. H. (1999). Propensities toward absorption are related to lapses in the monitoring of reasoning or discourse during the Adult Attachment Interview: A preliminary investigation. *Attachment and Human Development, 1,* 67–91.

Holmes, J. (1996). *Attachment, intimacy, autonomy: Using attachment theory in adult psychotherapy.* Northville, NJ: Jason Aronson.

Holmes, J. (2004). Disorganized attachment and borderline personality disorder: A clinical perspective. *Attachment and Human Development, 6,* 181–190.

Howell, E. F. (2005). *The dissociative mind.* London: Analytic Press.

Karpman, S. (1968). Fairy tales and script drama analysis. *Transactional Analysis Bulletin, 7,* 39–43.

Levy, K. N. (2005). The implications of attachment theory and research for understanding borderline personality disorder. *Development and Psychopathology, 17,* 959–986.

Levy, K. N., Meehan, K. B., Kelly, K. M., Reynoso, J. S., Weber, M., Clarkin, J. F., & et al. (2006). Change in attachment patterns and reflective function in a randomized control trial of transference-focused psychotherapy for borderline personality disorder. *Journal of Consulting and Clinical Psychology, 74,* 1027–1040.

Lichtenberg, J. D. (1989). *Psychoanalysis and motivation.* Hillsdale, NJ: Analytic Press.

Lieberman, A. F. (2004). Traumatic stress and attachment: Reality and internalization in disorders of infant mental health. *Infant Mental Health Journal, 25,* 336–351.

Linehan, M. M. (1993). *Cognitive-behavioral treatment of borderline personality disorder.* New York: Guilford Press.

Linehan, M. M., Comtois, K. A., Murray, A. M., Brown, M. Z., Gallopp, R. J., et al. (2006). Two-years randomized control trial and follow-up of dialectical behaviour therapy vs. therapy by experts for suicidal behaviours and borderline personality disorder. *Archives of General Psychiatry, 63,* 757–766.

Liotti, G. (1992). Disorganized/disoriented attachment in the etiology of the dissociative disorders. *Dissociation, 5,* 196–204.

Liotti, G. (1993). Disorganized attachment and dissociative experiences: An illustration of the developmental–ethological approach to cognitive therapy. In K. T. Kuehlvein & H. Rosen (Eds.), *Cognitive therapies in action* (pp. 213–239). San Francisco: Jossey-Bass.

Liotti, G. (1995). Disorganized/disoriented attachment in the psychotherapy of the dissociative disorders. In S. Goldberg, R. Muir, & J. Kerr (Eds.), *Attachment theory: Social, developmental, and clinical perspectives* (pp. 343–363). Hillsdale, NJ: Analytic Press.

Liotti, G. (1999). Understanding the dissociative processes: The contribution of attachment theory. *Psychoanalytic Inquiry, 19,* 757–783.

Liotti, G. (2004). Trauma, dissociation and disorganized attachment: Three strands of a single braid. *Psychotherapy: Theory, Research, Practice, Training, 41,* 472–486.

Liotti, G. (2006). A model of dissociation based on attachment theory and research. *Journal of Trauma and Dissociation, 7,* 55–74.

Liotti, G. (2007). Internal working models of attachment in the therapeutic relationship. In P. Gilbert & R. L. Leahy (Eds.), *The therapeutic relationship in the cognitive-behavioral psychotherapies* (pp. 143–162). London: Routledge.

Liotti, G., Cortina, M., & Farina, B. (2008). Attachment theory and the multiple integrated treatment of borderline personality disorder. *Journal of the American Academy of Psychoanalysis and Dynamic Psychiatry, 36,* 293–312.

Liotti, G., Pasquini, P., & the Italian Group for the Study of Dissociation. (2000). Predictive factors for borderline personality disorder: Patients' early traumatic experiences and losses suffered by the attachment figure. *Acta Psychiatrica Scandinavica, 102,* 282–289.

Lyons-Ruth, K. (1999). The two-person unconscious: Intersubjective dialogue, enactive relational representation, and the emergence of new forms of relational organization. *Psychoanalytic Inquiry, 19,* 576–617.

Lyons-Ruth, K. (2003). Dissociation and the parent–infant dialogue: A longitudinal perspective from attachment research. *Journal of the American Psychoanalytic Association, 51,* 883–911.

Lyons-Ruth, K., & Jacobvitz, D. (2008). Attachment disorganization: Genetic factors, parenting contexts and developmental transformations from infancy to adulthood. In J. Cassidy & P. R. Shaver (Eds.), *Handbook of attachment* (2nd ed., pp. 666–697). New York: Guilford Press.

Lyons-Ruth, K., Melnick, S., Patrick, M., & Hobson, R. P. (2007). A controlled study of hostile–helpless states of mind among borderline and dysthymic women. *Attachment and Human Development, 9,* 1–16.

Lyons-Ruth, K., Yellin, C., Melnick, S., & Atwood, G. (2005). Expanding the concept of unresolved mental states: Hostile/helpless states of mind on the Adult Attachment Interview are associated with disrupted mother–infant communication and infant disorganization. *Development and Psychopathology, 17,* 1–23.

Main, M. (1991). Metacognitive knowledge, metacognitive monitoring, and singular (coherent) versus multiple (incoherent) models of attachment. In C. M. Parkes, J. Stevenson-Hinde, & P. Marris (Eds.), *Attachment across the life cycle* (pp. 127–160). London: Routledge.

Main, M., & Hesse, E. (1990). Parents' unresolved traumatic experiences are related to infant disorganized attachment status: Is frightened and/or frightening parental behavior the linking mechanism? In M. T. Greenberg, D. Cicchetti, & E. M. Cummings (Eds.), *Attachment in the preschool years* (pp. 161–182). Chicago: University of Chicago Press.

Main, M., Kaplan, N., & Cassidy, J. (1985). Security in infancy, childhood and adulthood: A move to the level of representation. *Monographs of the Society for Research in Child Development, 50,* 66–104.

Main, M., & Morgan, H. (1996). Disorganization and disorientation in infant Strange Situation behavior: Phenotypic resemblance to dissociative states? In L. Michelson & W. Ray (Eds.), *Handbook of dissociation* (pp. 107–137). New York: Plenum Press.

Ogawa, J. R., Sroufe, L. A., Weinfield, N. S., Carlson, E. A., & Egeland, B. (1997).

Development and the fragmented self: Longitudinal study of dissociative symptomatology in a nonclinical sample. *Development and Psychopathology, 9,* 855–879.

Paris, J. (1995). Memories of abuse in borderline patients: True or false? *Harvard Review of Psychiatry, 3,* 10–17.

Pasquini, P., Liotti, G., Mazzotti, E., Fassone, G., Picardi, A., & the Italian Group for the Study of Dissociation. (2002). Risk factors in the early family life of patients suffering from dissociative disorders. *Acta Psychiatrica Scandinavica, 105,* 110–116.

Prunetti, E., Framba, R., Barone, L., Fiore, D., Sera, F., & Liotti, G. (2008). Attachment disorganization and borderline patients' metacognitive responses to therapists' expressed understanding of their state of mind: A pilot study. *Psychotherapy Research, 18,* 28–36.

Radke-Yarrow, M., Cummings, E. M., Kuczynski, L., & Chapman, M. (1985). Patterns of attachment in two- and three-year olds in normal families and families with parental depression. *Child Development, 56,* 884–893.

Schore, A. N. (2009). Attachment trauma and the developing right brain: Origins of pathological dissociation. In P. F. Dell & J. A. O'Neill (Eds.), *Dissociation and the dissociative disorders: DSM-V and beyond* (pp. 107–141). New York: Routledge.

Simeon, D. (2009). Depersonalization disorder. In P. F. Dell & J. A. O'Neill (Eds.), *Dissociation and the dissociative disorders: DSM-V and beyond* (pp. 435–444). New York: Routledge.

Sloman, L., Atkinson, L., Milligan, K., & Liotti, G. (2002). Attachment, social rank, and affect regulation. *Family Process, 41,* 479–493.

Solomon, J., & George, C. (1996). Defining the caregiving system: Toward a theory of caregiving. *Infant Mental Health Journal, 17,* 183–197.

Solomon, J., & George, C. (1999). The place of disorganization in attachment theory: Linking classic observations with contemporary findings. In J. Solomon & C. George (Eds.), *Attachment disorganization* (pp. 3–32). New York: Guilford Press.

Solomon, J., & George, C. (2006). Intergenerational transmission of dysregulated caregiving: Mothers describe their upbringing and child rearing. In O. Mayseless (Ed.), *Parenting representations: Theory, research, and clinical implications* (pp. 265–295). Cambridge, UK: Cambridge University Press.

Solomon, J., George, C., & De Jong, A. (1995). Children classified as controlling at age six: Evidence of disorganized representational strategies and aggression at home and school. *Development and Psychopathology, 7,* 447–464.

Steele, H., & Steele, M. (2003). Clinical uses of the Adult Attachment Interview. In M. Cortina & M. Marrone (Eds.), *Attachment theory and the psychoanalytic process* (pp. 107–126). London: Whurr.

Stern, D. N. (1985). *The interpersonal world of the infant.* New York: Basic Books.

Stern, D. N. (2004). *The present moment in psychotherapy and everyday life.* New York: Norton.

Teti, D. M., Gelfand, D. M., Messinger, D. S., & Isabella, R. (1995). Maternal depression and the quality of early attachment: An examination of infants, preschoolers and their mothers. *Developmental Psychology, 34,* 361–376.

Van der Hart, O., Nijenhuis, E. R., & Steele, K. (2006). *The haunted self.* New York: Norton.

Weiss, J. (1993). *How psychotherapy works.* New York: Guilford Press.

West, M., Adam, K., Spreng, S., & Rose, S. (2001). Attachment disorganization and dissociative symptoms in clinically treated adolescents. *Canadian Journal of Psychiatry, 46,* 627–631.

Index

AAI. *See* Adult Attachment Interview
AAP. *See* Adult Attachment Projective
Abandonment, fear of, 347
Abdicated care. *See also* Caregiving
  helplessness; Caregiving system;
  Segregated systems
  description of, 322–323
  double-bind situation and, 305
  experience of, 55
  psychological, 135
  segregated systems and, 350
  unsoothed fear and, 215
Absence of mother
  dysregulation markers for, 299, 302,
    303–304
  foster care, adoption, and, 9
Abuse, lack of resolution of, 29. *See also*
  Maltreatment
Academic performance, 67–68, 69–72
Adaptability, parent ratings of, 305
Adjustment problems and CHQ scales,
  156–157
Adolescence. *See also* Goal-Corrected
  Partnership in Adolescence Coding
  System
  assessment of attachment in, 209–212
  assessment of organized attachment
    strategies in, 219–222
  attachment patterns in, 207, 236–237
  attachment theory and, 208–209
  caregiving stances in, 231–232
  disorganized/controlling attachment
    strategies in, 222–224
  disoriented stances in, 235–236
  longitudinal trajectories of attachment
    disorganization from infancy to,
    213–219

overview of, 208
punitive stances in, 233–234
submissive stances in, 234–235
Adolescent Unresolved Attachment
  Questionnaire, 212
Adoption, 9, 294
Adrenocortical responses with attachment
  disorganization, 11, 112–113, 119
Adult Attachment Classification System, 28
Adult Attachment Interview (AAI). *See*
  also Cannot Classify; Unresolved
  classification
  adolescents and, 209–212
  associations with life events, 91–92
  associations with Strange Situation,
    80–81, 92, 102
  coherence discourse, 86, 91–92, 229–230
  continuity of classifications, 81, 101
  description of, 26–27, 34, 85–86, 344
  group classifications, 209
  longitudinal validity of GPACS in relation
    to, 227–231, 236–237
  socioeconomic status and, 82–83
  U classification based on, 83
Adult Attachment Interview (AAI) stability
  study
  case studies of instability in unresolved
    classification, 95–101
  classifications at Time 1 and Time 2,
    88–89, 90
  consistency of life event reporting, 89–90
  design, 84
  dismissing to unresolved classifications,
    99–101
  measures, 85–88
  methods of, 84–88
  overview of, 105–106

Adult Attachment Interview (AAI) stability study (*continued*)
  participants and procedure, 84–85
  results, 88–95
  secure to unresolved classifications, 97–99
  summary of cases rated unresolved, 93–95
  unresolved to dismissing classification, 96
  unresolved to secure classification, 96–97
Adult Attachment Projective (AAP)
  activation of medial temporal regions and, 391
  alone responses to, 360–363, 365–366, 369–371, 373–374, 375–376
  anxiety disorders clinical case example, 367–375
  attachment classification distributions, 354–355
  BPD clinical case example, 360–367
  classification system, 350, 351
  description of, 212, 310, 349–352
  dyadic responses to, 363–365, 366–367, 371–373
  fMRI study and, 365–367
  study using, 375–376
  traumatic dysregulation markers in patients with BPD and with anxiety disorders, 355–359
  validity in German population, 353–354
Adversative system, 389
Affect, dysregulated. *See also* Dysregulation; Regulation
  anger, 11–12, 281
  BPD and, 347
  caregiving helplessness and, 45
  description of, 11–12, 34–35
Agency, definition of, 36
Ainsworth's theory, 3, 7. *See also* Strange Situation
Aloneness, intolerance of, 347, 365
Alone responses to AAP
  anxiety disorder and, 369–371, 373–374, 376
  BPD and, 360–363, 365–366, 375–376
Alpha elements and function, 274, 283
AMBIANCE system, 6
Ambivalent attachment. *See* Insecure–ambivalent attachment
Anger
  dysregulated, 11–12, 281
  unavailability of caregiver and, 303
Anterior medial cingulate cortex, 358
Anxiety, management of, 331

Anxiety disorders
  AAP clinical case example, 367–375
  attachment studies of, 348–349
  dysregulation markers and, 354–355, 375–376
  symptoms of, 343
  traumatic dysregulation markers and, 355–359
Assaults
  to attachment, 345, 374
  to caregiving system, 137
Assessment. *See also specific instruments*
  of attachment in adolescence, 209–212
  of organized attachment strategies, 219–222
Attachment. *See also* Adult Attachment Interview; Adult Attachment Interview stability study; Adult Attachment Projective; Attachment disorganization; Attachment system; Attachment theory; Insecure–ambivalent attachment; Insecure–avoidant attachment; Unresolved attachment
  classifications of and gender, 37–38, 177–186
  coherence of patterns of, 111
  developmental approach to, 345–346
  ethological theory of, 3, 7, 134, 247
  insecure, 173–174, 343–344
  insecure–other, 139–140, 157
  insecure–resistant, 168, 321
  "maximizing" and "minimizing," 293
  preoccupied, 347, 349
  process of formation of, 110
  rare states of mind regarding, 228, 230–231
  secure, 3, 7, 168, 273
Attachment disorganization. *See also* Behaviorally disorganized pattern
  antecedents, features, and consequences of, 384–391
  biological processes associated with regulation in, 111–113
  causality, 14–16
  changes in beyond infancy, 54–57
  characteristics of, 25
  in childhood, 216–219
  clinical and research implications of, 16–18
  conditions likely to foster, 9–10
  extreme responses to separation and, 272–273

gene–environment interactions in, 122–125

genetic correlates of, 115–119, 120–121

in infancy, 213–216

lack of coherent strategy in, 111, 119

maltreatment of mothers and, 103–104

in normative and high-risk child-rearing contexts, 4–5

other contexts, observations of in, 7–9

risks of, 293, 387–388

sequelae of, 168–171

social and individual determinants of, 113–115, 121–122

Attachment Doll Play Assessment, 32

Attachment security (Ainsworth), 3, 7

Attachment status, 346

Attachment style, 346, 349

Attachment system

activation of, 390, 392

caregiving system compared to, 83–84

Circle of Security and, 320

dissociation contingent on activation of, 393–396

Attachment theory

adolescence and, 208–209

of Ainsworth, 3, 7

of Bowlby, 3, 7, 134, 247

regulation and, 119

Autonomy in adolescence, 208–209, 210

Avoidant attachment. See Insecure–avoidant attachment

B

Balanced relational processes and Circle of Security, 321

Balance in relationship system in adolescence, 219–220

Bayley Scales of Infant Development–Second Edition, 251

Beck Depression Inventory, 145

Behavioral control systems, 318. See also Caregiving system

Behaviorally disorganized pattern

description of, 53

externalizing problems, underachievement, and, 71–72

family history and, 218

marital dysfunction, parental hospitalization, and, 64–66

Behavior Assessment System for Children, 300–301

Behavior patterns. See also Behaviorally disorganized pattern; Controlling–caregiver behavior pattern; Controlling–punitive behavior pattern

controlling–containing, 224

hostile/capitulating, 226

leading/stifled, 226, 234–235

organized–avoidant, 258–259

Behavior problems. See Externalizing behavior problems; Internalizing behavior problems; School-age behavior problems; Social-emotional problems

Berkeley Puppet Interview, 176–177

Beta elements, 274, 280

Biobehavioral adaptational processes, dysregulation of, 9–13. See also Dysregulation; Regulation

Biological processes associated with regulation in disorganized infants, 111–113

Borderline defensive style, 325

Borderline personality disorder (BPD)

AAP clinical case example, 360–367

attachment studies of, 346–347

DBT for, 398, 407–408

dysregulation markers and, 354–355, 375–376

mentalization-based treatment for, 407

parallel interventions for, 401–407

symptoms of, 343

transference-focused psychotherapy of, 408

traumatic dysregulation markers and, 355–359

Boundary disturbances in family systems, 202

Bowlby's ethological theory of attachment, 3, 7, 134, 247

BPD. See Borderline personality disorder

Buffering, 36, 213–214, 269

"Building New Dreams" intervention, 248

C

Cannot Classify (AAI)

adolescent classifications and, 210, 212, 230–231

clinical samples and, 230

coding of, 391

criteria for, 211

unresolved classification on AAP and, 376 n. 1

Cardiac activation with attachment disorganization, 112, 119

Caregiving. *See also* Caregiving helplessness;
  Caregiving Interview; Caregiving
  system; Controlling–caregiver
  behavior pattern; Disorganized
  caregiving behavior; Intergenerational
  transmission of caregiving patterns;
  Maternal care
 as balancing act, 134
 disabled, 323
 emergence of disorganization and, 58–60
 representations of, 137–138
 suspended, 323
Caregiving–containing adolescent stances,
  226–227, 231–232
Caregiving–controlling behavior pattern. *See*
  Controlling–caregiver behavior pattern
Caregiving helplessness. *See also* Abdicated
  care; Caregiving Helplessness
  Questionnaire; Maternal helplessness
 gender of child and, 44–45
 hypotheses of study of, 30–31
 maternal loss related to rage events,
  40–41
 maternal rage pattern events and
  protection, 38–40
 methods of study of, 31–36
 overview of, 27–28, 41–47
 replication of earlier findings on, 36–
  38
Caregiving Helplessness Questionnaire
  (CHQ)
 construct approach and, 142
 convergent validity of, 149
 development of, 141–157
 development version of, 143–144
 discriminant validity of, 149, 150
 empirical structure of, 148
 exploratory analyses of, 151–154, 157
 factor structure of, 146–147, 148
 goals in development of, 141
 maternal depression and, 156
 measures, 143–145
 overview of, 151–152, 154–157
 participants and recruitment, 142–
  143
 predictive validity of, 149–150
 procedures, 143
 sample of, 164–166
 statistical analysis, 145–146
Caregiving Interview
 description of, 32, 144
 helplessness rating scale for, 33–34, 142
 mental representations and, 137
 scale correlations with CHQ, 154–155

Caregiving system. *See also* Segregated
  systems
 activation of, 389
 adult attachment system compared to,
  83–84
 disorganized caregiving and, 135–141
 goal of, 306, 319
 ineffectiveness of, 217–218
 interventions at level of, 307, 309
 in normative and high-risk child-rearing
  contexts, 4–5
 overactivation of, 247–248, 259–260
 overview of, 133–135
Cassidy, Marvin, and McArthur Working
  Group on Attachment classification
  system, 53
Causality, 14–16
Child Behavior Checklist, 145, 176, 304
Child Caregiving scale of CHQ, 146–152,
  154–157
"Childhood bipolar disorder," 17–18
Children. *See* Adolescence; Controlling/
  disorganized behavior in children;
  School-age behavior problems; Special
  needs, children with
CHQ. *See* Caregiving Helplessness
  Questionnaire
Chronic mourning, 344, 348, 350, 375
Circle of Security (COS). *See also* COS
  Protocol
 clinical illustration, 328–339
 defensive styles and, 324–326, 331
 description of, 318
 "formula" for parenting, 322–323
 graphic for, 319–320
 linchpin struggles and, 327, 332–338
 organizing feelings and, 320–321
 as organizing framework, 339–340
 safe haven and, 321
 segregated systems and, 323–324
 "Shark Music," 324, 330, 333, 336
Circle of Security Interview (COSI),
  326–327, 331
Classifications. *See also* Cannot Classify;
  Unclassifiable cases in Strange
  Situation; Unresolved classification
 from AAP, 350, 351
 of attachment, 32–33
 of attachment, gender and, 37–38,
  177–178
 of children with special needs, 245–
  256
 of controlling/disorganized behavior, 53
 Dismissing/Derogating, 228, 230, 231

"Disorganized Frightened" case
illustration, 307–311
Fearfully Preoccupied classification, 228,
230, 231
in patients with BPD and with anxiety
disorders, 354–355
stability of, and timing of AAI, 104–105
from Strange Situation, 81, 87
in study of maltreated children, using doll
play story stem technique, 296–298
Clinical and research implications
of attachment disorganization, 16–18
of dissociative responses, 391–393
of maternal containment issues, 288–
289
of presence of security and dysregulation
markers, 306–307
Clinical dialogue. See also Therapeutic
relationship
activation of attachment motivations
within, 394–396
drama triangle and, 396–397
fright without solution, 397–401
relational dilemmas and parallel
interventions, 401–407
Closet narcissistic personality, 331
Coding. See also Goal-Corrected Partnership
in Adolescence Coding System
Cannot Classify (AAI), 391
defensive processes, 350
Emotional Facial Action Coding System,
367
interview-wide indices of disorganization
on AAI, 211–212
Kobak Q-set method for coding AAI,
209–210
of life events, 34–35, 86–87
Cognitive disconnection, 13–14, 293, 298
Cognitive functioning, deficits in, 67–68,
69–70
Coherence discourse (AAI), 86, 91–92,
229–230
Coherence of attachment patterns, 111
Collapse of strategy, 55, 389–391, 393–
396
Communication, maternal disrupted, 59–60
Complicated loss
anxiety disorders and, 368, 374
child disorganization and, 40–41, 43
definition of, 35
Conduct disorder, 302–303, 304
Congenital anomaly. See Special needs,
children with
Constricted story stems, 298

Constriction
definition of, 304
dysregulation markers for, 300, 302, 304
examples of, 14
as manifestation of segregated systems
processing, 137–138
Construct approach and CHQ, 142
Contained, definition of, 274
Container, definition of, 273–274
Containment, 269, 273–274. See also
Maternal containment
Context, importance of, and maternal
behavior, 257. See also Marital context;
Visitation context of foster care
Controlling behaviors, role of, 332
Controlling–caregiver behavior pattern
CHQ scales and, 156–157
collapse of, and dissociation, 393–
396
description of, 52–53, 304
impact of loss on, 62–64
in internalizing boys, 193–196
internalizing problems and, 70–71,
170–171, 185, 217
mastery motivation and, 70–71
mothers and, 218
origins of, 200–201
signature of, 139
Controlling–containing behavior pattern,
224
Controlling/disorganized behavior in
children
caregiving and, 5–7
changes beyond infancy, 54–57
developmental risk and, 68–72
longitudinal study of, 56–57
overview of, 72–73
patterns of, 52–53
studies of, 58, 66–67
trajectories of, 57–66
Controlling–punitive behavior pattern
in adolescence, 226, 233–234
"baiting" and, 139
behavior problems, underachievement,
and, 69–70
CHQ scales and, 156
Circle of Security and, 330
collapse of, and dissociation, 395–396
description of, 5, 52, 53
"Disorganized Frightened" classification,
case illustration, 307–311
externalizing problems and, 170–171,
217
mothers and, 218

Controlling–punitive behavior pattern (*continued*)
  relational dilemmas, parallel interventions, and, 401–407
  role of maternal stress and caregiving in, 60–62
Controlling strategies
  in childhood, 216–219
  collapse of, 55, 393–396
  development of, 388–389
  development of social-emotional problems and, 170–171
  dissociation as collapse of, 389–391
  of role-reversal, 169–170
Convergent validity of CHQ, 149
Coping styles, gender differences in, 173
Coregulation, maternal, 10–11
Cortisol response, 213
COS. *See* Circle of Security
COS Project, 319
COS Protocol, 319, 326, 339–340

D

Danger and rescue/genuine reintegration markers, 298, 299
DBT (dialectic behavioral model of psychotherapy), 398, 407–408
Deactivating defenses, 13, 292–293, 298
Defensive processes. *See also* Segregated systems
  AAP coding system and, 350
  in caregiving system, 135
  dysregulation of, 298
  formation of, 323
  as related to theoretically relevant variables, 312
  separations and, 272, 285
  types of, 292–293
Defensive styles, 324–326, 331. *See also* Esteem-sensitivity
Deflecting/minimizing dyadic strategy, 225
Delight, need for and experience of, 319, 320
Depression, maternal
  attachment disorganization and, 140–141, 393
  CHQ scales and, 155–156
Developmental approach to attachment, 345–346
Developmental outcomes
  gender and, 171–174
  insecure attachment and, 343–344

Developmental risk
  controlling/disorganized behavior in children and, 68–72
  disorganized caregiving and, 140–141
  insecure attachment and, 343–344
Dialectic behavioral model of psychotherapy (DBT), 398, 407–408
Differential susceptibility model, 124
Disabled caregiving, 323
Discourse dysregulation, 344
Discriminant validity of CHQ, 149, 150
Disgust responses and unresolved attachment, 367
Dismissing/Derogating classification, 228, 230, 231
Disorganized attachment. *See* Attachment disorganization
Disorganized caregiving behavior
  developmental risk and, 140–141
  mother–child interaction and, 138–140
  overview of, 5–7, 135–137
  representations of caregiving and, 137–138
  types of, 322–323
Disorganized/controlling attachment strategies in adolescence, 222–224
Disorganized/disoriented category of children, 110–111, 321–322
"Disorganized Frightened" classification, case illustration, 307–311
Disoriented adolescent stance, 227, 235–236
Dissociative responses
  adult disorders and, 383–384
  attachment disorganization and, 387–388
  to child distress or anger, 61–62
  clinical implications of, 391–393
  as collapse of controlling strategies, 389–391
  contingent upon activation of attachment system, 393–396
  fright without solution and, 397–401
Divided-attention situations, 252, 255
Doll play story stem techniques
  case illustration, 308–309
  classification and, 296–298
  description of, 293–295
Dopaminergic system, 115–116
"Drama triangle" metaphor, 386, 392, 396–397
DRD4 gene, 116–118, 120–121, 123–124
Dual-risk model, 124
Dyadic responses to AAP
  anxiety disorder and, 371–373
  BPD and, 363–365, 366–367

Dyads
  deflecting/minimizing strategy of, 225
  entangled/oscillatory strategy of, 225–226
  hostile–helpless, 223
  lack of balance and asymmetry of power
    in, 200–201
  reciprocity and balanced emotional
    expression in, 54, 59
Dysregulation. *See also* Affect, dysregulated;
    Regulation
  of biobehavioral adaptational processes,
    9–13
  of defensive processes, 298
  discourse, 344
  fragmentation of self-experience and, 388
  at level of representation, 13–14, 344
  as manifestation of segregated systems
    processing, 137
  risk for, 169–170
Dysregulation markers. *See also* Traumatic
    dysregulation markers
  AAP and, 351–352
  attachment classification distributions
    and, 354–355
  in foster care, 307–311
  security and, 306–307
  study of, 302, 303–304, 352–353
  types of, 299–300

E

Early Head Start (EHS) Research and
    Evaluation Project, 84
Emotional dysregulation. *See* Dysregulation
Emotional expression, socialization of,
    172–173
Emotional Facial Action Coding System,
    367
Emotionally misattuned maternal care,
    196–199
Emotionally overinvolved maternal care,
    257–258, 259
Emotional unavailability, parental, 214,
    227
Emotion regulation. *See* Regulation
Entangled/oscillatory dyadic strategy,
    225–226
Environment–gene interactions, 117–118,
    122–125
Esteem-sensitivity, 325, 328, 330, 331
Ethological theory of attachment (Bowlby),
    3, 7, 134, 247
Evidence-based models of infant and child
    mental health intervention, 26
Exploration system, 319–320

Externalizing behavior problems
  boys with internalizing problems and,
    190–193
  controlling–punitive behavior pattern and,
    170–171, 217
  gender and, 184
  maternal caregiving representations and,
    304–305
  in school-age children, 66–67, 69, 71–72

F

Factor structure of CHQ, 146–147, 148
Failed protection, 135
"Failure to terminate" hypothesis, 385
Family systems, boundary disturbances in,
    202
Family violence, definition of, 34
Father–child interactions, 202
Fear. *See also* Fright
  of caregiver, 168–169
  children with special needs and, 248–250,
    258
  gender and, 171, 185–186
  separation from or loss of parent and,
    215–216
  in therapeutic relationship, 392
  unsoothed, history of in parents, 214–215
Fearfully Preoccupied classification, 228,
    230, 231
5HTT-LPR (SERT) serotonin transporter
    gene, 118–119, 120–121, 123
-521 C/T single nucleotide polymorphism,
    116–117, 120
"Flight or fight" behavior, 171, 200, 385
Foster care
  case illustration of dysregulation markers
    in, 307–311
  disorganized attachment classifications
    and, 9
  insecure–ambivalent attachment and,
    305–306
  maternal containment and, 284–289
  maternal containment case vignettes,
    275–284
  story stem technique and, 294–295
  visitation context of, 270–271
Fright. *See also* Fear
  experiences of, 42–43, 114, 215–216
  without solution, 10, 15, 385, 392,
    397–401
Frightened or frightening behavior of
    mothers (FR)
  development of attachment
    disorganization and, 114, 174

Frightened or frightening behavior of
    mothers (FR) (*continued*)
    disorganized caregiving and, 136–137
    dysregulation markers for, 300, 302, 303
    during foster care visits, 278–280
    gender, social-emotional problems, and,
        183, 185–186, 194–196
    solicitous behavior compared to, 258
Frightening material in play, 307

G

Gender
    attachment and, as predictors of
        social-emotional problems, 178–186,
        200–203
    attachment classifications and, 37–38,
        177–178
    caregiving helplessness and, 44–45
    developmental outcomes and, 171–174
    social-emotional problems and, 190–199
Gene–environment interactions, 117–118,
    122–125
Genetic correlates of disorganized
    attachment, 115–119, 120–121
Genetic variations in neurotransporter
    efficiency, 16
"Gifted," children described as, 328
Goal-Corrected Partnership in Adolescence
    Coding System (GPACS)
    caregiving stances, 231–232
    development of, 224–227
    dialogue examples from disorganized
        classifications, 231–236
    disorganized/unbalanced profiles,
        226–227
    disoriented stances, 235–236
    insecure but organized profiles, 225–226
    longitudinal validity study of, 227–231,
        236–237
    punitive stances, 233–234
    secure profile, 225
    submissive stances, 234–235
Goal-corrected partnerships, 135, 208, 219
"Good enough" parents, 249
GPACS. *See* Goal-Corrected Partnership in
    Adolescence Coding System

H

Haven of safety markers
    Circle of Safety and, 299, 301–303, 306
    description of, 298
    in therapy, 311
Helplessness. *See* Caregiving helplessness;
    Maternal helplessness

Holding, as essential parental function, 319
Homeostatic system, 10–11, 113, 119, 350
Hospitalizations, parental, and behaviorally
    disorganized pattern, 66
Hostile/capitulating behavior pattern, 226
Hostile–helpless relational processes in
    adolescence, 223
Hostile–Helpless (HH) state of mind,
    211–212
Hostile maternal care, 190–193, 278–280
Hypervigilance and unresolved attachment,
    367
Hypothalamic–pituitary–adrenal system, 11,
    112, 119

I

Imaginary friends, 281
Individual determinants of disorganized
    attachment, 113–115, 120, 121–122
Infant–parent psychotherapy (Fraiberg), 26
Insecure–ambivalent attachment
    in adolescents, 221–222
    cognitive disconnection and, 13–14, 298
    in infants, 8, 119
    prevalence of, 305–306
Insecure attachment, 173–174, 343–344
Insecure–avoidant attachment
    in adolescents, 221
    deactivation and, 13, 298
    description of, 8, 321
    in infants, 119, 168
Insecure–other children, 139–140, 157
Insecure–resistant attachment, 168, 321
Institutionalized children, 9
Intergenerational effects of trauma, 384–385
Intergenerational transmission of caregiving
    patterns
    hypotheses of study of, 30–31
    methods of study of, 31–36
    overview of, 26–28, 41–47
    results of study of, 36–41
    trauma, loss, and, 28–30, 384–385
Internalization of self-soothing reflective
    capacity, 273, 274, 286–287. *See also*
    Maternal containment
Internalized secure base markers, 298, 299,
    310–311
Internalizing behavior problems
    boys with, 193–196
    boys with externalizing problems and,
        190–193
    controlling–caregiver behavior pattern
        and, 170–171, 217
    gender and, 184–185

girls with, 196–199, 202
in school-age children, 67, 70
Internal working models (IWMs). *See also*
    Representations
in adolescence, 208–209
of caregiving, 134, 338
contradictory, 215
description of, 292, 323, 386
maternal containment and, 287
as multiple, incoherent, and
    compartmentalized, 386
as segregated from consciousness, 392
Intersubjective perspective on dissociative
    pathology, 391
Interventions. *See also* Clinical dialogue;
    Therapeutic relationship
attachment-based, 384
for BPD, 401–408
"Building New Dreams," 248
evidence-based models of, 17, 26
at level of caregiving system, 307, 309
Intra-AAI stability, 81
Intra-Strange Situation stability, 81
Intrusive maternal care, 190–193, 199
IWMs. *See* Internal working models

K

Knowing and being known, attempts at, 287
Kobak Q-set method for coding AAI,
    209–210

L

Leadership, parent ratings of, 305
Leading/stifled behavior pattern, 226,
    234–235
Life events
    activation of attachment system and, 393
    associations of AAI U ratings and
        coherence of mind with, 91–92,
        102–103
    associations with infant attachment, 93
    coding of, 34–35
    consistency of reporting of, 89–90
    emergence of disorganization and, 60
Life Events Coding Scale, 86–87
Linchpin moments in Circle of Security, 327,
    332–338
Loss. *See also* Complicated loss; Mourning;
    Trauma
    consistency of reporting of, 89–90
    intergenerational effects of, 384–385
    in lives of mothers of controlling–
        caregiving children, 62–64

of parent, 215–216
prenatal, 103
as separation, and pathology, 345
through death, definition of, 35
unresolved, and anxiety disorders,
    348–349
of "wished for" attachment figures, 374
Loss, lack of resolution of
AAI and, 93–95, 102
consistency of ratings of, 90–91
disorganized caregiving and, 28–30,
    40–41, 43, 136
ratings of, 86
in young, high-risk mothers, 105–106

M

MacArthur Story Stem Battery, 294
Maltreatment. *See also* Maltreatment,
    presence of markers of security and
    disorganization with
attachment disorganization and, 14–15,
    293
BPD and, 346–347
caregiving helplessness and, 42–43
of children with special needs, 247
consistency of reporting of, 89–90
defensive stance toward, and birth of first
    child, 104–105
doll play story stem techniques and,
    293–295
foster care and, 271
infant disorganization and, 103–104
lack of resolution of, 29, 136
Maltreatment, presence of markers of
    security and disorganization with
Behavior Assessment System for Children
    and, 300–301
case illustration, 307–311
clinical implications of, 306–307
dysregulation markers, 299–300
security markers, 299
study classification procedure, 296–298
study methods, 295–301
study participants, 295–296
study rationale, 295
study results, 301–306, 311–312
Marital context, 60, 64–66, 202
Mastery motivation, 70–71
Maternal care
    emotionally misattuned, 196–199
    emotionally overinvolved, 257–258, 259
    hostile, 190–193, 278–280
    intrusive, 190–193, 199
    representations of, 304–305, 322

Maternal containment
    attachment disorganization and, 286–287
    case vignettes, 275–284
    clinical services and, 288–289
    conditions for, 277
    examples of, 282–284
    foster care visits and, 270
    internal working models and, 287
    lack of, 276–282, 284–286
    overview of, 284–289
    quality of, 269–270
    rationale for study of, 274–275
Maternal helplessness, 28, 139–140. *See
    also* Abdicated care; Caregiving
    helplessness; Caregiving Helplessness
    Questionnaire
Maternal sensitivity, 5, 11, 16, 115, 273
"Maximizing" attachment, 293
Meanness, vacillating between weakness
    and, 329
Medial temporal regions, activation of with
    AAP, 391
Mentalization, 273, 388
Mentalization-based treatment for BPD, 407
Metacognitive functioning, 67–68, 70
"Minimizing" attachment, 293
Minnesota Longitudinal Study of Parents
    and Children, 210–211
Miscarriage, lack of resolution of, 30
Molecular-genetic research, 116–119,
    120–121, 125
Mother–Child Frightened scale of CHQ,
    146–152, 154–157
Mother Helpless scale of CHQ, 146–151,
    153–157
Mothers. *See also* Depression, maternal;
    Frightened or frightening behavior
    of mothers; Maternal care; Maternal
    containment; Maternal helplessness
    absence of, 9, 299, 302, 303–304
    behaviors of, and emergence of
        disorganization, 59–60
    descriptions of disorganized behavior of,
        6–7
    as disorganized in caregiving behavior,
        25–26
    maternal co-regulation, 10–11
Motivational dynamics of disorganized
    infants, 385–386
Motivational systems, 388–389, 406–407
Mourning
    chronic, 344, 348, 350, 375
    incomplete or "pathological," 29, 136,
        295, 344, 350

N

Narcissistic defensive style, 325, 331
Neural attachment activation patterns,
    358–359
Neuroendocrine responses to stress, 12–13
Neuroimaging study, 365–367
NICHD Early Child Care Research Network
    study, 246
Normative markers, 351–352

O

Organization discourse (AAI), 86
Organized attachment strategies, assessment
    of, 219–222
Organized–avoidant pattern, and solicitous
    parenting, 258–259
Organized–insecure attachment strategies in
    adolescence, 221
Out-of-context anger, 8–9, 11–12
Out-of-context behavior in adolescence,
    235–236

P

Panic disorder, 348
Parallel interventions, 401–407
Parental Stress Index (PSI), 144–145,
    151–154
Parent Development Interview, 144, 327
Parenting dimensions, studies of, 134
Parent out of control, definition of, 35–36
Parents. *See also* Marital context; Maternal
    care; Maternal containment; Maternal
    helplessness; Mothers; Partners and
    Parents Project; Solicitous parental
    behavior
    behavior ratings by, 305
    of children with special needs, 246–248,
        259–260
    in Circle of Security, 319
    emotionally unavailable, 214, 227
    fear of separation from or loss of,
        215–216
    "good enough," 249
    holding as essential function of, 319
    infant–parent psychotherapy, 26
    marital dysfunction and hospitalization
        of, 64–66
    unsoothed fear, history of in, 214–
        215
Partners and Parents Project
    description of, 174
    descriptive statistics, 177–178
    study 1 discussion, 184–186

study 1 methods, 175–177
study 1 results, 177–183
study 2 methods, 186–190
study 2 results, 190–199
Paths Over Time study, 227
Patterns. *See* Behaviorally disorganized
    pattern; Behavior patterns;
    Controlling–caregiver behavior pattern;
    Controlling–punitive behavior pattern;
    Intergenerational transmission of
    caregiving patterns
Peer groups, gender-segregated, 173
Predictive validity of CHQ scales, 149–150,
    155
Predictors of social-emotional problems,
    178–186
Preoccupied attachment, 347, 349
Protection
    emotional, for foster children, 311
    emphasis on in doll play, 309
    failed, and mother absence, 304
    as goal of caregiving system, 319
    rage pattern events and, 38–41
Protection-related ratings, 35–36, 38–40
Protective factors and caregiving
    helplessness, 41–42
PSI (Parental Stress Index), 144–145,
    151–154
Psychopathology
    disorganized infant–caregiver
        relationships and, 17–18
    dissociative responses to child distress or
        anger and, 383–384
    stress, activation of attachment system,
        and, 390
    unresolved attachment and, 343–
        344
    vulnerability to, 213–214
Punitive–controlling behavior pattern. *See*
    Controlling–punitive behavior pattern

Q

Q-set method for coding AAI (Kobak),
    209–210

R

Rage pattern events, 38–41
Ranking system, 389
Rare states of mind regarding attachment,
    228, 230–231
Reaction to Diagnosis Interview, 246
Reciprocity and balanced emotional
    expression in dyads, 54, 59

Regulation. *See also* Dysregulation
    attachment theory and, 119
    biological processes associated with, in
        disorganized infants, 111–113
    Circle of Security and, 320–321
    experience with, 249, 261
    internalization of self-soothing reflective
        capacity, 273, 274
    maternal coregulation, 10–11
Relatedness in adolescence, 208–209, 210
Relational dilemmas, 401–407
Relational processes
    balanced, 321
    hostile–helpless, 223
    unbalanced, 215–216, 223–224
Relational styles, 390
Repair after relationship rupture, 322
Representation, dysregulation at level of,
    13–14, 344
Representations. *See also* Internal working
        models; Maltreatment, presence of
        markers of security and disorganization
        with
    of caregivers and of self, 46–47, 306–307
    of caregiving, 137–138, 154, 322
    of caregiving system, 134–135
    contradictory, of self and attachment
        figures, 374–375
    of haven of safety, 303
    of maltreatment, 136
    of past of mothers, 27
    of relationships as dyadic, 215
    of relationships with children, 5–6, 27,
        31, 43–44
    in segregated systems, 14
    story stem techniques and, 293–294
    traumatic attachment, 324–325
Resolution, and AAP, 351
Retraumatization, 285
Reunion behavior in Strange Situation, 138
Reverie, state of, 274, 282, 286–287
Risks. *See also* Developmental risk
    of attachment disorganization, 293,
        387–388
    dual-risk model, 124
    for dysregulation, 169–170
Role-reversal. *See also* Controlling–caregiver
        behavior pattern; Controlling–punitive
        behavior pattern
    in adolescence, 231–232
    behaviorally disorganized pattern and, 65
    chronic mourning and, 375
    Circle of Security and, 330, 332, 335
    controlling strategies of, 169–170

Role-reversal (*continued*)
  developmental costs of, 156–157
  loss and, 63
  school performance and, 69–70

S

Safety-sensitivity, 325
Scaffolding
  as caregiving function, 321
  in cognitive development, 287
Schizoid defensive style, 325
School-age behavior problems. *See also*
    Externalizing behavior problems;
    Internalizing behavior problems
  development of, 66–67
  representational attachment constructs
    and, 307–311
School performance, 67–68, 69–72
Secure attachment
  Ainsworth and, 3, 7
  description of, 168
  maternal behavioral sensitivity and, 273
Secure base behavior in adolescence,
    219–221
Segregated systems. *See also* Abdicated care;
    Caregiving system
  AAP and, 350–351
  case vignettes, 275–284
  CHQ and, 154
  conditions for emergence and
    maintenance of, 285, 307, 323–324
  description of, 13, 45, 272, 293, 350
  disorganized caregiving and, 135–136
  extreme responses to separation and,
    272–273
  representations in, 14
Self-activation, 326, 334–335
Selfhood, growth of, 287
Self-perceptions, multiple, 397
Sensitivity
  esteem-sensitivity, 325, 328, 330, 331
  maternal, 5, 11, 16, 115, 273
  ratings of, 252
  safety-sensitivity, 325
  separation-sensitivity, 325
Separation Anxiety Test, 390
Separation distress, 252–253, 257
Separations
  in adolescence, 215–216
  extreme responses to, 271–274, 285
  pathology and, 345
  reunion behavior and, 8–9
Separation-sensitivity, 325
Separation threat and anxiety, 348

SERT serotonin transporter gene, 118–119,
    120–121, 123
7-repeat allele of dopamine receptor D4,
    116, 117–118, 120, 123–124
"Shark Music," 324, 330, 333, 336
Sleep, feigning, to shut off intense feelings,
    276–278
Social determinants of disorganized
    attachment, 113–115, 121–122
Social-emotional problems. *See also*
    Externalizing behavior problems;
    Internalizing behavior problems
  case studies of, 186–199
  disorganized attachment and gender as
    predictors of, 178–186
  overview of, 167–168, 200–203
  risk for development of, 169–170
Social problems, definition of, 174
Social skills, parent ratings of, 305
Solicitous parental behavior
  attachment disorganization and, 248–250,
    256–261
  ratings of, 252
  study measures and procedures, 251–253
  study methods, 250–253
  study participants, 250–251
  study results, 253–256, 257
"Special," children described as, 328
Special needs, children with. *See also*
    Solicitous parental behavior
  attachment classification in, 245–246
  attachment disorganization and, 248–
    250
  parental adaptation to, 246, 259–260
  parental overprotection, overinvolvement,
    and, 246–248
State of mind
  Hostile–Helpless, 211–212
  with regard to attachment, 86, 344
  reverie, 274, 282, 286–287
Stereotypes, gender-role, 172–174
Story stem techniques
  case illustration, 308–309
  classification and, 296–298
  description of, 293–295
Strange Situation (Ainsworth)
  associations with AAI, 80–81, 92, 102
  children with special needs and, 251
  classifications, 81, 87
  COS protocol and, 326
  description of, 110
  indices of disorganization in, 7–8
  reunion behavior in, 138
  unclassifiable cases in, 4–5, 139–140, 157

Stress
    activation of attachment system, psychopathology, and, 390
    buffering from, 3, 213–214, 269
    controlling behaviors and, 55–56, 60–62
    cortisol response to, 213
    of foster care, 271
    homeostatic response to, 10–11, 113, 119, 350
    maternal, 60–62, 141
    neuroendocrine responses to, 12–13
    parenting children with special needs and, 246–247
    during pregnancy, 122
    responses to, and gender, 171–172
Stress arousal model, 112
Submissive stances in adolescence, 226, 234–235
Substance abuse, definition of, 35
Suspended caregiving, 323

T

"Temper dysregulation disorder with dysphoria," 17–18
"Tending and befriending" behavior, 171, 200
Thematic integration markers, 298, 299
Therapeutic relationship. *See also* Clinical dialogue
    activation of attachment system in, 392
    balance in, 393
    fear in, 392
    transformation from passive to active within, 401
Therapeutic strategies, attachment-based, 384
Thought problems, definition of, 174
Timing of AAI, and stability of classifications, 104–105
Transference-focused psychotherapy of BPD, 408
"Transmission block," 211
"Transmission gap," 82, 83
Trauma. *See also* Loss
    caregiving helplessness and, 41
    consistency of reporting of, 89–90
    defensive stance toward, and birth of first child, 104–105
    early relational, 385–386
    emergence of disorganization and, 60
    feelings of anger and helplessness with experiences of, 288

intergenerational effects of, 384–385
lack of resolution of, and disorganized caregiving, 28–30
Traumatic dysregulation markers
    anxiety disorders and, 355–359
    BPD and, 355–359, 376
    clinical case example, 360–367, 371, 373–374
    description of, 351–352
    study of, 352–353
Two-therapist intervention model, 401–407

U

Unbalanced relational processes, 215–216, 223–224
Unclassifiable cases in Strange Situation, 4–5, 139–140, 157
    maternal helplessness and
Uncomplicated loss, definition of, 35
Unintegrated self, 135
Unresolved attachment
    AAP-fMRI paradigm and, 365–366
    BPD and, 347
    Cannot Classify on AAI and, 376 n. 1
    disgust responses and, 367
    hypervigilance and, 367
    psychiatric symptoms and, 343–344
Unresolved classification (AAI)
    adolescents and, 210
    case studies of instability in, 95–101
    coherence of mind, life events, and, 91–92, 102–103
    frightening behavior and, 196
    HH states of mind and, 212
    patterns of interaction and, 230
    summary of cases rated, 93–95
Unresolved loss. *See* Loss, lack of resolution of

V

Validity of AAP in German population, 353–354
Visitation context of foster care
    case vignettes, 275–284
    maternal containment and, 284–289
    overview of, 270–271

W

Weakness, vacillating between meanness and, 329
Working Group on Attachment classification system, 53